Interpretation of Complex Arrhythmias: A Case-Based Approach

Editor

MELVIN SCHEINMAN

CARDIAC ELECTROPHYSIOLOGY CLINICS

www.cardiacEP.theclinics.com

Consulting Editors
RANJAN K. THAKUR
ANDREA NATALE

March 2016 • Volume 8 • Number 1

ELSEVIER

1600 John F. Kennedy Boulevard • Suite 1800 • Philadelphia, Pennsylvania, 19103-2899

http://www.theclinics.com

CARDIAC ELECTROPHYSIOLOGY CLINICS Volume 8, Number 1
March 2016 ISSN 1877-9182, ISBN-13: 978-0-323-39555-7

Editor: Lauren Boyle
Developmental Editor: Susan Showalter

Cardiac Electrophysiology Clinics (ISSN 1877-9182) is published quarterly by Elsevier Inc., 360 Park Avenue South, New York, NY 10010-1710. Months of issue are March, June, September, and December. Subscription prices are $205.00 per year for US individuals, $318.00 per year for US institutions, $225.00 per year for Canadian individuals, $359.00 per year for Canadian institutions, $285.00 per year for international individuals, $384.00 per year for international institutions and $100.00 per year for US, Canadian and international students/residents. To receive student/resident rate, orders must be accompanied by name of affilliated institution, date of term, and the signature of program/residency coordinator on institution letterhead. Orders will be billed at individual rate until proof of status is received. Foreign air speed delivery is included in all Clinics subscription prices. All prices are subject to change without notice. **POSTMASTER:** Send address changes to Cardiac Electrophysiology Clinics, Elsevier Health Sciences Division, Subscription Customer Service, 3251 Riverport Lane, Maryland Heights, MO 63043. **Customer Service: 1-800-654-2452 (US and Canada). From outside of the US and Canada, call 314-477-8871. Fax: 314-447-8029. E-mail: JournalsCustomerService-usa@elsevier.com (for print support); JournalsOnlineSupport-usa@elsevier.com (for online support).**

Reprints. For copies of 100 or more of articles in this publication, please contact the Commercial Reprints Department, Elsevier Inc., 360 Park Avenue South, New York, NY 10010-1710. Tel.: 212-633-3874; Fax: 212-633-3820; E-mail: reprints@elsevier.com.

Cardiac Electrophysiology Clinics is covered in *MEDLINE/PubMed (Index Medicus)*.

Contributors

CONSULTING EDITORS

RANJAN THAKUR, MD, MPH, MBA, FACC, FHRS
Professor of Medicine and Director, Arrhythmia Service, Thoracic and Cardiovascular Institute, Sparrow Health System, Michigan State University, Lansing, Michigan

ANDREA NATALE, MD, FACC, FHRS
Texas Cardiac Arrhythmia Institute, St. David's Medical Center; Dell Medical School, University of Texas, Austin, Texas; MetroHealth Medical Center, Case Western Reserve University School of Medicine, Cleveland, Ohio; Division of Cardiology, Stanford University, Stanford, California; Electrophysiology and Arrhythmia Services, California Pacific Medical Center, San Francisco, California; Division of Cardiovascular Diseases, Scripps Clinic, La Jolla, California

EDITOR

MELVIN SCHEINMAN, MD
Director of the Genetic Arrhythmia Program, University of California San Francisco Medical Center, San Francisco, California

SECTION EDITORS

NITISH BADHWAR, MD, FHRS –
Supraventricular Tachycardia
Section of Cardiac Electrophysiology, Division of Cardiology, Department of Medicine, University of California San Francisco; Professor of Medicine, UCSF Medical Center San Francisco, San Francisco, California

HENRY H. HSIA, MD, FACC, FHRS –
Ventricular Tachycardia
Chief, Arrhythmia Service, VA San Francisco; Health Science Professor of Medicine, University of California San Francisco, San Francisco, California

EDWARD P. GERSTENFELD, MD – *Atrial Fibrillation and Flutter*
Professor of Medicine; Chief, Cardiac Electrophysiology, Section of Cardiac Electrophysiology, Division of Cardiology, Department of Medicine, University of California San Francisco, San Francisco, California

BYRON LEE, MD – *Troubleshooting Device Function*
Professor, University of California San Francisco School of Medicine, San Francisco, California

RONN TANEL, MD – *Adult Congenital Cardiac Disease*
Electrophysiologist, Department of Pediatrics, Pediatric and Congenital Arrhythmia Center, UCSF Benioff Children's Hospital, University of California San Francisco, San Francisco, California

MARWAN M. REFAAT, MD, FACC, FAHA, FHRS, FASE, FESC, FACP, FAAMA –
Arrhythmias in Patients with Genetic Arrhythmia Syndromes
Section of Cardiac Electrophysiology, Cardiology Division, Department of Internal Medicine; Department of Biochemistry and Molecular Genetics, American University of Beirut Medical Center, Beirut, Lebanon; Assistant Professor of Medicine, Cardiac Electrophysiology, Cardiology, Department of Internal Medicine, American University of Beirut Faculty of Medicine and Medical Center, New York, New York

AUTHORS

BERNARD ABI-SALEH, MD, FHRS
Section of Cardiac Electrophysiology, Division of Cardiology, Department of Internal Medicine, American University of Beirut Medical Center, Beirut, Lebanon

RYAN G. ALEONG, MD
Section of Cardiac Electrophysiology, Division of Cardiology, University of Colorado, Denver, Aurora, Colorado

MARIAM ARABI, MD
Department of Pediatrics and Adolescent Medicine, American University of Beirut Medical Center, Beirut, Lebanon

NITISH BADHWAR, MD, FHRS
Section of Cardiac Electrophysiology, Division of Cardiology, Department of Medicine, University of California San Francisco; Professor of Medicine, UCSF Medical Center San Francisco, San Francisco, California

SHERRIE JOY BAYSA, MD
Electrophysiology Fellow, Division of Cardiology, The Heart Program, Nicklaus Children's Hospital, Miami Children's Hospital Health System, Miami, Florida

FADI F. BITAR, MD
Department of Pediatrics and Adolescent Medicine, American University of Beirut Medical Center, Beirut, Lebanon

RYAN T. BORNE, MD
Electrophysiology Fellow, Cardiac Electrophysiology, University of Colorado, Denver, Aurora, Colorado

SCOTT R. CERESNAK, MD
Professor, Department of Pediatrics, Division of Pediatric Cardiology, Stanford University, Palo Alto, California

AKASH DADLANI
Division of Electrophysiology, Department of Medicine, University of California San Francisco, San Francisco, California

JERMEY DOCEKAL, MD
Section of Electrophysiology, Division of Cardiology, Queens Medical Center, Honolulu, Hawaii

JONATHAN W. DUKES, MD
Division of Electrophysiology, Department of Medicine, University of California San Francisco, San Francisco, California

MOHAMMAD ELBABA, MD
Section of Cardiac Electrophysiology, Division of Cardiology, Department of Internal Medicine, American University of Beirut Medical Center, Beirut, Lebanon

THOMAS FAGAN, MD
Associate Professor, The Children's Hospital and University of Colorado, Denver, Aurora, Colorado

AKL C. FAHED, MD
Department of Genetics, Harvard Medical School; Department of Medicine, Massachusetts General Hospital, Boston, Massachusetts

PAUL GARABELLI, MD
Assistant Professor, Department of Medicine,
Heart Rhythm Institute, University of Oklahoma
Health Sciences Center, Oklahoma City,
Oklahoma

EDWARD P. GERSTENFELD, MD
Professor of Medicine; Chief, Cardiac
Electrophysiology, Section of Cardiac
Electrophysiology, Division of Cardiology,
Department of Medicine, University of
California San Francisco, San Francisco,
California

JAIME E. GONZALEZ, MD
Electrophysiology Fellow, Cardiac
Electrophysiology, Cardiology Division,
University of Colorado, Denver, Aurora,
Colorado

DANIEL W. GROVES, MD
Fellow, Division of Cardiology, Cardiac
Electrophysiology, University of Colorado,
Denver, Aurora, Colorado

LEA EL HAGE, MD
Division of Cardiology, Department of
Medicine, University of California San
Francisco Medical Center, San Francisco,
California

FREDERICK T. HAN, MD, FACC, FHRS
Assistant Professor of Medicine, Section of
Cardiac Electrophysiology, Division of
Cardiovascular Medicine, University of Utah
Health Sciences Center, Salt Lake City, Utah

NASSIER HARFOUCH, BS
University of South Florida College of
Medicine, Tampa, Florida

SYLVANA HASSANIEH, BS
Department of Biochemistry and Molecular
Genetics, American University of Beirut
Medical Center, Beirut, Lebanon

MOSTAFA HOTAIT, MD
Cardiology Division, Department of Internal
Medicine, American University of Beirut
Medical Center, Beirut, Lebanon

HENRY H. HSIA, MD, FACC, FHRS
Chief, Arrhythmia Service, VA San
Francisco; Health Science Professor of
Medicine, University of California San
Francisco, San Francisco, California

RONALD J. KANTER, MD
Division of Cardiology, The Heart
Program, Nicklaus Children's Hospital,
Miami Children's Hospital Health System,
Miami, Florida; Director, Electrophysiology;
Professor Emeritus, Duke University
School of Medicine, Durham,
North Carolina

JOSEPH KAY, MD
Associate Professor of Medicine, Cardiology
Division, University of Colorado and
Children's Hospital Colorado, Aurora,
Colorado

AMBER D. KHANNA, MD
Adult Congenital Heart Disease, Division of
Cardiology, University of Colorado, Denver,
Aurora, Colorado

MAURICE KHOURY, MD
Section of Cardiac Electrophysiology,
Division of Cardiology, Department of
Internal Medicine, American University
of Beirut Medical Center, Beirut,
Lebanon

SAURABH KUMAR, BSc(Med), MBBS, PhD
Arrhythmia Service, Cardiovascular Division,
Brigham and Women's Hospital, Boston,
Massachusetts

PUI-YAN KWOK, MD, PhD
Institute for Human Genetics, University of
California San Francisco, San Francisco,
California

LEILA LARROUSSI, MD
Section of Cardiac Electrophysiology,
Division of Cardiology, Department of
Medicine, University of California San
Francisco, San Francisco, California

DAVID LIN, MD
Associate Professor of Medicine,
Cardiovascular Division, Hospital of the
University of Pennsylvania, Philadelphia,
Pennsylvania

FRANCIS E. MARCHLINSKI, MD
Richard T. and Angela Clark President's
Distinguished Professor, Cardiovascular
Division, Hospital of the University of
Pennsylvania, Philadelphia, Pennsylvania

KARA S. MOTONAGA, MD
Clinical Assistant Professor, Division of
Pediatric Cardiology, Department of
Pediatrics, Stanford University, Palo Alto,
California

BABAK NAZER, MD
Cardiac Electrophysiology, University of
California San Francisco, San Francisco,
California

WILLIAM P. NELSON, MD
Retired

GEORGES NEMER, PhD
Department of Biochemistry and Molecular
Genetics, American University of Beirut, Beirut,
Lebanon

DUY THAI NGUYEN, MD
Assistant Professor of Medicine, Cardiac
Electrophysiology, Cardiology Division,
University of Colorado, Denver, Aurora,
Colorado

AKIHIKO NOGAMI, MD, PhD
Professor, Cardiovascular Division, Faculty of
Medicine, University of Tsukuba, Tsukuba,
Japan

ADAM C. OESTERLE, MD
Section of Cardiac Electrophysiology, Division
of Cardiology, Department of Medicine,
University of California San Francisco, San
Francisco, California

AKASH PATEL, MD
Electrophysiologist, Department of Pediatrics,
Pediatric and Congenital Arrhythmia Center,
UCSF Benioff Children's Hospital, University of
California San Francisco, San Francisco,
California

C. THOMAS PETER, MD
Division of Electrophysiology, Queens
Heart Physicians Practice, Honolulu, Hawaii

SUNNY S. PO, MD, PhD
Professor of Medicine and Warren Jackman
Chair of Cardiac Electrophysiology; Director,
Clinical Electrophysiology, Department of
Medicine, Heart Rhythm Institute, University of
Oklahoma Health Sciences Center, Oklahoma
City, Oklahoma

SALMAN RAHMAN, BS
Section of Cardiac Electrophysiology, Division
of Cardiology, Department of Medicine,
University of California San Francisco, San
Francisco, California

**MARWAN M. REFAAT, MD, FACC, FAHA,
FHRS, FASE, FESC, FACP, FAAMA**
Section of Cardiac Electrophysiology,
Cardiology Division, Department of Internal
Medicine; Department of Biochemistry and
Molecular Genetics, American University of
Beirut Medical Center, Beirut, Lebanon;
Assistant Professor of Medicine, Cardiac
Electrophysiology, Cardiology, Department of
Internal Medicine, American University of
Beirut Faculty of Medicine and Medical Center,
New York, New York

JASON D. ROBERTS, MD
Section of Cardiac Electrophysiology, Division
of Cardiology, Department of Medicine,
University of California San Francisco, San
Francisco, California

EMILY SUE RUCKDESCHEL, MD
Adult and Pediatric Cardiology Fellow,
University of Colorado and Children's Hospital
Colorado, Aurora, Colorado

PASQUALE SANTANGELI, MD
Assistant Professor of Medicine,
Cardiovascular Division, Hospital of the
University of Pennsylvania, Philadelphia,
Pennsylvania

WILLIAM H. SAUER, MD
Associate Professor of Medicine, Cardiac
Electrophysiology, Cardiology Division,
University of Colorado, Denver, Aurora,
Colorado

MELVIN SCHEINMAN, MD
Director of the Genetic Arrhythmia Program,
University of California San Francisco Medical
Center, San Francisco, California

NICOLE SCHMITT, MSc, PhD
Department of Biomedical Sciences, Faculty
of Health and Medical Sciences, Danish
National Research Foundation Centre for
Cardiac Arrhythmia, University of Copenhagen,
Copenhagen, Denmark

JOSEPH SCHULLER, MD
Assistant Professor of Medicine, Cardiac
Electrophysiology, University of Colorado,
Denver, Aurora, Colorado

CHRISTINE E. SEIDMAN, MD
Department of Genetics, Harvard Medical
School; Division of Cardiology, Howard
Hughes Medical Institute, Brigham and
Women's Hospital, Boston, Massachusetts

JONATHAN G. SEIDMAN, PhD
Department of Genetics, Harvard Medical
School, Boston, Massachusetts

DAVID K. SINGH, MD
Assistant Professor, Section of Cardiac
Electrophysiology, Division of Cardiology,
Departments of Medicine and Internal
Medicine, Queens Medical Center, Honolulu,
Hawaii

HADI SKOURI, MD
Department of Internal Medicine, American
University of Beirut, Beirut, Lebanon

STAVROS STAVRAKIS, MD, PhD
Assistant Professor, Department of Medicine,
Heart Rhythm Institute, University of Oklahoma
Health Sciences Center, Oklahoma City,
Oklahoma

ANNETTE BUUR STEFFENSEN, MSc, PhD
Department of Biomedical Sciences, Faculty of
Health and Medical Sciences, Danish National
Research Foundation Centre for Cardiac
Arrhythmia, University of Copenhagen,
Copenhagen, Denmark

WILLIAM G. STEVENSON, MD
Arrhythmia Service, Cardiovascular Division,
Brigham and Women's Hospital, Boston,
Massachusetts

AHMED KARIM TALIB, MD, PhD
Cardiac Electrophysiology Fellow,
Cardiovascular Division, Faculty of

Medicine, University of Tsukuba, Tsukuba,
Japan

RONN TANEL, MD
Electrophysiologist, Department of Pediatrics,
Pediatric and Congenital Arrhythmia Center,
UCSF Benioff Children's Hospital, University of
California San Francisco, San Francisco,
California

PAUL TANG, PhD
Institute for Human Genetics, University of
California San Francisco, San Francisco,
California

USHA B. TEDROW, MD
Arrhythmia Service, Cardiovascular Division,
Brigham and Women's Hospital, Boston,
Massachusetts

WENDY TZOU, MD
Assistant Professor of Medicine, Cardiac
Electrophysiology, Cardiology Division,
University of Colorado, Denver, Aurora,
Colorado

PAUL VAROSY, MD
Section of Cardiac Electrophysiology, Division
of Cardiology, University of Colorado, Denver,
Aurora, Colorado

JULIANNE WOJCIAK, MS
Division of Cardiology, Department of
Medicine, University of California San
Francisco Medical Center, San Francisco,
California

EUGENE WOLFEL, MD
Professor of Medicine, Cardiology Division,
University of Colorado, Aurora, Colorado

MATTHEW M. ZIPSE, MD
Electrophysiology Fellow, Section of Cardiac
Electrophysiology, Division of Cardiology,
University of Colorado, Denver, Aurora,
Colorado

Contents

Despite unprecedented advances in technology, the electrocardiogram (ECG) remains essential to the practice of modern electrophysiology. Since its emergence at the turn of the nineteenth century, the form of the ECG has changed little. What has changed is our ability to understand the complex mechanisms that underlie various arrhythmias. In this article, the authors review several important principles of ECG interpretation by providing illustrative tracings. The authors also highlight several important concepts that be can used in ECG analysis. There are several fundamental principles that should be considered in ECG interpretation.

The atrioventricular (AV) bridge is vulnerable to many circumstances that depress conduction. Abnormal impulse transmission may be caused by drugs, autonomic effects, or destructive processes. Type 1 (Wenckebach) AV block is owing to depressed AV nodal conduction and is recognized by a prolonging PR interval ending in a "dropped beat". Type II (Mobitz) AV block is owing to abnormal infranodal conduction, and is usually accompanied by bundle branch block. Second-degree AV block with 2:1 conduction can be a difficult problem. Third-degree (complete) AV block is a diagnosis too often rendered and too often incorrect.

Section 1: Supraventricular Tachycardia
Editor: Nitish Badhwar

Atrioventricular reciprocating tachycardia is a common cause of undifferentiated supraventricular tachycardia. In patients with manifest or concealed accessory pathways, it is imperative to assess for the presence of other accessory pathways. Multiple accessory pathways are present in 4% to 10% of patients and are more common in patients with structural heart disease. In rare cases, multiple accessory pathways can act as the anterograde and retrograde limbs of the tachycardia.

Contents

tachycardia initiation with atrial extrastimulus as well as on the response to progressive decremental atrial extrastimuli. The progressive increase in A2H2′ and H2H2′ in response to atrial extrastimuli favors reentry as the mechanism of the tachycardia. This is a novel mechanistic differentiation of AVNRT from focal JT.

A 13-year-old boy had a positive P wave in V1 with a negative P wave in lead I, aVL, and aVR, as well as a positive P wave in the inferior leads, which correlated with a left atrial appendage (LAA) atrial tachycardia (AT) focus. P-wave morphologies can provide clues regarding an AT's origin, and this P-wave negative in lead I favored LAA AT. Careful mapping along the atria and coronary sinus to determine the earliest site of activation for the surface P wave is a reliable method for precisely localizing the AT origin as a target for catheter ablation.

Section 2: Ventricular Tachycardia
Editor: Henry H. Hsia

Ventricular tachyarrhythmia is an important cause of morbidity and sudden death. Although implantable cardioverter-defibrillator (ICD) reduces the risk of arrhythmic death, ICD therapies are associated with an increased mortality and worsening quality of life. Antiarrhythmic drugs may be effective in preventing arrhythmia recurrences but have increased adverse effects and non-cardiac mortality. Catheter ablation has evolved into an effective intervention in patients with and without structural heart disease. This monograph is a collection of thought-provoking challenging case scenarios. These cases emphasize important electrocardiographic and anatomic features, illustrating crucial diagnostic maneuvers, mapping techniques, imaging integration, as well as formulating the ablation strategies.

Distinguishing premature ventricular contractions/ventricular tachycardia from the right ventricular outflow tract versus the left ventricular outflow tract can be difficult by electrocardiogram findings alone. A thorough understanding of the outflow tract anatomy and a systematic and meticulous approach to mapping of the ventricular outflow regions and great vessels increases the success rate and decreases the risk of damage to adjacent structures and the conduction system. The use of multimodality imaging, particularly real-time intracardiac echocardiographic guidance, is essential for defining anatomy, ensuring adequate catheter contact, and minimizing risks.

Ventricular arrhythmias arising from the region of the left ventricular summit can be challenging for catheter-based percutaneous ablation. A detailed knowledge of the anatomy of this region and the need of high-density mapping of surrounding structures are critical in ensuring safe and effective ablation. This case-based review focuses on the particular challenges with ablation in this region.

Multi-modality imaging and detailed electroanatomic mapping demonstrated two predominant regional scar distributions: basal inferolateral and basal anteroseptal locations. Among the latter group, patients with predominantly septal scar pose a particularly difficult subset. Careful and systemic mapping is required to define the VT substrate. Aggressive ablations are often required from both sides of the septum to achieve arrhythmia control.

Patients with ventricular noncompaction are susceptible to developing ventricular tachycardia. Commonly, the origin of ventricular tachycardia is endocardial; however, epicardial origins and scar cannot be excluded and should be considered when poor endocardial mapping is present. Other cardiomyopathies, such as arrhythmogenic right ventricular cardiomyopathy, can coexist with ventricular noncompaction and should be excluded in these patients.

Section 3: Atrial Fibrillation and Flutter
Editor: Edward P. Gerstenfeld

Variant pulmonary venous anatomy is common and its pre-procedural recognition through cardiac imaging facilitates a personalized approach to ablation tailored to the individual patient. Close juxtaposition of the right and left pulmonary veins is an anatomic variation that serves as an ideal substrate for creation of a single box lesion set that concomitantly isolates the pulmonary veins and posterior wall. Isolation of the posterior wall may serve as an adjunctive ablative strategy in addition to pulmonary vein isolation that facilitates maintenance of sinus rhythm among patients with persistent atrial fibrillation.

The electrophysiologic nature of atrial fibrillation (AF) and related atrial arrhythmias in Friedreich ataxia has not previously been characterized. In the presented case, dense atrial scar had progressed to the point of acquired pulmonary vein (PV) isolation before the delivery of a single radiofrequency lesion. AF was induced, and ultimately organized spontaneously into a microreentrant atrial tachycardia. Other atrial tachycardias were also identified near scar border zones; these potentially served as triggers for AF in this patient, independent of the PVs. This case emphasizes the need to address non-PV substrate in some patients undergoing catheter ablation of AF.

Clinicians must be mindful of the left ventricular lead when cannulating the coronary sinus with a decapolar catheter or an ablation catheter. Left atrial catheter ablation for the treatment of atrial fibrillation in patients with a mechanical mitral valve, when approached carefully, can be performed safely and effectively. Block across linear

Section 5: Adult Congenital Cardiac Disease
Editor: Ronn Tanel

mapping and entrainment maneuvers, are important to identify and successfully treat arrhythmias. This case was unique in that the lack of femoral venous access required transhepatic venous access and bidirectional block was attained with ablation lesions along the cavotricuspid isthmus on both sides of the baffle.

Ventricular Tachycardia Following Surgical Repair of Complex Congenital Heart Disease

Sherrie Joy Baysa and Ronald J. Kanter

A nine year old boy with complex congenital heart disease requiring right ventricular outflow tract surgery and palpitations had inducible monomorphic ventricular tachycardia at 300 bpm by programmed ventricular stimulation. He was treated with enteral phenytoin. With a therapeutic plasma level, repeat electrophysiological study was negative for inducible ventricular tachycardia using an aggressive pacing protocol. An insertable loop recorder was implanted, and the family was prescribed an automatic external defibrillator. The decision to not place an implantable cardioverter-defibrillator was based upon anticipated need for serial cardiac MRI scans to monitor the effect of progressive outflow tract stenosis and regurgitation.

Ventricular Tachycardia in Congenital Pulmonary Stenosis

Emily Sue Ruckdeschel, Joseph Schuller, and Duy Thai Nguyen

With modern surgical techniques, there is significantly increased life expectancy for those with congenital heart disease. Although congenital pulmonary valve stenosis is not as complex as tetralogy of Fallot, there are many similarities between the 2 lesions, such that patients with either of these conditions are at risk for ventricular arrhythmias and sudden cardiac death. Those patients who have undergone surgical palliation for congenital pulmonary stenosis are at an increased risk for development of ventricular arrhythmias and may benefit from a more aggressive evaluation for symptoms of palpitations or syncope.

Section 6: Arrhythmias in Patients with Genetic Arrhythmia Syndromes
Editor: Marwan M. Refaat

Twin Atrioventricular Nodal Reentrant Tachycardia Associated with Heterotaxy Syndrome with Malaligned Atrioventricular Canal Defect and Atrioventricular Discordance

Akash Patel and Ronn Tanel

There are limited data on the experience of transbaffle access for catheter ablation in patients who have undergone a Fontan palliation for complex congenital heart. Nevertheless, these issues will be encountered more frequently, because patients who have undergone Fontan palliation continue to survive into adulthood and develop a variety of arrhythmias that may be refractory to medical therapy.

Arrhythmogenic Right Ventricular Cardiomyopathy Caused by a Novel Frameshift Mutation

Marwan M. Refaat, Paul Tang, Nassier Harfouch, Julianne Wojciak, Pui-Yan Kwok, and Melvin Scheinman

Arrhythmogenic right ventricular cardiomyopathy is a rare cardiomyopathy that might be asymptomatic or symptomatic, causing palpations or syncope, and might lead to sudden cardiac death. It is recommended that physical exertion be reduced. It is also recommended that those with syncope and ventricular tachycardia/ventricular fibrillation have an implantable cardioverter-defibrillator placed. β-Blockers, antiarrhythmic drugs, and radiofrequency ablation should be used to control the ventricular arrhythmia burden in arrhythmogenic right ventricular cardiomyopathy.

Hypertrophic cardiomyopathy (HCM) is a familial cardiac disease manifested in a wide phenotype and diverse genotype and, thus, presenting unpredictable risks mainly in young adults. Extensive studies are being conducted to categorize patients and link phenotype with genotype for a better management and control of the disease with all its complications. Because the full mechanisms behind HCM are still not revealed, therapeutics are not definitive. Further research is to be conducted for the generation of a complete picture and directed therapy for HCM.

Catecholaminergic polymorphic ventricular tachycardia (CPVT) is a challenging and serious disease with a high incidence of sudden cardiac deaths. Patients with CPVT should not be exposed to physical or emotional exertion that might induce ventricular tachycardia. This article presents a case with CPVT and discusses the clinical features of the disease, its genetic background, and the management of CPVT.

Brugada syndrome might stay undetected in patients until surviving cardiac arrest. Despite the prominent advances in exploring the disease in the past 2 decades, many questions remain unanswered and the controversies continue. Despite all mutations identified to be associated with the disease, two-thirds of cases have a negative genetic test. Future studies should be more directed on modulating factors and their impact on patients' risk for sudden death to help physicians in risk stratifying their patients and optimally implementing an implantable cardioverter defibrillator to prevent sudden cardiac death.

The authors present a unique case of torsades de pointes in a β-thalassemia patient with early iron overload in the absence of any structural abnormalities as seen in hemochromatosis. Genetic testing showed a novel *KCNQ1* gene mutation 1591C >T [Gln531Ter(X)]. Testing of the gene mutation in *Xenopus laevis* oocytes showed loss of function of the IKs current. The authors hypothesize that iron overload combined with the *KCNQ1* gene mutation leads to prolongation of QTc and torsades de pointes.

CARDIAC ELECTROPHYSIOLOGY CLINICS

FORTHCOMING ISSUES

June 2016
Cardiac Potassium Channel Disorders
Mohammad Shenasa and Stanley Nattel, *Editors*

September 2016
Ventricular Arrhythmias in Apparently Normal Hearts
Frank M. Bogun, Thomas Crawford, and Rakesh Latchamsetty, *Editors*

December 2016
The His-Purkinje System
Masood Akhtar, *Editor*

RECENT ISSUES

December 2015
Cardiac Resynchronization Therapy: State of the Art
Luigi Padeletti, Martina Nesti, and Giuseppe Boriani, *Editors*

September 2015
Controversies in Electrophysiology
Emile G. Daoud and Raul Weiss, *Editors*

June 2015
Arrhythmias in Cardiomyopathies
Mohammad Shenasa, Mark S. Link, and Martin S. Maron, *Editors*

ISSUE OF RELATED INTEREST

Cardiology Clinics, November 2014 (Vol. 32, No. 4)
Atrial Fibrillation
Hakan Oral, *Editor*
Available at: http://www.cardiology.theclinics.com/

THE CLINICS ARE AVAILABLE ONLINE!
Access your subscription at:
www.theclinics.com

Foreword

Interpretation of Complex Arrhythmias: A Case-Based Approach

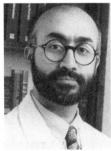

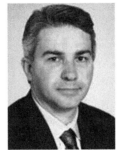

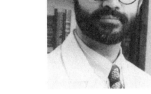
Ranjan Thakur, MD, MPH, MBA, FACC, FHRS   Andrea Natale, MD, FACC, FHRS
Consulting Editors

Imitation is not just the sincerest form of flattery—it's the sincerest form of learning
—George Bernard Shaw,
Irish writer (1856–1950)

Case reports are probably the oldest form of medical literature and a time-honored teaching tool. Observations made on a single patient with a rare/new condition add to our understanding of a disease, but even for common conditions, they add up to the education of trainees and physicians at all stages of their careers. Being clinicians, our daily job revolves around individual patients, and what we learn from them helps us in treating other patients. As we learn from most of our cases, we can learn from the cases of the others. Through their peculiar narrative, case reports allow us to get an insight of a colleague's diagnostic and therapeutic reasoning, and they can have a big impact, as we can use others' experience to solve future clinical problems.

In this issue of *Cardiac Electrophysiology Clinics*, Dr Melvin Scheinman has selected interesting case studies focused on electrocardiography. The cases range from supraventricular tachycardia to genetic arrhythmia syndromes, and whose take-home points serve an important role for everyday practice. To discuss these cases, he has selected well-known teachers of electrocardiography.

We hope that the readers will enjoy reading these cases, giving them an opportunity to challenge or improve their knowledge in some of the common and less common clinical conditions as presented through the expertise of this issue's contributors.

Ranjan Thakur, MD, MPH, MBA, FACC, FHRS
Sparrow Thoracic and Cardiovascular Institute
Michigan State University
1200 East Michigan Avenue, Suite 585
Lansing, MI 48912, USA

Andrea Natale, MD, FACC, FHRS
Texas Cardiac Arrhythmia Institute
Center for Atrial Fibrillation at
St. David's Medical Center
1015 East 32nd Street, Suite 516
Austin, TX 78705, USA

E-mail addresses:
thakur@msu.edu (R. Thakur)
andrea.natale@stdavids.com (A. Natale)

Card Electrophysiol Clin 8 (2016) xix
http://dx.doi.org/10.1016/j.ccep.2015.12.003
1877-9182/16/$ – see front matter © 2016 Published by Elsevier Inc.

Preface
Challenging Cases, Match Wits with the Masters

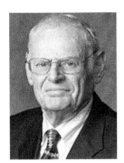

Melvin Scheinman, MD

Editor

I am proud and delighted to present the third issue of case studies for *Cardiac Electrophysiology Clinics*. We are indeed fortunate to have contributing authors who are both expert electrophysiologists and superb teachers. I am also indebted to the Section Editors for their tireless work and diligence. I am happy that the case presentation format allows the reader to match wits with the experts and remains an important and exciting educational tool. I hope the readers agree, and I would, of course, appreciate your valued and constructive input.

Melvin Scheinman, MD
University of California
San Francisco Medical Center
San Francisco
500 Parnassus Avenue, MUE 436
San Francisco, CA 94143-1354, USA

E-mail address:
Melvin.Scheinman@ucsf.edu

Card Electrophysiol Clin 8 (2016) xxi
http://dx.doi.org/10.1016/j.ccep.2015.12.002
1877-9182/16/$ – see front matter © 2016 Published by Elsevier Inc.

Use of the Surface Electrocardiogram to Define the Nature of Challenging Arrhythmias

David K. Singh, MD*, C. Thomas Peter, MD

KEYWORDS

- Electrocardiogram • Arrhythmias • Intracardiac tracings

KEY POINTS

- A methodical approach to ECG analysis is essential for dissecting complex tracings.
- The use of a ladder diagram can be a useful tool to analyze and communicate the principles underlying a complex ECG.
- The surface ECG continues to be indispensible and relevant tool to the modern practice of electrophysiology.

INTRODUCTION

Despite unprecedented advances in technology, the electrocardiogram (ECG) remains essential to the practice of modern electrophysiology. Indeed since its emergence at the turn of the nineteenth century, the form of the ECG has changed little. What has changed is our ability to understand the complex mechanisms that underlie various arrhythmias. These advances have introduced a deeper understanding about the power of the ECG as a tool to both diagnose and treat cardiac rhythm disturbances.

In this article, the authors review several important principles of ECG interpretation by providing illustrative tracings. Although a comprehensive review of ECG analysis is beyond the scope of this article, the authors highlight several important concepts that be can used in ECG analysis. There are several fundamental principles that should be considered in ECG interpretation.

BE METHODICAL

Even the most seasoned clinician can miss important findings on an ECG. An interventional cardiologist may miss complete heart block in the setting of an acute myocardial infarction. An electrophysiologist might make exactly the opposite mistake. Using a systematic approach is particularly important in the setting of complex arrhythmias.

THE PROCESS IS MORE IMPORTANT THAN THE ANSWER

Analyzing a complex ECG is analogous to solving a puzzle. Like many puzzles there may be more than one solution. Thinking about multiple explanations for any given tracing can only strengthen one's ability to analyze an ECG. Even the most sophisticated readers may disagree about the mechanisms underlying a particular ECG. Moreover, it is often impossible to prove or disprove one theory over the other. The magic of ECG interpretation is in the journey. How did one arrive at a conclusion? Can it be defended using the principles of electrophysiology? How likely is the proposed explanation? An ECG with normal sinus rhythm could theoretically be interpreted as complete heart block with isorhythmic atrioventricular (AV)

Division of Electrophysiology, Queens Heart Physicians Practice, 550 South Beretania Street, Suite 601, Honolulu, HI 96813, USA
* Corresponding author.
E-mail address: dsingh@queens.org

Card Electrophysiol Clin 8 (2016) 1–24
http://dx.doi.org/10.1016/j.ccep.2015.10.021
1877-9182/16/$ – see front matter © 2016 Elsevier Inc. All rights reserved.

cardiacEP.theclinics.com

dissociation and junctional escape complexes. The authors would say that, although this explanation is possible, it is not probable. It is important to seek out the most probable explanation when analyzing a tracing.

In this article, the authors share many tracings and provide what they think to be the most probable explanation in order to illuminate various principles of ECG analysis. The reader may disagree with their explanation or even suggest a more plausible one. The authors welcome them. Some of these tracings in this article have been shared hundreds of times over the years. The authors continue to make new discoveries about them all the time.

USE A LADDER DIAGRAM

It may feel antiquated to use a pen or pencil to construct a ladder diagram, but it can be immensely helpful in deconstructing complex tracings. It is also a powerful communication tool. It is often easier to share a theory about a tracing using a ladder diagram than by doing so through the use of language. In this article, the authors rely heavily on ladder diagrams to explain the basis of a given arrhythmia.

TAKE THE TIME TO NURTURE YOUR PRACTICE

Many of us were drawn toward electrophysiology through our passion for the ECG interpretation. With the demands of modern medicine, we are frequently confronted with a challenging ECG but lack the time to dwell on it and recognize that unlocking its mystery may not impact our clinical decision. Although it is not realistic to perseverate on every challenging ECG that comes across one's desk, take a few minutes each week and retire to a quiet room with some calipers and a few

tracings. ECG interpretation is a lifelong pursuit that needs to be nurtured with patience and practice.

DISORDERS OF IMPULSE CONDUCTION: WHAT IS THE MECHANISM AND LOCATION OF THE BLOCK?

Karel Frederik Wenckebach first described Wenckebach periodicity in 1893, before the invention of the ECG. Through analysis of the radial pulse in his patient, he was able to describe a predictable pattern of pauses now known to be the result of block in the AV node. Typical AV nodal Wenckebach or Mobitz I block is associated with the following findings.

- There is a constant input rate (eg, sinus node, atrial tachycardia, and so forth). In practical terms, this is rare, even though most of the following statements are critically linked to the p-p intervals being constant.
- There is progressive lengthening of the PR interval followed by a dropped beat (QRS complex).
- The shortest PR interval follows the dropped beat.
- The largest absolute increase in the PR interval typically occurs on the second beat following the dropped QRS. Although the PR interval continues to prolong, it prolongs to a lesser degree with each subsequent p wave (**Fig. 1**).
- Shortening output intervals: As a result of decreasing incremental delay in AV nodal conduction, the R-R intervals typically shorten.
- As a result of decreasing incremental delay in AV nodal conduction, the R-R interval encompassing the nonconducted beat is less the 2 times the input rate.

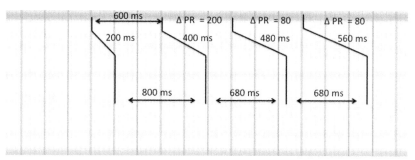

Fig. 1. Classic Wenckebach physiology. The RR interval = the sinus rate + the PR interval − the preceding PR interval. The second beat marks the largest delta (Δ) PR (200 milliseconds). The subsequent delta PRs are 80 milliseconds. The RR shortens on the third beat from 800 milliseconds to 680 milliseconds because the delta PR has shortened. Because the delta PR remains constant between the third and fourth beats, the RR interval remains constant.

- There is a grouped beating with p/QRS ratios that may vary (3:2, 4:3, 5:4).

Any input to the AV node can result in Mobitz 1 physiology. **Fig. 2** demonstrates AV nodal Wenckebach in the setting of atrial flutter. Although the flutter waves can be difficult to discern, the presence of a grouped beating should alert the reader to the presence of Wenckebach phenomena. Note that in the first portion of the tracing there is 4:3 Wenckebach followed by a period of 3:2 Wenckebach.

It is also important to recognize that Wenckebach physiology does not always follow the rules outlined earlier. In general, however, the pause is almost always less than twice the basic pacemaker cycle length. The return PR interval is also usually shorter than the PR interval preceding the dropped beat.

Mobitz 2 AV block is associated with the following characteristics.

- There is a constant input rate.
- There is an unchanging PR interval followed by a sudden loss of AV conduction and a dropped QRS complex.
- The RR interval encompassing the nonconducted beat is 2 times the input rate.

Mobitz 1 and Mobitz 2 block can take place anywhere along the conduction system, including the sinus node, AV node, His bundle, bundle branches, and fascicles. Moreover, both forms of block can be seen in the setting of rhythms associated with enhanced automaticity, such as atrial tachycardia and idiopathic ventricular tachycardia. In this case, exit block from the focus can exhibit Mobitz 1 or Mobitz 2 physiology. **Fig. 3**A demonstrates a patient with right bundle branch block (RBBB), left anterior fascicular block (LAFB), and **Fig. 3**B demonstrates a typical alternating 3:2 and 4:3 Wenckebach pattern. Intracardiac recordings in the same patient reveal Wenckebach in the His bundle with preserved AV nodal conduction.[1]

In Mobitz 1 or Mobitz 2 AV block, the input is generally visible on the ECG. In the case of sinus rhythm with Mobitz 1 AV block, the input to the AV node is the surface p wave and prolongation

of the AV interval manifests through PR prolongation. Depending on the site of block, however, the input may not be visible. In the case of sinoatrial (SA) block, the input (sinus node discharge) is electrocardiographically silent. Only the output phase of the block is visible and is represented by p waves on the surface ECG. Nonetheless, the presence of Wenckebach periodicity can be inferred based on the behavior of the output.

Fig. 4 reveals a patient with Mobitz I SA block. Note the subtle decrease in the output interval that is shortening of the p-p interval before the dropped beat. Also note that the interval encompassing the dropped beat is less than twice the sinus rate. Both of these features should alert the reader to the presence of Wenckebach phenomena. It is also important to recognize that SA Wenckebach should be suspected whenever a pause is less than twice the p-p interval even if the p-p intervals remain the same or even increase before the pause. Such a scenario can result because the incremental increases in the SA conduction times may remain the same or even increase.

Fig. 5 demonstrates an unusual scenario in which multiple sites of block can be observed. The initial portion of the ECG reveals sinus rhythm with RBBB.

Following the fourth conducted QRS complex, a PAC marks the onset of an atrial tachycardia. The p wave morphology suggests a focus in the crista terminalis (upright p wave morphology with negative terminal deflection in V1). There is gradual PR prolongation followed by a dropped beat consistent with Wenckebach in the AV node. Close inspection of the morphology of the p wave on the return beat suggests persistence of the atrial tachycardia. Note that within the pause there is a missing p wave (blue/red circle). The p-p interval is approximately 2 times the rate of the atrial tachycardia implying Mobitz 2 exit block from the tachycardia focus.

Fig. 6A illustrates that Mobitz I and II block can originate in the bundle branches and fascicles. In this case, the patient has an acute anterior myocardial infarction. The first two QRS complexes are conducted down the right bundle (RB)

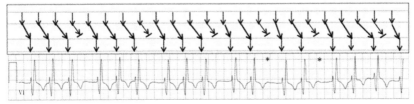

Fig. 2. AV nodal Wenckebach in the setting of atrial flutter. A 4:3 Wenckebach is observed with periods of 3:2 Wenckebach (*asterisks*).

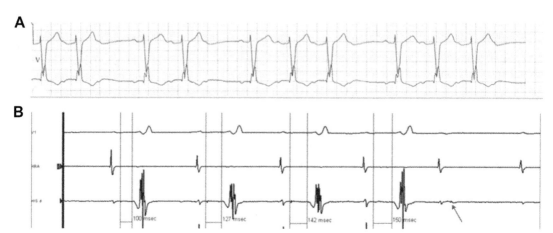

Fig. 3. (A) Patient with RBBB and left anterior fascicular block and a typical alternating 3:2 and 4:3 Wenckebach pattern. (B) Intracardiac recordings reveal Wenckebach in the His bundle with preserved AV nodal conduction. (*From* Tandon A, Simpson L, Assar MD. Unusual origin of type 1 atrioventricular block with comments on Wenckebach's contribution. Proc (Bayl Univ Med Cent) 2011;24(1):9–12; with permission.)

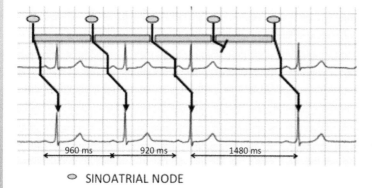

SINOATRIAL NODE

Fig. 4. SA exit block. Note the shortening of the p-p interval before the dropped p wave. Also note that the pause is less than 2× the sinus rate. Both of these findings support the diagnosis of SA Wenckebach.

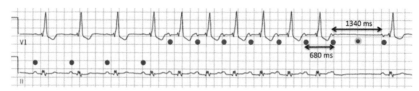

Fig. 5. Sinus rhythm with RBBB. Following the fourth conducted QRS complex a premature atrial beat marks the onset of an atrial tachycardia. There is gradual PR prolongation followed by a dropped beat consistent with Wenckebach in the AV node. Close inspection of the morphology of the p wave on the return beat suggests persistence of the atrial tachycardia. If this is the case, then there appears to be exit block from the ectopic focus as evidenced by the absence of a p wave (*blue circle*). The pause is approximately 2× the rate of the atrial tachycardia suggesting Mobitz 2 exit block from the tachycardia focus.

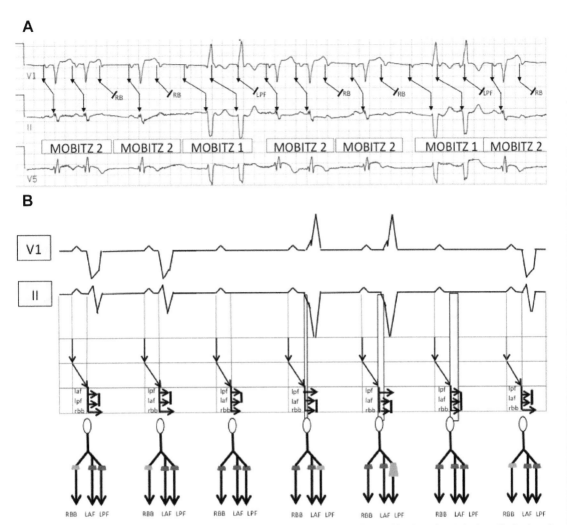

Fig. 6. (A) Patient with anterior myocardial infarction demonstrating Mobitz 2 block in the right bundle (RB) and Mobitz I block in the left posterior fascicle (LPF). (B) Diagram depicting Mobitz 2 block in right bundle branch (RBB) and Mobitz 1 block in LPF. laf, left anterior fascicle.

with left bundle branch block (LBBB) morphology. The PR interval does not prolong and is followed by a nonconducted p wave suggesting Mobitz 2 block of the RB. The subsequent p wave is conducted to the ventricle with a prolonged PR interval and a RBBB LAFB pattern. Conduction to the ventricle is, therefore, via the left posterior fascicle (LPF). The subsequent PR interval is slightly prolonged (best seen in lead V1), followed by a nonconducted p wave. This pattern implies Mobitz 1 block in the LPF. **Fig. 6**B illustrates this pattern in cartoon form.

CONCEALED CONDUCTION

Early descriptions of concealed conduction revolutionized our ability to explain many phenomena related to cardiac conduction.[2,3] The term

concealed conduction refers to the effects of impulses on conduction that are not visible on the surface ECG. These effects on impulse propagation and formation are the result of either antero- grade or retrograde penetration of various elements of the cardiac conduction system. Con- cealed conduction can be used to explain other- wise unexpected findings on a surface ECG and can often be proven with invasive electrophysi- ology studies (where they are not concealed). Because concealed conduction is by definition not visible on a surface ECG, its presence can only be inferred as an underlying mechanism. Manifestations of concealed conduction include.[4]

- Unexpected prolongation of conduction
- Unexpected failure of propagation
- Unexpected facilitation of conduction

Fig. 7 illustrates the concept of retrograde concealed conduction. The patient has ventricular trigeminy and preexisting LBBB. Note prolongation of the PR interval that always follows the ventricular beat. This implies retrograde concealed conduction into the right bundle, AV node or AV nodal fast pathway. The result is prolongation of the PR on the subsequent sinus beat.

Fig. 8A illustrates a similar concept. At first glance, one might be tempted to conclude that the ECG illustrates 2:1 AV block with a premature ventricular contraction (PVC) or junctional beat toward the end of the tracing. Note, however, that there is mild prolongation of the PR interval following the first nonconducted P wave. An even longer PR follows the second nonconducted P wave. This longer PR should alert the reader to another potential explanation. The PR interval should generally shorten or stay the same following a nonconducted P wave in the setting of AV block. Fig. 8B demonstrates the intracardiac electrogram for the same patient. In this tracing, one can observe the presence of pseudo-AV block as a result of His-extrasystoles. In this case, the first two His-extrasystoles (arrow with asterisk) are not conducted to the atrium or the ventricle creating the appearance of AV block. The third His-extrasystole is conducted through the LB. The H-H coupling interval is slightly longer than previous H-H intervals likely resulting in recovery of the LB and subsequent conduction.

Finally, the prolongation of the PR in the second and third conducted beats can be explained by concealed conduction into the AV node from the His-extrasystole. Note that the atrial-His (AH) interval following the His-extrasystole is directly related to the preceding H-H interval. A longer preceding H-H interval results in more delayed concealed conduction into the AV node and, thus, longer antegrade AH conduction time in the subsequent beat.

This tracing illustrates an important concept: when confronted by apparent Mobitz I or Mobitz II AV block and the presence of junctional premature beats or wide complexes with a typical aberrancy pattern, always consider His extrasystoles as a possible mechanism.

Fig. 9 is a challenging tracing characterized by a wide complex escape rhythm, a dissociated sinus rhythm (red bar), and a trigeminy pattern. What is the origin of the LBBB escape rhythm? Does the rhythm arise from the junction or the ventricle? Note that the junctional escape cycle length can be inferred from the J1 interval where there are 2 successive LBBB conducted complexes. The interval from the RBBB/LAFB complex to the LBBB complex is labeled as J2. Note the lack of a full compensatory pause following this beat. This finding implies that the focus, wherever its origin, has been reset. One can infer the presence of concealed conduction from the RBBB complex into the LBBB escape focus.

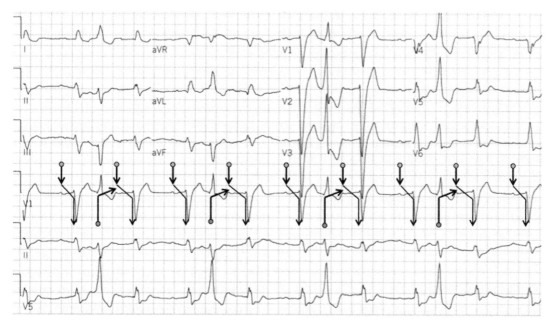

Fig. 7. Ventricular trigeminy with retrograde concealed conduction resulting in PR prolongation following each premature ventricular complex.

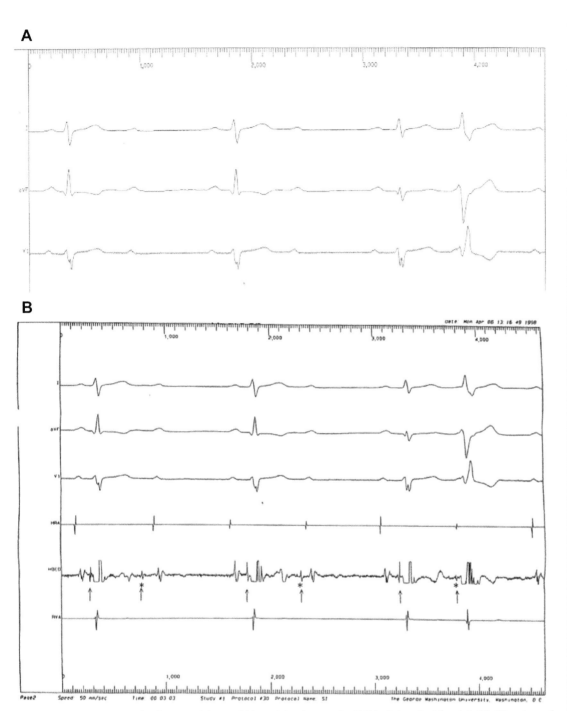

Fig. 8. (*A, B*) His-extrasystoles (*arrow with asterisk*) resulting in pseudo-AV block (see text for details). (*Courtesy of Dr Steven Singh, Washington, DC.*)

Working backwards, one can derive the point of reset by using the J1 interval. The red arrows mark the point of reset, which occurs before the onset of the RBBB complex. This would imply that the point of reset must have occurred in the junction proving the LBBB complex must be junctional in origin. If this is the case, the mechanism underlying the trigeminy pattern must be the result of escape-capture and depends on the presence of dual AV nodal pathways. The junction likely penetrates one AV pathway in the retrograde fashion, turns around, and traverses a second AV nodal pathway

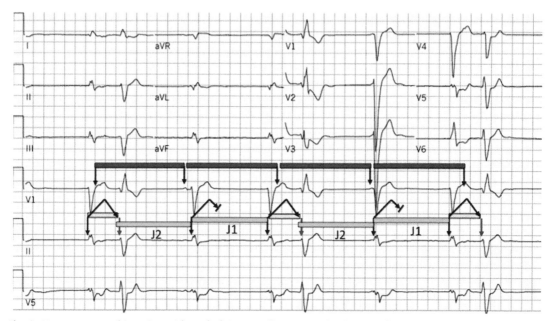

Fig. 9. Escape capture bigeminy with underlying AV dissociation (*red bars indicate sinus rate*). J1 refers to the LBBB escape rate. J2 refers to the interval between the RBBB echo beat and the subsequent LBBB escape. Is the wide QRS complex ventricular or junctional in origin? The answer lies in the timing of the reset. Note the lack of full compensatory pause following the RBBB echo beat (ie, J2 <2× J1). The red arrows indicate the point of reset that occurs at the onset of the QRS. Thus, the escape rhythm must have been reset before ventricular depolarization, which could have only occurred in the junction. Therefore, the wide QRS complex must be junctional in origin. If the point of reset had occurred following the echo beat, the origin of the escape would likely have arisen in the ventricle. Note that the third and sixth QRS complexes are not associated with an echo beat. This finding suggests that the sinus node conceals into the AV nodal slow pathway rendering it refractory to retrograde conduction from the junctional beat, thus preventing the echo.

resetting the junctional focus in the process and finally transmitting to the ventricle via the LPF.

The junctional escape complex not associated with an echo beat is likely the result of concealed conduction from the sinus impulse into the AV nodal pathway involved in the echo circuit. This concealed conduction interrupts the circuit, preventing the echo beat from arising. This observation is critical in establishing that the LBBB beat is an echo beat and not ventricular in origin. A ventricular beat would not be interrupted by the presence of a critically timed p wave that occurs before the onset of the preceding QRS complex. In contrast, an echo beat arising from a circuit involving an AV nodal pathway most certainly could be affected by a critically timed p wave. Finally the echo beat occurs because there is a unidirectional block with respect to antegrade conduction into the AV node. The echo circuit is manifest when retrograde penetration of the AV nodal pathway occurs and the antegrade conduction from the sinus p wave is blocked.

Thus, several take-home points can be derived from this complex tracing:

1. The wide QRS rhythm with LBBB morphology was identified as junctional in origin because the point of reset of the junctional pacemaker occurred *before* the onset of the echo QRS complex.
2. The RBBB QRS complex was identified as an echo beat, not ventricular in origin, because critically timed p waves were observed to interrupt the echo circuit. A p wave occurring just before a junctional beat would not be expected to interrupt a circuit arising in the ventricle.
3. The presence of the echo beat is associated with antegrade unidirectional block in the AV node with respect to the sinus p wave.

Dual Atrioventricular Nodal Physiology

The term *dual AV nodal pathways* is used to describe the highly complex physiology surrounding conduction inputs to the compact AV node. The posterior inferior input to the AV node is commonly referred to as the slow pathway, whereas the anterior superior input to the AV node is commonly referred to as the fast pathway. Although these are probably not discrete structures, this nomenclature can be useful to explain various ECG and intracardiac phenomena. In addition, although dual AV nodal pathways provide the substrate for reentrant arrhythmias, such as typical and atypical atrioventricular reentrant tachycardia, they can be associated with other ECG anomalies that can be easily missed.

The presence of varying PR intervals of fixed length should alert the reader to the presence of dual AV nodal physiology with alternating slow and fast pathway conduction. **Fig. 10** illustrates this concept. There is an underlying sinus mechanism with apparent variation in the PR intervals as well as nonconducted p waves. On closer inspection, there seem to be 2 distinct PR intervals. The first measures approximately 520 milliseconds and likely represents conduction down the slow pathway. The second measures approximately 200 milliseconds and likely represents conduction down the fast pathway. Thus, there seems to be alternating conduction down the slow and fast pathways. In other instances, both the fast and slow pathways are blocked resulting in nonconducted p waves.

Fig. 11 reveals an ECG from a patient with a prior diagnosis of atrial fibrillation. Although the rhythm is irregular, there is a clear underlying sinus mechanism. The ECG represents a relatively uncommon manifestation of dual AV nodal physiology known as a double fire whereby a double ventricular response is observed following a single atrial depolarization. This manifestation occurs because the atrial stimulus conducts down both the fast and slow AV nodal pathways. The result is a nonreentrant tachycardia originally referred to as paroxysmal nonreentrant tachycardia.[5] Ablation of the AV nodal slow pathway resulted in elimination of the patient's tachycardia.

Fig. 12 demonstrates the double-fire mechanism in retrograde fashion. The patient has an underlying junctional rhythm. Each junctional beat is followed by a conducted beat preceded by a superior axis p wave. Although the axis of the p wave might suggest the presence of an ectopic atrial focus, the more likely explanation is that the p wave is conducted in retrograde fashion via the AV nodal slow pathway. The impulse then turns around and conducts down the AV nodal fast pathway producing the subsequent echo beat.

FROM NARROW TO WIDE

The presence of alternating or transient patterns of bundle branch/fascicular block is frequently the mechanism underlying a widening QRS morphology. The most common cause of transient block in the cardiac conduction system is phase 3 block or aberrancy. In phase 3 block (or aberrancy), a premature impulse arises during the refractory period of some portion of the conduction system. **Fig. 13** demonstrates this concept. The underlying rhythm is atrial bigeminy. Note that the QRS following each ectopic p wave is characterized by left anterior fascicular block. The left anterior fascicle is refractory at the time of the premature beat giving rise to the typical LAFB pattern. This pattern can be explained by the phase 3 block in the left anterior fascicle.

Fig. 14 is a marvelous tracing that illustrates several important concepts. The underlying rhythm is atrial trigeminy (2 sinus beats followed by a premature atrial beat in a repetitive pattern). There are also alternating QRS morphologies. The beats following sinus impulses are characterized by an incomplete RBBB and LAFB pattern. The beats following the premature atrial beat are an LBBB pattern. Conduction following the sinus beats is, therefore, achieved chiefly through

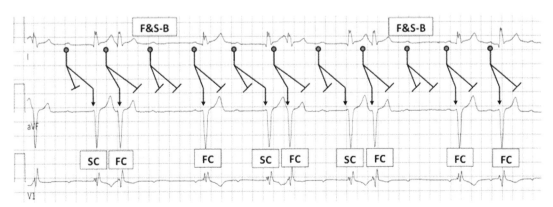

Fig. 10. Sinus rhythm with alternating conduction between AV nodal slow and fast pathways. At times, both fast and slow pathways are blocked resulting in a nonconducted p wave. F&S-B, block in both fast and slow pathways; FC, conduction via fast pathway; SC, conduction via slow pathway.

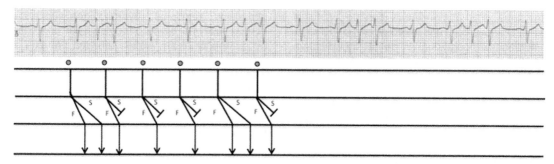

Fig. 11. Double-fire mechanism in a patient with dual AV nodal physiology. Note that throughout the tracing one p wave intermittently results in 2 QRS complex as a result of conduction down both fast (F) and slow (S) pathways.

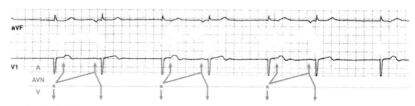

Fig. 12. Retrograde double fire. A junctional beat (*asterisk*) results in retrograde conduction up to the atrium via both fast and slow AV nodal pathways. Retrograde conduction up the slow pathway results in an echo beat.

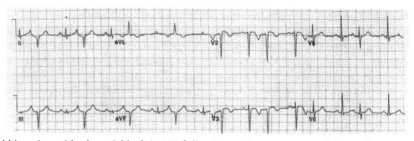

Fig. 13. Atrial bigeminy with phase 3 block in LPF following each premature atrial complex.

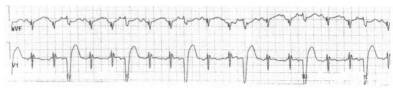

Fig. 14. Atrial trigeminy. Sinus beats are conducted primarily via the LPF (incomplete RBBB/LAFB); the PAC is conducted via the RBB (LBBB).

conduction via the LPF. Moreover, it is important to recognize that the presence of incomplete RBBB suggests that most of the right ventricle (RV) is activated via transseptal conduction from the left ventricle with only a minor portion of RV activated by the delayed impulse from the RBB.

Following the premature atrial beat, the QRS morphology changes to an LBBB pattern. Because we know left anterior fascicle (LAF) is diseased from the sinus beats, the LBBB pattern is likely the result of phase 3 block in the LPF (**Fig. 15**). If this explanation is true, then it is worth considering what would happen to the His-ventricular (HV) interval (if were it available) during the LBBB beats. If the RBBB is slower to conduct than the LPF as established during sinus beats, then it follows that conduction exclusively via the RBB during the premature beats should result in a longer HV interval. From this tracing one can infer the presence of a highly diseased conduction system that may require permanent pacing in the future.

Several other mechanisms can be responsible for the transient appearance of bundle branch or fascicular block. Acceleration-dependent bundle branch block is seen with increases in heart rate. In patients with advanced conduction disease, bundle branch block may seem to relatively slow heart rates. **Fig. 16** displays a patient with sinus rhythm and LBBB. There is normalization of the QRS complex following a PVC-related compensatory pause. This normalization suggests that there is rate-related (phase 3) block in the LBBB. The recovery of left bundle branch (LBB) following the pauses suggests that the LBB could conceivably conduct at slower heart rates in this patient.

Bradycardia-dependent block is also referred to as phase 4 block and can be seen in all areas of the conduction system, including the bundle branches. One of the earliest descriptions of this phenomenon came from Massumi[6] in 1968.

Fig. 17 is a tracing demonstrating sinus tachycardia with a 3:2 Wenckebach pattern. Note that the QRS complex following the blocked beat is always characterized by LBBB. This is an excellent example of a bradycardia-dependent block in the LBB.

The mechanism of phase 4 block remains elusive. Under normal circumstances, phase 4 depolarization is a normal property of the conduction system that accounts for the automaticity associated with the sinus node, AV node, His bundle, and bundle branches. Phase 4 block typically occurs when a diseased portion of the conduction system is confronted with a supraventricular impulse during phase 4 of the action potential.[7] During this time, sodium channels are inactive and, thus, incapable of depolarization.

Fusion between conduction arising in the His-Purkinje system and ventricular conduction can also result in widening of the QRS complex. In individuals with fixed preexcitation due to an accessory pathway, each ventricular complex represents fusion between conduction via the His-Purkinje system and the accessory pathway. In patients with intermittent preexcitation, wider QRS complexes may represent contribution from the accessory pathway, whereas narrow complexes may mark the absence of pathway conduction. Consider **Fig. 18** that demonstrates a patient with an underlying sinus tachycardia. The 2nd, 15th, and 18th beats display a shortened PR interval with slurring of the QRS complex suggesting the possibility of intermittent preexcitation. An alternative explanation for these beats is fusion between AV nodal conduction and a late diastolic PVC. It is important to observe that the p-delta wave interval in the second beat is longer that the p-delta intervals in the 15th and 18th beats. For most accessory pathways, irrespective of AV nodal contribution to ventricular depolarization, the p-delta wave interval should not vary. That is,

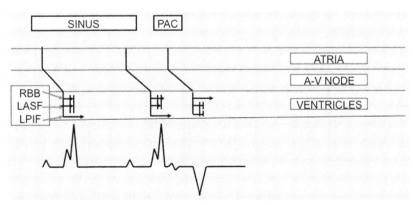

Fig. 15. Atrial trigeminy; note that sinus beats are conducted primarily via the LPF, and the premature atrial beat (PAC) is conducted via the right bundle branch (RBB).

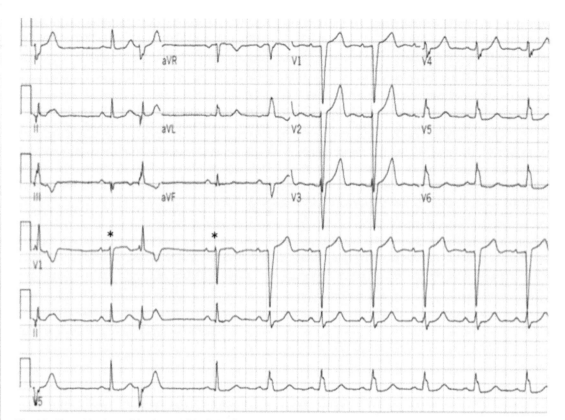

Fig. 16. Sinus Rhythm with phase 3 block in the LBB.

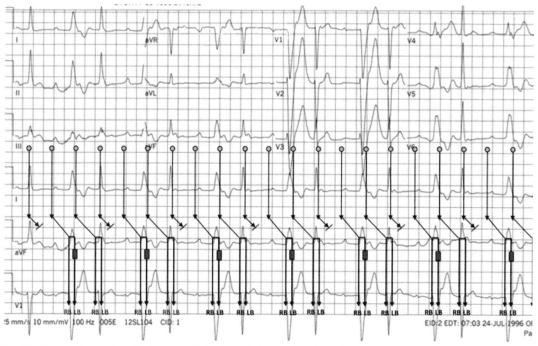

Fig. 17. Sinus tachycardia with 3:2 Wenckebach and phase 4 block in the left bundle (LB) branch. Note that all beats conducted after the pause are characterized by LBBB. Red boxes indicate block in the LBBB. Blue circles indicate sinus beats. Red bars indicate conduction block.

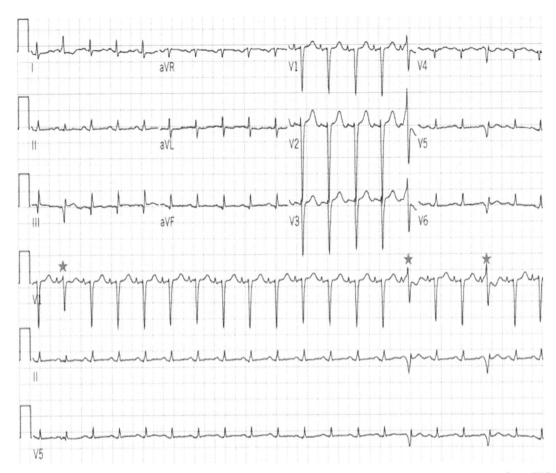

Fig. 18. Sinus tachycardia with intermittent shortening of PR interval (*asterix*). Note the variation in the p-QRS duration in these complexes. This finding argues against the presence of intermittent preexcitation.

the time from atrial depolarization to the onset of pathway activation remains fixed (exceptions to this would include decremental accessory pathways, manifest nodofascicular and nodoventricular pathways, and fasciculoventricular pathways). In this tracing, because the p-delta wave interval seems variable, these beats are not likely to be the result of intermittent preexcitation. A more likely explanation is fusion between normal conduction and late diastolic PVCs.

FROM WIDE TO NARROW

The presence of a narrow QRS complex in the presence of an otherwise wide complex rhythm can be attributed to several underlying mechanisms. **Fig. 19**A demonstrates a wide-complex rhythm, which can be attributed to preexcitation via a right-sided accessory pathway. The third QRS complex is narrower and does not seem to be preceded by a p wave. What are the possible mechanisms for this finding? One possibility is

the presence of dual AV nodal physiology and a double fire. That is, the first impulse conducts down both the fast pathway and the accessory pathway. The second impulse is the result of slow pathway conduction from the preceding sinus beat. At this time the accessory pathway is refractory and does not contribute anything to the QRS complex.

Another possibility, however, is the presence of a premature fascicular beat likely arising from the LPF. Following ablation of the accessory pathway, the patient presented with the ECG displayed in **Fig. 19**B. Note the presence of identical premature beats in complexes 4 and 8. Does the nature of their appearance narrow the differential diagnosis? Note that the coupling interval between beats 3 and 4 is different than the coupling interval between beats 7 and 8. This difference would argue against a double-fire mechanism. It is unlikely that the transit time down the slow pathway would vary this much. Thus, the more likely explanation for the narrow complex in

A

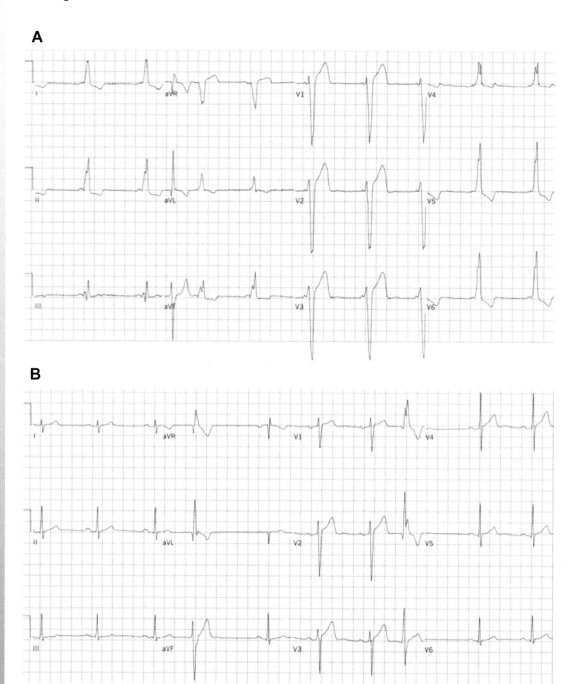

B

Fig. 19. (*A*) Normal sinus rhythm with preexcitation. The third QRS complex is narrow. The origin of this beat could be the result of a double fire from the preceding p wave or a fascicular premature beat. (*B*) Following ablation, premature beats of identical morphology are seen. Note the lack of a fixed coupling interval between the premature beat and the preceding p wave. The origin of these beats is, therefore, more likely due to the presence of fascicular premature beats rather than a double-fire mechanism.

Fig. 19A is the presence of a fascicular premature beat.

When wavefronts from opposite regions of the heart collide, the resulting fusion is often associated with QRS narrowing. Consider **Fig. 20** which demonstrates a patient with high-grade AV block. The third, fifth, and sixth beats are conducted with LBBB (R3, R5, and R6). There appears to be a ventricular escape rhythm characterized by RBBB that therefore, likely originates in the left ventricle.

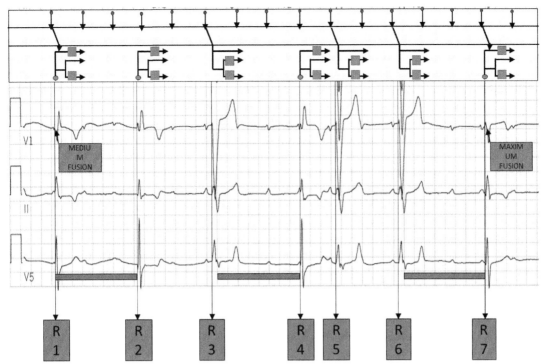

Fig. 20. Complex bradycardia involving high-degree AV block, (probably infranodal, ie, Mobitz-2), idioventricular escape rhythm originating in the LV in the left posterior fascicle distribution (R1, R2, R4 & R7), and sinus capture with normal PR and complete LBBBB (R3, R5, and R6). Two examples of fusion in the ventricles are seen: one with incomplete RBBB pattern (R2, medium degree of fusion) and one with normal QRS (R7, maximum degree of fusion) in lead V1. Note that the idioventricular focus is reset by the sinus QRS with LBBB late in the QRS and not earlier in the QRS or before it. The variation in the degree of fusion is explained by the timing of the p wave in relation to the idioventricular rhythm. The earlier the p wave with respect to the idioventricular QRS, the greater the degree of fusion and more narrow QRS.

The first beat R1 is actually a fusion beat between the ventricular escape complex and conduction via the RB from the preceding p wave. Note that the p wave originates relatively close to the onset of the QRS. There is, therefore, less contribution from conduction via the His-Purkinje system; the resulting complex is more similar in morphology to the escape focus. The seventh beat (R7) is the narrowest beat on the tracing and represents balanced fusion between the ventricular escape focus and conduction through the RBB. In this case, fusion between 2 contralateral wavefronts produces a relatively narrow QRS complex.

Fig. 21 displays a similar concept in a patient with underlying sinus rhythm and a ventricular pacemaker. Note the varying degrees of fusion between the paced ventricular beats (LBBB) and conduction via the His-Purkinje system via the LBB (RBBB). The second and third QRS complexes (R2 and R3) are the result of native conduction via the LBB producing an RBBB pattern. R1, R4, and R6-10 are fully paced ventricular beats producing an LBBB pattern. R5 and R7 are both fusion beats. Note the relationship between the p

wave and the QRS in these beats. In R7, the p-QRS interval is relatively short and the QRS complex is primarily the result of ventricular pacing with a small contribution from native LBB conduction. In the fifth QRS complex (R5), the p-QRS interval is slightly longer allowing for greater contribution from LBB conduction and more balanced fusion. The balanced activation from contralateral wavefronts results in a relatively narrow QRS. There are, of course, many other mechanisms that can result in narrowing of the QRS, including peeling back refractoriness, equal delay in both bundle branches, gap phenomena, and supernormal conduction (see section on supernormal conduction later).

REENTRY VERSUS PARASYSTOLE

When premature complexes of identical morphology are linked to a preceding complex with identical coupling intervals (such as in the case of ventricular bigeminy or trigeminy) the presumed mechanism is believed to be the result of reentry (**Fig. 22**).[8]

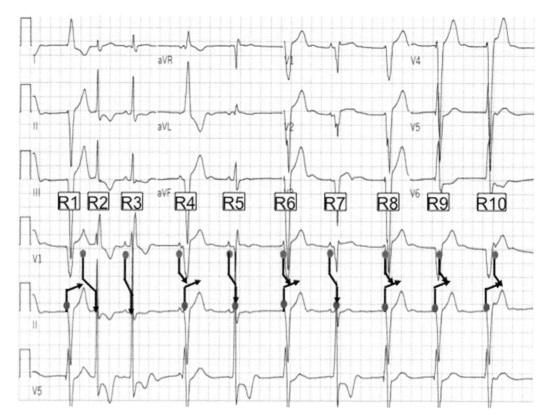

Fig. 21. A patient with underlying sinus rhythm and a ventricular pacemaker. Note the varying degrees of fusion between the paced ventricular beats (LBBB) and conduction via the His-Purkinje system via the LBB (RBBB).

Although patterns of trigeminy or bigeminy can be easy to identify, there are instances whereby the pattern may break because of exit block from the reentrant circuit producing the extrasystole. In this scenario, the bigeminal pattern is manifest only some of the time. **Fig. 23** demonstrates a tracing with sinus rhythm and extrasystoles that appear in an unpredictable pattern. The coupling interval of the PVC to sinus beat remains constant suggesting reentry as the putative mechanism. One important observation in this tracing is the fact that there is always an odd number of sinus beats interposed between the PVCs. This phenomenon is referred to as concealed bigeminy whereby the number of intervening sinus beats = 2n − 1, where n is any positive integer

(1, 3, 5, 7, and so forth).[9] Another phenomenon known as concealed trigeminy (**Fig. 24**) can be inferred when the number of intervening sinus beats = 3n − 1 (eg, 2, 5, 8, 11).[9]

It is also possible to develop Wenckebach or Mobitz II block in the reentrant circuit responsible for an extrasystole. Consider **Fig. 25** that demonstrates an alternating pattern of ventricular bigeminy and a sinus beat coupled with 2 PVCs of identical morphology. The coupling interval between the sinus beat and the extrasystoles and the coupling interval between the extrasystoles remains fixed, which would suggest the presence of reentry. The alternating pattern can be explained by the presence of a 2:1 block in the reentrant circuit.

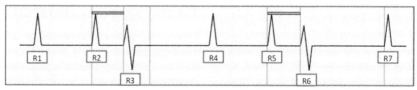

Fig. 22. Ventricular trigeminy marked by the presence of identical premature complexes with fixed coupling intervals (*horizontal bars*). The presumed mechanism for this phenomenon is reentry.

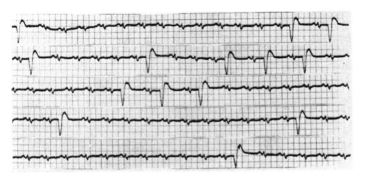

Fig. 23. Sinus rhythm with numerous PVCs at a fixed coupling interval. The number of intervening sinus beats is always odd suggesting the presence of concealed ventricular bigeminy. (*From* Schamroth L, Marriott HJ. Concealed ventricular extrasystoles. Circulation 1963;27:1043–9; with permission.)

More rarely, one can observe the presence of Wenckebach in the setting of reentry-dependent extrasystoles. Consider **Fig. 26** that demonstrates a pattern of interpolated ventricular bigeminy. After the third PVC, however, there is abrupt cessation of the bigeminal pattern. On closer inspection, however, there is a subtle prolongation of the coupling interval before the dropped PVC suggesting the presence of Wenckebach. This rare tracing underscores the importance of meticulous analysis when approaching a tracing with an unusual pattern.

The hallmark of parasystole is automaticity, which is the ability of cardiac cells to generate spontaneous action potentials. Parasystole is characterized by the presence of 2 pacemakers, a dominant pacemaker that is often the sinus node and a secondary pacemaker that can arise in the atria, AV node, fascicles, or ventricular myocardium. In its classic form, a parasystolic focus is shielded from surrounding impulses (entrance block) and, therefore, will discharge at a predictable rate (**Fig. 27**). Occasionally, variations in the parasystolic rate can be observed under several conditions, including the following:

1. Physiologic exit block whereby the focus fires at a time during which the surrounding tissue is refractory
2. Nonphysiologic exit block, whereby the focus itself exhibits either Wenckebach or Mobitz II behavior

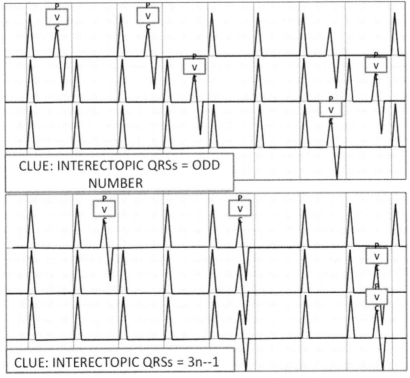

CLUE: INTERECTOPIC QRSs = ODD NUMBER

CLUE: INTERECTOPIC QRSs = 3n--1

Fig. 24. Concealed ventricular reentry: bigeminy (*top*) and trigeminy (*bottom*).

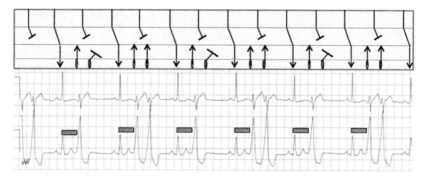

Fig. 25. Alternating pattern of ventricular bigeminy and a sinus beat coupled with 2 PVCs of identical morphology. Note also that the coupling interval between the sinus beat and the extrasystoles and the coupling interval between the extrasystoles remain fixed. The alternating pattern can be explained by the presence of 2:1 block in the reentrant circuit.

3. Modulated parasystole whereby entrance block is absent or incomplete and impulses from the dominant pacemaker or surrounding tissue can penetrate and reset the focus

Fig. 28 displays a patient with atrial parasystole likely arising from the floor of the left atrium. In the tracing there are examples of both physiologic and true exit block from the parasystolic focus. The eighth beat also displays fusion between the parasystolic focus and the sinus node. Also note that the seventh beat has the shortest coupling interval resulting in block in the left anterior fascicle and right bundle. There is also a likely delay through the AV node given the prolongation of the PR interval.

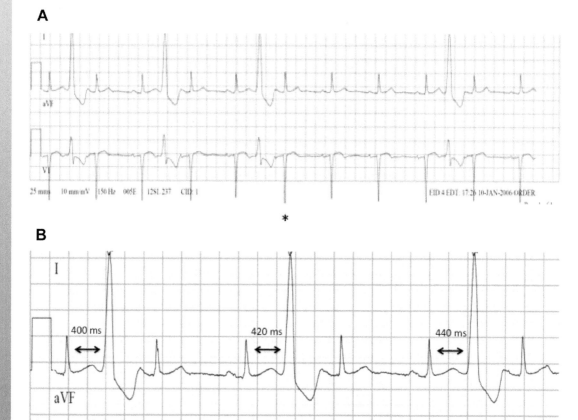

Fig. 26. (*A*) Ventricular trigeminy with abrupt cessation of the PVC following the sixth sinus complex (*asterisk*). (*B*) Enlarged view demonstrating subtle increases in the coupling interval before the dropped PVC.

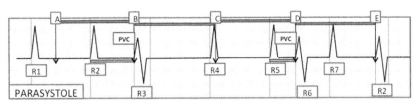

Fig. 27. Ventricular parasystole characterized by extrasystoles with variable coupling intervals. A, true exit block; B, D, and E, manifest parasystole; C, physiologic exit block. Note that the B-D interval is a multiple of the D-E interval. In addition, the junctional QRS and the parasystolic focus do not invade and reset each other. Red lines indicate parasystolic rate. Blue lines indicate coupling intervals.

Fig. 29 demonstrates a similar phenomenon from a parasystolic focus likely arising in the fascicular system. The first beat likely arises from the parasystolic focus and is coupled to a PVC. On the seventh and eighth QRS complexes, a conducted sinus beat is followed by a PVC. The rate of the parasystolic focus can be assessed by taking the shortest parasystolic intervals that appear on the tracing, in this case the first and third QRS complexes. After the fourth QRS complex, there appears to be exit block from the focus as evidenced by the absence of a QRS complex at its expected time of discharge. This observation is most likely due to a nonphysiologic exit block, as the ventricle would not be expected to be refractory at this time. After the seventh QRS complex, the block from the focus appears to be physiologic, that is, it occurs during a period when the ventricle is refractory and does not represent true block from the focus.

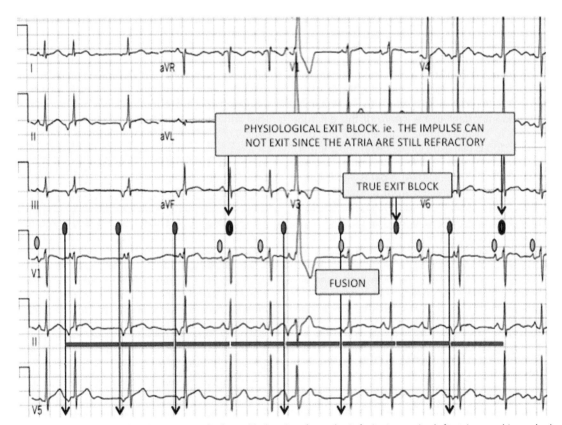

Fig. 28. Atrial parasystole. The parasystolic focus likely arises from the inferior/posterior left atrium and is marked by the red ovals and bars. Sinus beats are marked with blue ovals. Note the presence of physiologic and nonphysiologic exit block. The seventh QRS complex seems to be conducted with aberrancy. There is fusion between the parasystolic focus and discharge from the sinus node on the eighth p wave.

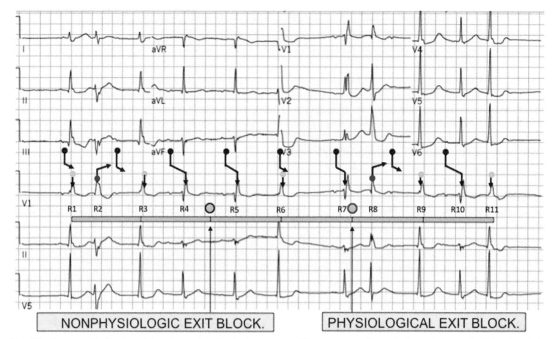

NONPHYSIOLOGIC EXIT BLOCK.   PHYSIOLOGICAL EXIT BLOCK.

Fig. 29. Parasystole likely arising from the fascicular system. The parasystolic cycle length is marked by the light blue bars and circles. PVCs are seen on the second and eighth beats (*red circles*). There is an underlying sinus rhythm (*dark blue circles*) with intermittent conduction to the ventricle with RBBB (R1, R5, R7, R10). Note the presence of physiologic and nonphysiologic block from the parasystolic focus.

The interplay between a dominant pacemaker and a parasystolic focus can be difficult if not impossible to prove in any given tracing. Nonetheless, it is important to be aware of the different manners in which a dominant pacemaker and parasystolic focus can exert influence on one another. **Fig. 30** demonstrates 3 different hypothetical scenarios. In the first scenario (*A*), a parasystolic focus is not completely isolated from surrounding impulses. In this case, the parasystolic focus is reset by the second junctional beat. The point of reset can be inferred from assessing the parasystolic rate and measuring backwards from third PVC. In the second scenario (*B*), a junctional rhythm is reset by a parasystolic focus. The third scenario (*C*) demonstrates how a junctional rhythm and parasystolic focus can exert mutual influence on one another.

TRIGGERED ACTIVITY AND TORSADE DE POINTES

If parasystolic activity is the result of automaticity, triggered activity relates to after-depolarizations that can lead to atrial or ventricular arrhythmias. Early after-depolarizations (EADs) occur during phase 2 or phase 3 of the cardiac action potential, whereas delayed after-depolarizations occur

following complete repolarization. One of the most common ventricular arrhythmias related to triggered activity is torsades de pointes (TDP). This arrhythmia is typically associated with congenital or acquired long QT syndrome (LQTS). Increases in transmural dispersion of repolarization combined with the formation of EADs form the basis of arrhythmic substrate in TDP.[10] It is hypothesized that EADs exceeding the activation threshold can result in action potential formation and ultimately PVC's that occur during the vulnerable period of ventricular repolarization triggering TDP.[10]

The presence of U waves has also been observed as a common feature among patients with LQTS and TDP. The origin of the U wave remains controversial. However, one prevailing hypothesis is that the U wave is an electrocardiographic manifestation of EADs. The basis of this theory stems from studies using monophasic action potential recordings that demonstrated close correlation between the timing of U waves and EADs occurring at a cellular level.[11] Whether or not this theory accounts for the origin of U waves, there are clinical data to support a temporal relationship between the presence of augmented U waves and the onset of TDP.[12]

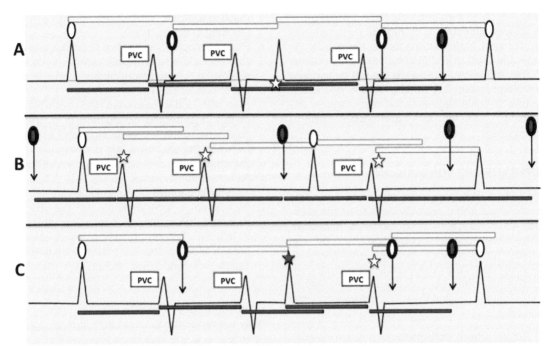

Fig. 30. (A) Junctional pacemaker invades and resets the parasystolic focus; the junction itself is not reset. Blue bars indicate the junctional rate. Red bars indicate the parasystolic focus rate. The point of reset is indicated by the star. Red ovals indicate nonphysiologic exit block from the parasystolic focus; thick white ovals represent physiologic exit block from the junction. White ovals indicate conducted junctional beat. (B) Parasystolic focus invades and resets the junctional focus. The ventricular focus is not reset. Blue bars indicate the junctional rate. Red bars indicate the parasystolic focus rate. The points of reset are indicated by the stars. Red ovals indicate nonphysiologic exit block from the parasystolic focus. White ovals indicate conducted junctional beat. (C) Junctional beats invade and reset parasystolic focus, and parasystolic focus invades and resets junction. Blue bars indicate the junctional rate. Red bars indicate the parasystolic focus rate. White star indicates parasystolic focus resetting junction. Red star indicates junction resetting parasystolic focus. Thick white ovals represent physiologic exit block from the junction. Red ovals indicate nonphysiologic exit block from the parasystolic focus. White ovals indicate conducted junctional beat.

Consider **Fig. 31** demonstrating a patient with prominent U waves. Note that the amplitude of the U wave in the last beat is larger following a prolonged diastolic interval. Because the action potential duration is affected predominantly by the preceding diastolic interval, repolarization following a pause is prolonged. This phenomenon may lead to the formation of enhanced EAD activity and augmented U waves. This finding also underscores the pause-dependent nature of TDP whereby pauses lead to prolonged repolarization on the subsequent

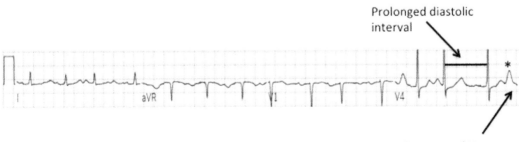

Prolonged diastolic interval

Augmented U wave

Fig. 31. Patient with prominent U waves. Note U wave augmentation following a pause (*asterisk*).

beat, which in turn promotes the formation of EADS and ultimately TDP. **Fig. 32** demonstrates this concept. Note that the longer the pause, the larger the U wave and the more likely the chance of TDP. Although all U waves are not considered pathologic, giant T-U complexes and postextrasystolic U-wave augmentation may suggest impending TDP in the appropriate clinical environment.

SUPERNORMAL CONDUCTION

The notion of supernormal conduction remains controversial and is typically defined as the presence of conduction when block is expected. When unanticipated conduction can be explained by alternative factors, supernormality does not need to be invoked. Supernormal conduction can often be explained by a variety of physiologic explanations including[4] the following:

1. The gap phenomena proximal delay in the conduction system that allows for recovery of the distal conduction system and subsequent conduction.
2. "Peeling back refractoriness" (Retrograde preexcitation of the conduction system resulting in a refractory period that ends earlier in the cycle length than expected. This leadis to a greater recovery time of the in region of block and subsequent conduction.)
3. Shortening of the refractory period due to changes in the preceding cycle length (The duration of the refractory period is directly proportional to the preceding cycle length; thus, shortening of the preceding cycle length can

result in a shorter subsequent refractory period resulting in conduction.)
4. Phase 4 block (The absence of conduction due to phase 4 diastolic depolarization can be preempted by a premature stimulus and subsequent conduction.)
5. Dual AV nodal pathways (An example includes unexpected conduction of a premature atrial complex resulting from a switch between the slow and fast pathway.)
6. Summation of subthreshold responses (Closely timed subthreshold stimuli can fuse producing a stimulus capable of excitation.)
7. Wenckebach phenomenon in the bundle branches (Progressive concealed delay in a bundle branch resulting in a bundle branch block pattern is followed by normalization of conduction during the recovery cycle.)

Although supernormality has not been definitively proven in the human heart, it is thought to be the result of enhanced excitability during phase 3 of the action potential.[13] During this period, the cell has recovered enough to respond to a stimulus. However, because the membrane potential has not fully recovered, less depolarization is required to bring the cell to threshold. Thus, a relatively small stimulus can result in an action potential. The same stimulus applied earlier or later in the cycle would not be expected to produce the same result. Only impulses that decrease during the critical phase of repolarization are thought to result in supernormal excitability.

Consider **Fig. 33**A that demonstrates a wide complex rhythm with complete heart block. The asterisk marks a premature beat with a different QRS morphology. What is the origin of this beat? Although it may represent a premature ventricular complex, an alternate explanation is that the beat is conducted as a result of supernormal excitability (**Fig. 33**B). Evidence in favor of this was found on a subsequent ECG whereby the patient was found to have a 2:1 block (see **Fig. 33**C). The morphology of the QRS complex in this tracing is identical to the QRS complex, strongly supporting the theory that the premature beat on the prior tracing was the result of supraventricular conduction.

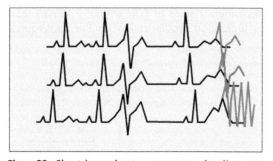

Fig. 32. Short-long-short sequence leading to torsade. Note the U-wave augmentation is directly proportional to the length of the preceding diastolic interval. Longer pauses can lead to increased dispersion of repolarization, the formation of EADs, and the presence of giant U waves triggering TDP.

SUMMARY

Analysis of complex ECG tracings requires both imagination and keen knowledge about the patterned behaviors of the cardiac conduction

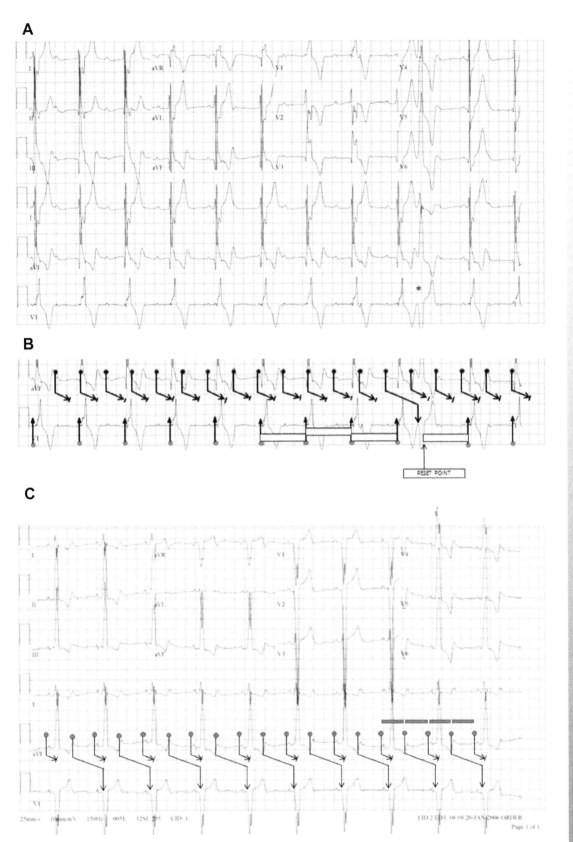

Fig. 33. (A) Wide QRS rhythm with RBBB and LPFB pattern and CHB; the asterisk marks a premature complex with LBBB pattern. (B) Ladder diagram suggesting that the premature beat is the result of supernormal conduction through the AV node or His-Purkinje system. Note that the premature beat resets the escape rhythm. (C) Sinus tachycardia in the same patient with 2:1 block. Note that the QRS morphology is identical to the premature QRS complex in (B).

systems and myocardium. The authors have attempted to highlight some of these patterns in this article and demonstrate how similar patterns can appear in various locations in the heart. Every anomaly on an ECG can theoretically be explained by applying one's knowledge of these patterns to construct a defensible explanation for the phenomena. In the absence of intracardiac tracings, it is often not possible to prove one's hypothesis. However, as mentioned toward the beginning of this article, the process is more important than the outcome. When dissecting complex tracings, one should ask whether one's explanation makes sense, whether it is probable, and whether there are competing explanations. The surface ECG continues to be indispensible and a relevant tool because it offers a portal into the electrical behavior of the heart. One's ability to discern this behavior, whether mundane or complex, is a skill that will be essential for many years to come.

REFERENCES

1. Tandon A, Simpson L, Assar MD. Unusual origin of type 1 atrioventricular block with comments on Wenckebach's contribution. Proc (Bayl Univ Med Cent) 2011;24:9–12.
2. Langendorf R, Pick A. Concealed conduction further evaluation of a fundamental aspect of propagation of the cardiac impulse. Circulation 1956;13:381–99.
3. Langendorf R. Concealed A-V conduction; the effect of blocked impulses on the formation and conduction of subsequent impulses. Am Heart J 1948;35:542–52.
4. Josephson ME. Clinical cardiac electrophysiology. Philadelphia: Lippincott Williams & Wilkins; 2008.
5. Csapo G. Paroxysmal nonreentrant tachycardias due to simultaneous conduction in dual atrioventricular nodal pathways. Am J Cardiol 1979;43:1033–45.
6. Massumi RA. Bradycardia-dependent bundle-branch block. A critique and proposed criteria. Circulation 1968;38:1066–73.
7. Lee S, Wellens HJJ, Josephson ME. Paroxysmal atrioventricular block. Heart Rhythm 2009;6:1229–34.
8. Langendorf R, Pick A. Mechanisms of intermittent ventricular bigeminy. II. Parasystole, and parasystole or re-entry with conduction disturbance. Circulation 1955;11:431–9.
9. Schamroth L, Marriott HJ. Concealed ventricular extrasystoles. Circulation 1963;27:1043–9.
10. Antzelevitch C, Burashnikov A. Overview of basic mechanisms of cardiac arrhythmia. Card Electrophysiol Clin 2011;3:23–45.
11. el-Sherif N. Early afterdepolarizations and arrhythmogenesis. Experimental and clinical aspects. Arch Mal Coeur Vaiss 1991;84:227–34.
12. Kirchhof P, Franz MR, Bardai A, et al. Giant T-U waves precede torsades de pointes in long QT syndrome: a systematic electrocardiographic analysis in patients with acquired and congenital QT prolongation. J Am Coll Cardiol 2009;54:143–9.
13. Zipes DP, Jalife J. Cardiac electrophysiology: from cell to bedside. Philadelphia: Elsevier Health Sciences; 2013.

Diagnostic and Prognostic Implications of Surface Recordings from Patients with Atrioventricular Block

William P. Nelson, MD

KEYWORDS

- Atrioventricular block • Wenckebach block • Mobitz block • Complete AV block

KEY POINTS

- Classic type 1 (Wenckebach) atrioventricular (AV) block is owing to depressed AV nodal conduction and is recognized by a prolonging PR interval ending in a "dropped beat."
- Type II (Mobitz) AV block is owing to abnormal *infranodal* conduction, and is usually accompanied by bundle branch block.
- Second-degree AV block with 2:1 conduction can be a difficult problem.
- Third-degree (complete) AV block is a diagnosis too often rendered and too often incorrect.

ATRIOVENTRICULAR BLOCK

The atrioventricular (AV) bridge is vulnerable to many circumstances that depress conduction. Abnormal impulse transmission may be caused by drugs, autonomic effects, or destructive processes. The familiar separation into 3 degrees is useful, but occasionally insufficient.

First-Degree Atrioventricular Block

First-degree AV block is actually an incorrect term, because there is merely *delay* and not block of any sinus impulse (**Fig. 1**).

Second-Degree Atrioventricular Block

Classic type 1 (Wenckebach) AV block is owing to depressed AV nodal conduction and is recognized by a prolonging PR interval ending in a dropped beat. It is frequently owing to drugs that depress conduction through the AV node (digitalis, β-blockers, and calcium channel blockers.) It is frequently seen with inferior wall myocardial infarction (**Fig. 2**).

Fig. 3 illustrates the effect on AV conduction as successive atrial impulses (1–5) arrive in the AV junction earlier and earlier in it refractory period. The light stippling is the relative refractory period an the dark stippling is absolute refractory period.

Fig. 4 depicts the basis of type 1 AV block. The earlier the P wave is, in the wake of the preceding complex, the longer the PR interval will be. Ultimately, the P wave encounters the absolute refractory period and cannot be conducted.

Type II (Mobitz) AV block is owing to abnormal infranodal conduction, and is usually accompanied by bundle branch block. All conducted impulses share the same PR intervals (usually normal). The dropped beats appear without warning and may be sporadic or several in a row. Type II block may be seen with anterior infarction, but is not related to drugs in current use. A pacemaker is usually required (**Fig. 5**).

E-mail address: wpan747@gmail.com

Card Electrophysiol Clin 8 (2016) 25–35
http://dx.doi.org/10.1016/j.ccep.2015.10.031
1877-9182/16/$ – see front matter © 2016 Elsevier Inc. All rights reserved.

cardiacEP.theclinics.com

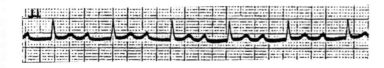

Fig. 1. First-degree atrioventricular block. The PR interval exceeds 0.20 seconds.

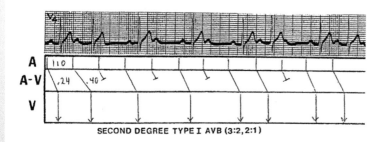

SECOND DEGREE TYPE I AVB (3:2, 2:1)

Fig. 2. A typical example of Wenckebach block is shown. AVB, atrioventricular block.

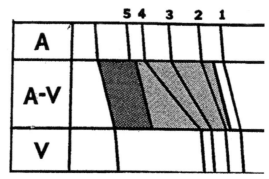

Fig. 3. The effect on atrioventricular (AV) conduction as successive atrial impulses (1–5) arrive in the AV junction earlier and earlier in it refractory period.

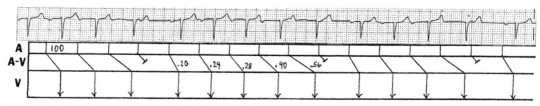

Fig. 4. The basis of type 1 atrioventricular (AV) block.

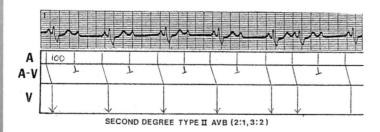

SECOND DEGREE TYPE II AVB (2:1, 3:2)

Fig. 5. Second-degree type II atrioventricular block (AVB; 2:1, 3:2).

Second-degree AV block with 2:1 conduction can be a difficult problem. Of importance, this ratio of conduction has little meaning unless the atrial rate is provided. For example, in patients with atrial flutter, there are approximately 300 impulses available for AV transmission. It is evident that if all were conducted, the ventricular rate would be life-threatening. In this circumstance, a conduction ratio of 2:1 is a boon, and represents physiologic refractoriness rather than AV block. Conversely, if the atrial rate is 70 bpm, a 2:1 conduction would be a disaster and represent pathologic AV block. Often, 2:1 conduction is said to represent type II block. Although this is sometimes correct, many cases are owing to 2:1 AV nodal block (type I). Clues for this diagnosis would be the absence of bundle branch block and prolonged PR interval of the conducted beats.

Fig. 6 illustrates how an increase in atrial rate, without change in the refractory period, can alter the conduction ratio from 1:1 to 2:1. The first 2 cycles represent a rate of 60 bpm; the last 5 cycles, a rate of 78 bpm. As the rate increases, the alternating P waves encounter the refractory period set up by the prior transmitted impulse and are not conducted. Shaded areas represent an unchanging refractory period (see **Fig. 6**).

Third-degree (Complete) Atrioventricular Block

Third-degree (complete) AV block is a diagnosis too often rendered and too often incorrect. There is a common definition: If no P waves are conducted, complete AV block is present. This simplistic concept leads to major errors and inappropriate management. It is evident that, to be conducted, an atrial impulse must have an opportunity for conduction. Thus, to diagnose complete heart block:

1. P waves should not occur in the absolute refractory period of a preceding activation.
2. P waves should not be in lockstep (isochronic dissociation) with a competing junctional or ventricular pacemaker.
3. There must be an adequate number of P waves sampling different portions of the cardiac cycle and none are conducted.
4. The rate of an escaping focus should be slow enough (<45 bpm?) to permit conduction of a dissociated P wave.

5. There should never be an early QRS complex indicating a capture beat. If one is present, it would require that the AV bridge be intact (**Fig. 7**).

An example of complete AV block is shown in **Fig. 7**.

Computer: Third-Degree Atrioventricular Block

The computer frequently confuses AV dissociation and AV block. In this example, there is marked sinus bradycardia at 30 bpm. An escape junctional focus assumes command at 43 bpm. It is conducted with right bundle branch block and Q waves of inferior wall infarction. The dissociated P waves gradually occur later and later after the QRS complexes. When the refractory period from the junctional discharge lessens, the impulse is conducted and captures the ventricles (**Fig. 8**, *arrow*). The next atrial impulse is conducted with only a slight PR prolongation. The capture beat proves that the AV bridge is intact and denies third-degree AV block. The problem is owing to the default of the sinus node, rather than AV block (see **Fig. 8**).

Computer: short QT interval
Note that, during the pauses after the premature ventricular contractions, there are convincing P waves (**Fig. 9**, *arrows*). The P–P cycle is regular at 80 bpm and bears a constant relation to the QRS complexes. The PR interval is prolonged to 0.44 sec, an example of first-degree AV block (see **Fig. 9**).

In **Fig. 10**, this 70-year-old woman has sustained an acute inferior–posterior myocardial infarction and has activated the Bezold–Jarisch reflex. Receptors for this are located in the inferior wall of the left ventricle and, when stimulated by stretch, prompt a variable, and at times, marked vagatonic suppression of AV nodal conduction, causing type 1 AV block. The prolonging PR intervals and dropped beats indicate Wenckebach AV block. This is common with inferior wall infarcts and is responsive to atropine.

In **Fig. 11**, a 55-year-old man was known to have left bundle branch block, but he presented with chest pain and ST elevation in lead II, not previously present. He has an acute inferior myocardial infarction with variable Wenckebach AV block.

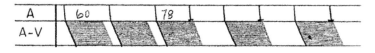

Fig. 6. Ladder diagram illustrates how an increase in atrial rate, without a change in the refractory period, can alter the conduction ratio from 1:1 to 2:1. A-V, atrioventricular.

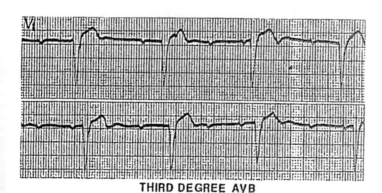

Fig. 7. Third-degree atrioventricular block (AVB).

THIRD DEGREE AVB

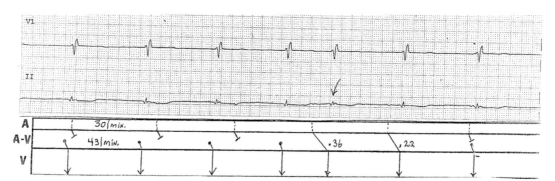

Fig. 8. Many atrial impulses are not conducted, but the early QRS complex (*arrow*) indicates that it is a "capture beat" and proves that the A-V bridge is capable of conducting. This is an example of A-V dissociation due to sinus bradycardia resulting in the "escape" of a junctional focus.

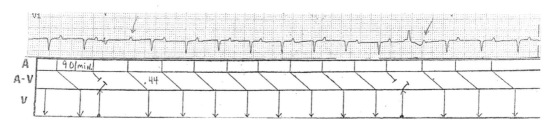

Fig. 9. A first-degree atrioventricular (AV) block.

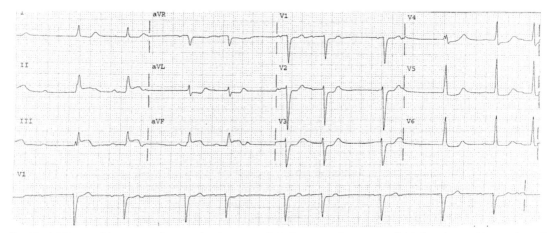

Fig. 10. A 70-year-old woman who sustained an acute inferior–posterior myocardial infarction and has activated the Bezold–Jarisch reflex. Receptors for this are located in the inferior wall of the left ventricle and, when stimulated by stretch, prompt a variable, and at times, marked vagatonic suppression of atrioventricular (AV) nodal conduction, causing type 1 AV block. The prolonging PR intervals and "dropped beats" indicate Wenckebach AV block. This is common with inferior wall infarcts and is responsive to atropine.

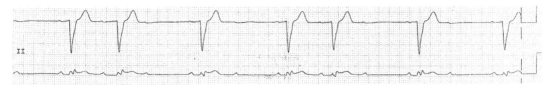

Fig. 11. A 55-year-old man known to have left bindle branch block presented with chest pain and ST elevation in lead II, not previously present. He has an acute inferior myocardial infarction with variable Wenckebach atrioventricular block. This is another example of the Bezold–Jarisch reflex. Atropine returned conduction to normal.

This is another example of the Bezold–Jarisch reflex. Atropine returned conduction to normal.

The computer interpretation is sorely lacking in **Fig. 12**! The atrial rhythm is regular at 165 bpm and, as depicted in the ladder diagram, there is progressive PR interval prolongation culminating in a dropped beat. This is a classic example of atrial tachycardia with Wenckebach AV block, representing serious digitalis intoxication.

The computer is mostly wrong in **Fig. 13**! The rhythm is atrial flutter. There is right bundle branch block and, although there is a right axis of the pre-blocked forces, there is no evidence of right ventricular hypertrophy. This rhythm is a common finding in patients with atrial flutter. Obviously, it would be foolhardy to conduct 300 stimuli per minute. The physiologic refractoriness of the AV node blocks alternate impulses and the patient usually presents with 2:1 AV conduction and an effective rate of 150 bpm. Two possibilities exist: all of the conductible stimuli may be transmitted, or they may be transmitted with gradual prolongation (Wenckebach AV block). This phenomenon has

been termed bilevel AV block, that is, 2:1 block at an upper level of the AV Junction, and Wenckebach block at a lower level (see **Fig. 13**).

A single premature atrial contraction (**Fig. 14**, *arrow*) disturbs an otherwise regular sinus rhythm at 90 bpm. Subsequently, the atrial impulses are transmitted in peculiar fashion. Some are not conducted; some are conducted with left bundle branch block morphology, and some with right bundle branch block. The varying bundle branch conduction has been termed bilateral bundle branch block, and signals the imminent demise of the intraventricular pathways, and justifies the insertion of an electronic pacemaker (see **Fig. 14**).

The interpretation is correct, but incomplete in **Fig. 15**. A significant omission is that the final P wave is not conducted. This is an unusual example of AV "block." Note that the rhythm begins at 75 bpm with a PR interval of 0.16. The rate gradually slows to 50 bpm and the PR interval prolongs to 0.26 seconds. This phenomenon can be seen during a marked vagotonic state, resulting in both sinus node depression and

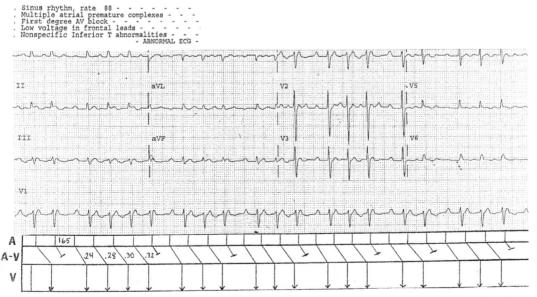

```
. Sinus rhythm, rate 88 - - - - - - -
. Multiple atrial premature complexes - - -
. First degree AV block - - - - - - - -
. Low voltage in frontal leads - - - - - -
. Nonspecific Inferior T abnormalities - - -
                        - ABNORMAL ECG -
```

Fig. 12. A progressive PR interval prolongation culminating in a dropped beat. This is a classic example of atrial tachycardia with Wenckebach atrioventricular (AV) block representing serious digitalis intoxication.

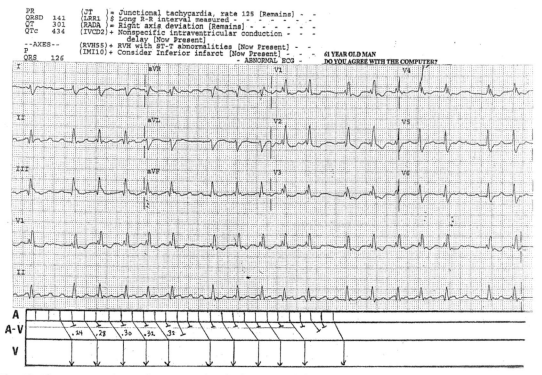

Fig. 13. The computer is mostly wrong! The rhythm is atrial flutter. There is right bundle branch block and, although there is a right axis of the "preblocked forces," there is no evidence of right ventricular hypertrophy. This rhythm is a common finding in patients with atrial flutter.

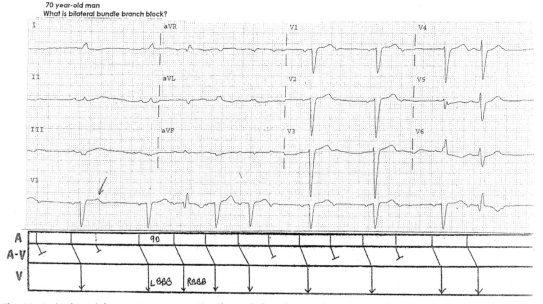

Fig. 14. A single atrial premature contraction (*arrow*) disturbs an otherwise regular sinus rhythm at 90 bpm. Subsequently, the atrial impulses are transmitted in peculiar fashion. Some are not conducted; some are conducted with left bundle branch block (LBBB) morphology and some with right bundle branch block (RBBB). The varying bundle branch conduction has been termed "bilateral bundle branch block," and signals the imminent demise of the intraventricular pathways, and justifies the insertion of an electronic pacemaker.

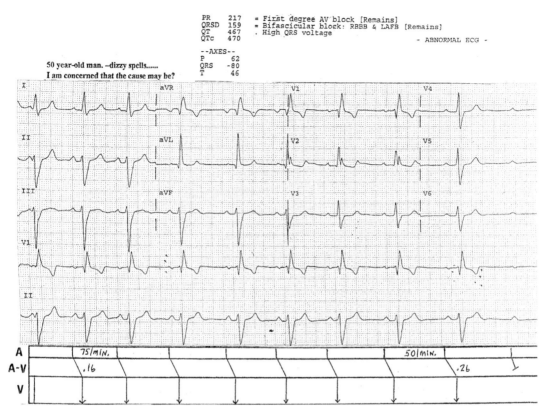

```
PR      217    = First degree AV block [Remains]
QRSD    159    = Bifascicular block: RBBB & LAFB [Remains]
QT      467    . High QRS voltage
QTc     470
                                              - ABNORMAL ECG -
--AXES--
P        62
QRS     -80
T        46
```

50 year-old man. –dizzy spells......
I am concerned that the cause may be?

Fig. 15. This is an unusual example of atrioventricular (AV) "block." Note that the rhythm begins at 75 bpm with a PR interval of 0.16. The rate gradually slows to 50 bpm and the PR interval prolongs to 0.26 seconds. This phenomenon can be seen during a marked vagotonic state, resulting in both sinus node depression and increased AV node refractoriness. It is possible that the last P wave is not conducted because of the markedly prolonged recovery time of the AV node. However, the patient's symptoms are concerning and the bifascicular block and nonconducted P wave may be owing to type 2 infranodal block.

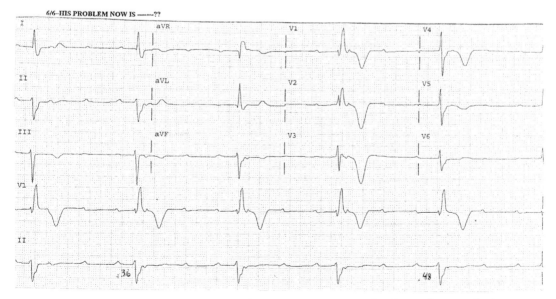

6/6–HIS PROBLEM NOW IS ——-??

Fig. 16. The PR intervals look constant, but careful measurement proves that is not the case. The P waves are dissociated from the QRS complexes due to complete A-V block. Now this man really needs a pacemaker!

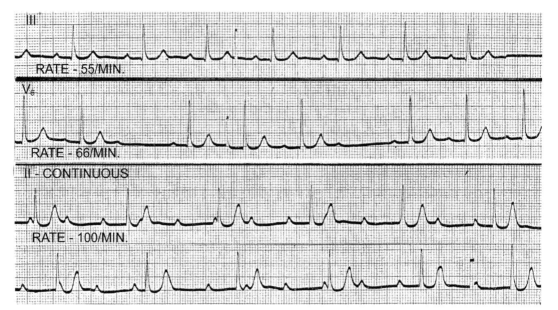

Fig. 17. A 55-year-old woman who presented with "passing out spells." The leads were recorded over several minutes and are an example of the effect of changing heart rate when there is a long refractory period of the AV node or distal pathways.

increased AV node refractoriness. It is possible that the last P wave is not conducted because of the markedly prolonged recovery time of the AV node. However, the patient's symptoms are concerning and the bifascicular block and non-conducted P wave may be owing to type 2 infranodal block (see **Fig. 15**).

Two days later, complete heart block has developed. A simple exercise to help clarify the relationship of the P waves and QRS complexes is to ask a series of 3 questions: (1) Is the P–P cycle regular? (2) Is the R–R cycle regular? (3) Is the PR interval constant? If the answer to all 3 questions is "yes," the atrial and ventricular events are related as cause and effect. However, if the P–P and R–R cycles are regular, but the PR interval is not constant, the P waves and the QRS complexes

are *dissociated*. In this example, dissociation is present and is owing to third-degree AV block.

Now this young man really needs a pacemaker (**Fig. 16**)!

Fig. 17 refers to a 55-year-old woman who presented with "passing out spells." The leads were recorded over several minutes and are an example of the effect of changing heart rate when there is a long refractory period of the AV node or distal pathways. At a rate of 55 bpm, all impulses are conducted with a PR interval of 0.30, or first-degree block. When the rate increases to 66 bpm, the PR remains the same but 2 P waves are blocked, indicating second-degree type 2 infranodal block. At a rate of 100 bpm, none of the atrial impulses can conduct—complete AV block. The narrow QRS morphology of the escape focus

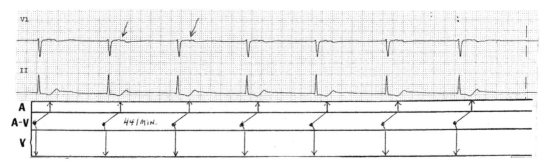

Fig. 18. P waves are present, but follow and are linked to the QRS complexes. The rhythm is owing to a slow, escaping junctional focus with a retrograde atrial activation (*arrows*). No P waves are available for anterograde conduction and, therefore, no judgment can be made about atrioventricular (AV) block.

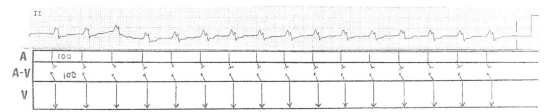

Fig. 19. P waves are saddled next to an accelerated junctional focus, both firing at 100 bpm. This is an example of "isochronic" atrioventricular (AV) dissociation, owing to an enhanced junctional pacemaker. Although none of the P waves is conducted, there is no opportunity for conduction because of the short PR interval, and there is likely no AV block.

suggest that it arises in the His bundle. A ventricular pacemaker was inserted.

SOME FOOLERS

P waves are present, but follow and are linked to the QRS complexes. The rhythm is owing to a slow, escaping junctional focus with a retrograde atrial activation (arrows). No P waves are available for anterograde conduction and, therefore, no judgment can be made about AV block (**Fig. 18**).

P waves are saddled next to an accelerated junctional focus, both firing at 100 bpm. This is an example of isochronic AV dissociation, owing to an enhanced junctional pacemaker. Although none of the P waves is conducted, there is no opportunity for conduction because of the short PR interval, and there is likely no AV block (**Fig. 19**).

In analyzing rhythm abnormalities, sometimes it is instructive to start at the end rather than the beginning of the tracing. **Fig. 20** is such an example. Note that the P waves appear in the fifth beat from the last, and the measurement of the P–P cycle becomes available. The final portion of the tracing shows atrial tachycardia at 120 bpm with P–R prolongation typical of type I AV block.

Looking "backward," it is evident that the P wave is retreating into the preceding T wave and is invisible for most of the tracing. The shortening interval of the R to the following P wave provides evidence that the P–R interval is prolonging (see **Fig. 20**).

The P wave configuration is stable in **Fig. 21**, but there is variation in the P–P cycle, with the sinus rate varying from 55 to 65 bpm. There are numerous single uniform premature ventricular contractions with a consistent "coupling" of 0.44 seconds. There are prolonging PR intervals with dropped beats, consistent with type 1 AV block. Note, however, that the PR intervals of sinus beats, without an accompanying premature ventricular contractions, are stable at 0.20 seconds. The ladder diagram is an explanation of this phenomenon. The premature ventricular contractions are conducted retrogradely into the AV junction, and establish a refractory zone of absolute and relative refractoriness. When a P wave encounters the relative refractory interlude, it is conducted, with a long PR interval. When the P wave lands in the absolute refractory period, it is not conducted. Thus, there is probably nothing wrong with the AV junctional bridge and this phenomenon represents pseudo-Wenckebach AV block (see **Fig. 21**).

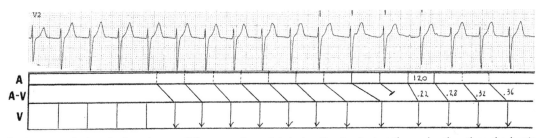

Fig. 20. In analyzing rhythm abnormalities, sometimes it is instructive to start at the end rather than the beginning of the tracing. This is such an example. Note that the P waves appear in the fifth beat from the last, and the measurement of the P–P cycle becomes available. The final portion of the tracing shows atrial tachycardia at 120 bpm with P–R prolongation typical of type I AV block. Looking backward, it is evident that the P wave is retreating into the preceding T wave and is invisible for most of the tracing. The shortening interval of the R to the following P wave provides evidence that the P–R interval is prolonging.

What "type" of AV Block ??

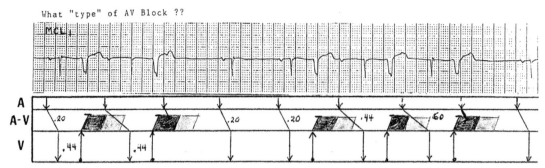

Fig. 21. The premature ventricular contractions are conducted retrogradely into the atrioventricular (AV) junction, and establish a refractory zone of absolute and relative refractoriness. When a P wave encounters the relative refractory interlude, it is conducted, with a long PR interval. When the P wave lands in the absolute refractory period, it is not conducted. Thus, there is probably nothing "wrong" with the AV junctional bridge and this phenomenon represents pseudo-Wenckebach AV block.

The computer is partially correct in **Fig. 22**. The atrial rate is 110 bpm and there is an accelerated junctional focus at 85 bpm. However, it ignored the acute inferior wall infarction, and concluded that the dissociation of the P waves and QRS complexes was owing to complete heart block. It is agreed that there must be "some degree" of AV block, or the atrial rate of 110 would be in command of ventricular activation. The ladder diagram depicts the solution. The repetitive discharge of the accelerated junctional focus and the resulting refractory period prevents transmission of *all* atrial

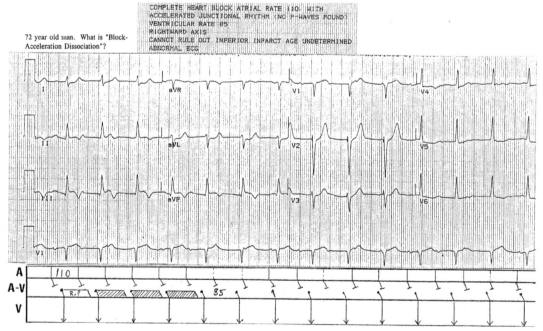

Fig. 22. The computer is partially correct. The atrial rate is 110 bpm and there is an accelerated junctional focus at 85 bpm. However, it ignored the acute inferior wall infarction, and concluded that the dissociation of the P waves and QRS complexes was owing to complete heart block. It is agreed that there must be some degree of atrioventricular (AV) block, or the atrial rate of 110 would be in command of ventricular activation. The ladder diagram depicts the solution. The repetitive discharge of the accelerated junctional focus and the resulting refractory period (R.P.) prevents transmission of all atrial stimuli. The dissociated P waves "leap frog" over the QRS–ST–T of the accelerated junctional pacemaker, but are unable to find a "window" that would permit AV passage. Thus, there is a combination of AV block (probably minor) and an enhanced junctional pacemaker. A descriptive term for this could be block-acceleration dissociation.

stimuli. The dissociated P waves "leap frog" over the QRS–ST–T of the accelerated junctional pacemaker, but are unable to find a "window" that would permit AV passage. Thus there is a combination of AV block (*probably* minor) and an enhanced junctional pacemaker. A descriptive term for this could be "block– dissociation" (see **Fig. 22**).

Section 1: Supraventricular Tachycardia

Editor: Nitish Badhwar

Antidromic Atrioventricular Reciprocating Tachycardia Using a Concealed Retrograde Conducting Left Lateral Accessory Pathway

Jaime E. Gonzalez, MD, Matthew M. Zipse, MD,
Duy T. Nguyen, MD, William H. Sauer, MD*

KEYWORDS

- Catheter ablation • Accessory pathways • Wolf Parkinson White

KEY POINTS

- Atrioventricular reciprocating tachycardia is a common cause of undifferentiated supraventricular tachycardia.
- In patients with manifest or concealed accessory pathways, it is imperative to assess for the presence of other accessory pathways.
- In rare cases, multiple accessory pathways can act as the anterograde and retrograde limbs of the tachycardia.

CLINICAL PRESENTATION

A 35-year-old man with a history of palpitations and preexcitation underwent prior electrophysiologic study and ablation. He had a reported ablation of a pathway in the coronary sinus as well as a left-sided para-Hisian pathway that was not successfully ablated. Since then the patient has had recurrent documented supraventricular tachycardia with symptoms of dizziness and palpitations that have been refractory to beta-blockers and flecainide. He was referred for a repeat electrophysiologic study and possible ablation.

ELECTROPHYSIOLOGY STUDY

Venous access was obtained in the left and right femoral veins; under fluoroscopic guidance, catheters were placed in the right atrium, His bundle region, right ventricle, and coronary sinus. Baseline electrocardiogram showed evident preexcitation with a left bundle morphology and left indeterminate axis (**Fig. 1**). Baseline intracardiac electrograms showed a negative His-Ventricular (HV) interval (**Figs. 2** and **3**). The Halo catheter (Biosense-Webster, Diamond Bar, CA) was placed with Halo 1-2 close to the coronary sinus, Halo 7-8 in the right lateral free wall, and Halo 11-12 in the high right atrium. Ventricular pacing demonstrated earliest activation in the lateral coronary sinus and right free wall (**Fig. 4**). Programmed ventricular and atrial extrastimulation easily induced tachycardia with manifest preexcitation and with earliest atrial activation in the distal coronary sinus. Ventricular overdrive pacing of the tachycardia demonstrated a V-A-V-A response

Cardiac Electrophysiology, Cardiology Division, University of Colorado, Denver, Anschutz Medical Campus, 12401 East 17th Avenue, B-132, Aurora, CO 80045, USA
* Corresponding author.
E-mail address: william.sauer@ucdenver.edu

Card Electrophysiol Clin 8 (2016) 37–43
http://dx.doi.org/10.1016/j.ccep.2015.10.001
1877-9182/16/$ – see front matter © 2016 Elsevier Inc. All rights reserved.

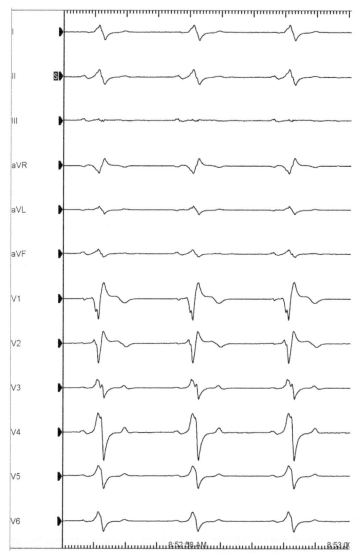

Fig. 1. Resting 12-lead electrocardiogram showing manifest preexcitation.

consistent with atrioventricular reciprocating tachycardia (AVRT) (**Fig. 5**).

QUESTION

What is the diagnosis and mechanism of the arrhythmia?

DISCUSSION

The electrograms illustrate an AVRT using a right free wall pathway as the anterograde limb and a left lateral free wall pathway as the retrograde limb. The evidence for this lies in the presence of manifest preexcitation without a His electrogram in tachycardia as well as retrograde activation via a left lateral pathway. The V-A-V response to overdrive pacing excludes an atrial tachycardia

originating from the left atrium.[1] A paced atrial premature beat during tachycardia demonstrates anterograde conduction through the AV node and His bundle. Anterograde AV nodal conduction during tachycardia is likely not present because of the retrograde invasion of the His bundle during tachycardia with a long refractory period due to conduction slowing in the His-Purkinje system.

CLINICAL COURSE

Electroanatomic mapping of the right free wall pathway was performed by assessing for earliest retrograde atrial and anterograde ventricular signals. Earliest atrial activation was performed with ventricular pacing. Earliest ventricular activation was performed with atrial pacing and during

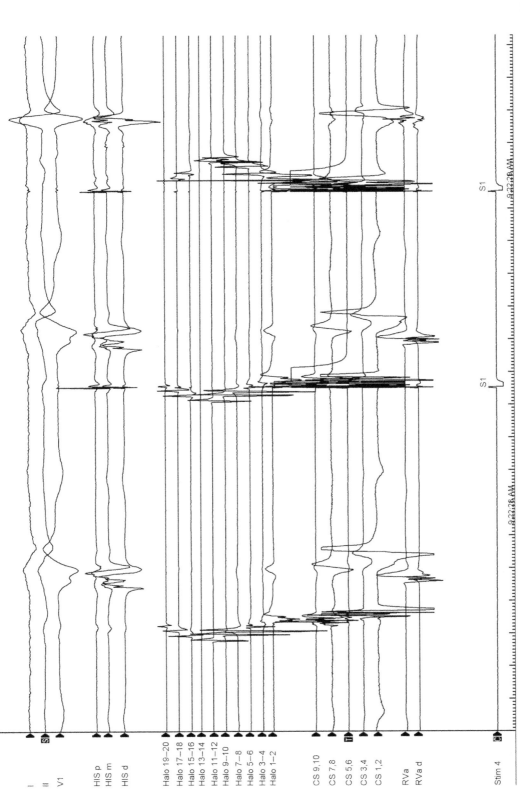

I
II
V1

HIS p
HIS m
HIS d

Halo 19–20
Halo 17–18
Halo 15–16
Halo 13–14
Halo 11–12
Halo 9–10
Halo 7–8
Halo 5–6
Halo 3–4
Halo 1–2

CS 9,10
CS 7,8
CS 5,6
CS 3,4
CS 1,2

RVa
RVa d

Stim 4

Fig. 2. Baseline intracardiac with manifest preexcitation and a negative HV interval followed by atrial pacing in the coronary sinus with loss of preexcitation and an HV interval of 69 milliseconds.

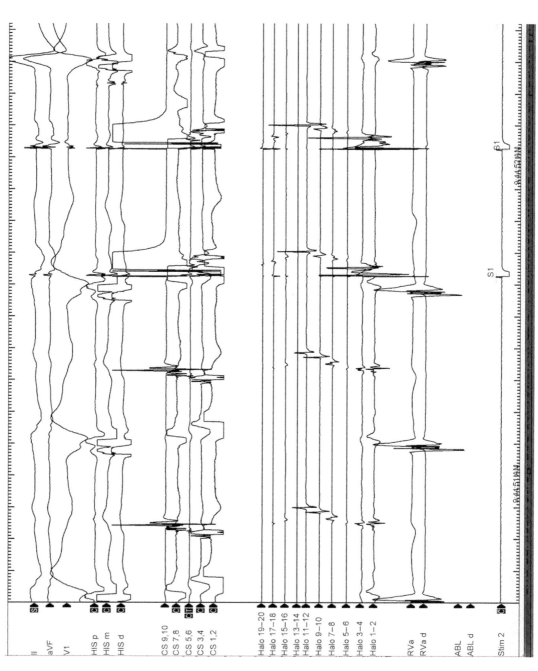

Fig. 3. Atrial pacing during tachycardia demonstrating a clear His signal and loss of preexcitation.

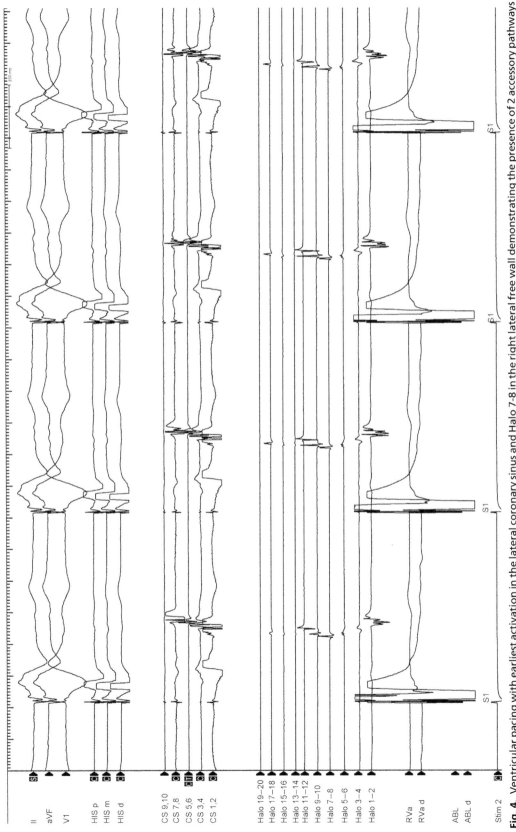

Fig. 4. Ventricular pacing with earliest activation in the lateral coronary sinus and Halo 7-8 in the right lateral free wall demonstrating the presence of 2 accessory pathways with retrograde conduction.

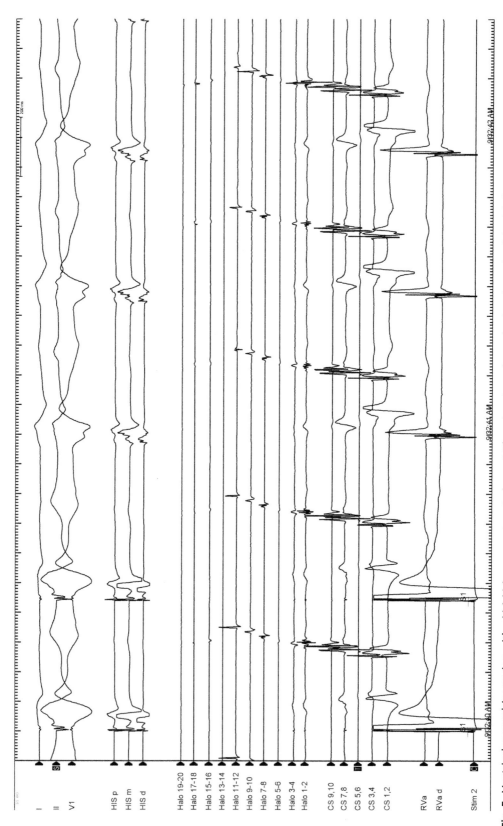

Fig. 5. Ventricular overdrive pacing with a V-A-V-A response to entrainment. There is antegrade conduction down the right-sided accessory pathway as evidenced by the left bundle morphology without a His signal. There is also earliest retrograde activation at the lateral coronary sinus observed during tachycardia.

tachycardia. There were no fascicular potentials noted on the ventricular insertion site excluding an atrio-fascicular pathway. The area of earliest atrial activation was noted to be quite broad, consistent with multiple insertion sites. A medium curl Agilis sheath (St. Jude Medical, St Paul, MN) was used for stability in the right lateral free wall and after several radio frequency (RF) lesions, the right free wall pathway was successfully ablated. After transseptal access, the left lateral free wall pathway was then mapped during ventricular pacing and the earliest atrial insertion was found at 5 o'clock on the mitral annulus. Several RF lesions were delivered at the site of earliest activation with elimination of this pathway. After ablation of these two pathways, no other pathways or tachycardias were noted or induced. Manifest preexcitation was not present. The atrial-His interval was 130 milliseconds; the HV was prolonged at 69 milliseconds, likely because of injury from a previous ablation of a para-Hisian accessory pathway. VA conduction was midline, concentric, and decremental. Para-Hisian pacing was consistent with an AV nodal response. Since ablation, the patient has had no recurrence of symptoms.

SUMMARY

AVRT is a common cause of undifferentiated supraventricular tachycardia. In patients with manifest or concealed accessory pathways, it is imperative to assess for the presence of other accessory pathways. Multiple accessory pathways are present in 4% to 10% of patients and are more common in patients with structural heart disease.[2,3] In rare cases, multiple accessory pathways can act as the anterograde and retrograde limbs of the tachycardia.

REFERENCES

1. Knight BP, Ebinger M, Oral H, et al. Diagnostic value of tachycardia features and pacing maneuvers during paroxysmal supraventricular tachycardia. J Am Coll Cardiol 2000;36:574–82.
2. Iturralde P, Guevara-Valdivia M, Rodríguez-Chávez L, et al. Radiofrequency ablation of multiple accessory pathways. Europace 2002;4:273–80.
3. Zachariah JP, Walsh EP, Triedman JK, et al. Multiple accessory pathways in the young: the impact of structural heart disease. Am Heart J 2013;165:87–92.

Supraventricular Tachycardia in a Patient with an Interrupted Inferior Vena Cava

 CrossMark

Jaime E. Gonzalez, MD, Duy Thai Nguyen, MD*

KEYWORDS

- Supraventricular tachycardia • Inferior vena cava • Cardiac • Azygous vein • Atrial tachycardia
- Ablation

KEY POINTS

- The noncoronary cusp and aortomitral continuity should be evaluated for early atrial activation when atrial tachycardias are noted to arise near the His bundle region, especially when the activation is diffuse around the His and when the P-wave morphology predicts a left atrial focus.
- In patients with congenital anomalies, alternate routes for catheter position need to be explored, including retrograde access for left atrial tachycardias and positioning of intracardiac echocardiography in the azygous vein for visualization of intracardiac structures.
- Consideration of remote magnetic navigation, if available, is another approach.

CLINICAL PRESENTATION

A 27-year-old woman with a history of an interrupted inferior vena cava (IVC) and previous ablation for atrioventricular (AV) node reentry tachycardia presents with recurrent tachycardia. She experiences daily palpitations with presyncope and has failed treatment with β-blockers and calcium channel blockers. She is referred for another electrophysiology study and possible ablation.

CLINICAL QUESTION

How should vascular access be approached in patients with an interrupted IVC?

ELECTROPHYSIOLOGY STUDY

Preparation was made for possible transhepatic access with interventional radiology.[1] A superior access approach was attempted but not successful because of anatomic challenges. Venous access was then obtained in the left femoral vein and, under fluoroscopic guidance, 2 decapolar catheters were inserted through the left femoral vein, azygous vein, and superior vena cava, and into the right atrium, His bundle region, right ventricle, and coronary sinus (**Fig. 1**). These catheters were exchanged through the study for an ablation catheter and a duodecapolar catheter that was placed through the right atrium into the coronary sinus. At baseline, the patient was in normal sinus rhythm with a normal AH interval of 62 milliseconds and a prolonged HV interval of 65 milliseconds (**Fig. 2**).

Ventricular pacing at baseline showed complete ventriculoatrial (VA) dissociation. Atrial extrastimulation did not reveal the presence of a slow pathway. VA conduction was present on isoproterenol and para-Hisian pacing was consistent with a nodal response. Atrial burst pacing on isoproterenol reliably induced a tachycardia with a variable cycle length up to 280 milliseconds (**Fig. 3**). The septal VA time in tachycardia was greater than 70 milliseconds. Ventricular overdrive pacing was performed multiple times. It was unable to accelerate

Cardiac Electrophysiology, Cardiology Division, Anschutz Medical Campus, University of Colorado, Denver, 12401 East 17th Avenue, B-132, Aurora, CO 80045, USA
* Corresponding author.
E-mail address: duy.t.nguyen@ucdenver.edu

Card Electrophysiol Clin 8 (2016) 45–50
http://dx.doi.org/10.1016/j.ccep.2015.10.002

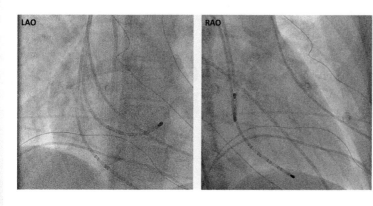

Fig. 1. Left anterior oblique (LAO) and right anterior oblique (RAO) projection of the 2 decapolar catheters coming up the azygous vein and into the heart.

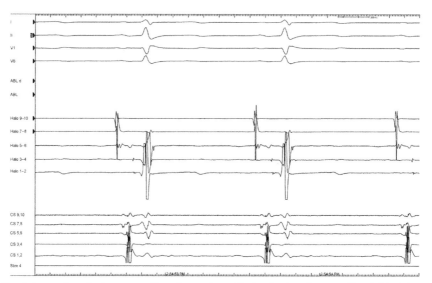

Fig. 2. Baseline intracardiac electrograms. One decapolar catheter is placed across the right atrium, His bundle electrogram, and right ventricle, and the other into the coronary sinus.

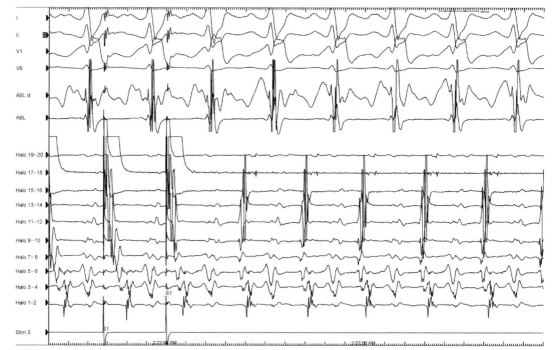

Fig. 3. Initiation of tachycardia. A duodecapolar catheter is in the right atrium (Duo 17–18 in high right atrium) and the distal electrodes are in the coronary sinus. The mapping catheter is located in the ventricle.

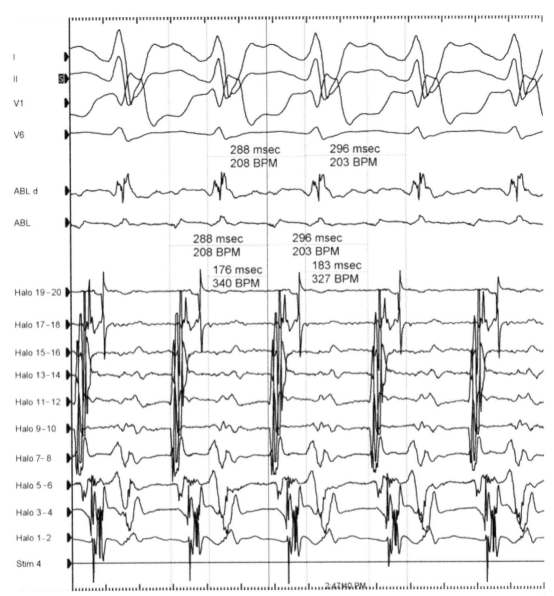

Fig. 4. Change in VA relationship (176 milliseconds vs 183 milliseconds) with the change in A-A timing (288 milliseconds vs 296 milliseconds) driving the change in V-V timing. BPM, beats per minute.

the atrial electrograms, but dissociated the atria and the ventricles with continuation of tachycardia (**Fig. 4**). Tachycardia was also noted to spontaneously have variable VA relationship with the change in A-A intervals driving the change in V-V intervals (see **Fig. 4**). The AH interval in tachycardia was similar to the AH interval in sinus rhythm. The P wave in tachycardia was positive in lead II and lead V1 and had an initial negative deflection followed by a larger positive deflection in lead I (**Fig. 5**). Electroanatomic mapping (activation mapping) was performed in the right atrium with diffuse earliest activation near the His region.

QUESTION

What is the diagnosis? How should the clinician proceed in the treatment of this tachycardia?

DISCUSSION

AV dissociation during tachycardia and with ventricular overdrive pacing excludes the possibility of AV reciprocating tachycardia. The septal VA time of greater than 70 milliseconds also excludes the typical form of AVNRT (atrioventricular nodal reentrant tachycardia). The variable VA timing

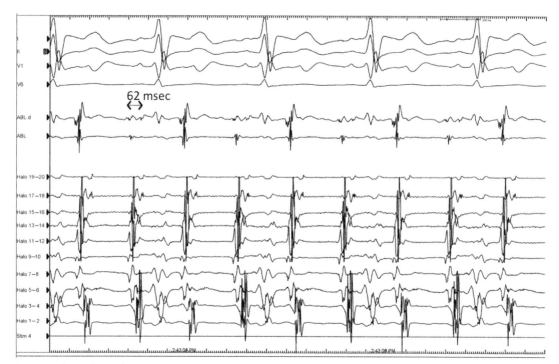

Fig. 5. Tachycardia with spontaneous 2:1 AV relationship. The AH in tachycardia is similar to the AH in sinus rhythm and the P-wave morphology is negative positive in lead I, positive in lead II, and positive in lead V1.

and AH in tachycardia being similar to the AH in sinus rhythm are highly suggestive of an atrial tachycardia. A high to low atrial activation in tachycardia with a P-wave morphology that was positive in II and V1 suggest a superior and posterior origin of the tachycardia, and the negative positive P wave in lead I is most consistent with an atrial tachycardia with a left-sided focus.[2]

Electroanatomic mapping of atrial tachycardias to the AV node/His bundle region is common. Because ablation at this site carries a high risk of AV block, it is prudent to evaluate non–right atrial structures such as the aortic cusps and the mitral annulus for earlier activation, especially considering the P-wave morphology and the more diffuse activation near the His region. The noncoronary cusp is located near the His bundle, is easily accessible retrograde, and delivery of radiofrequency energy at this site carries a much lower risk of AV block.[3] Retrograde access is also more feasible in patients with an interrupted IVC because the lack of an IVC makes standard transseptal puncture more challenging.

The introduction of catheters via a retrograde approach carry the risk of causing injury to the coronary arteries and angiography has been useful in

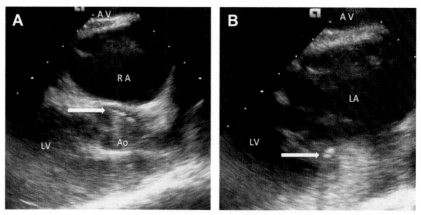

Fig. 6. ICE images from the azygous vein (AV) showing the catheter in the noncoronary cusp (*arrow* in *A*) and in the aortomitral continuity (*arrow* in *B*). Ao, aorta; LA, left atrium; LV, left ventricle; RA, right atrium.

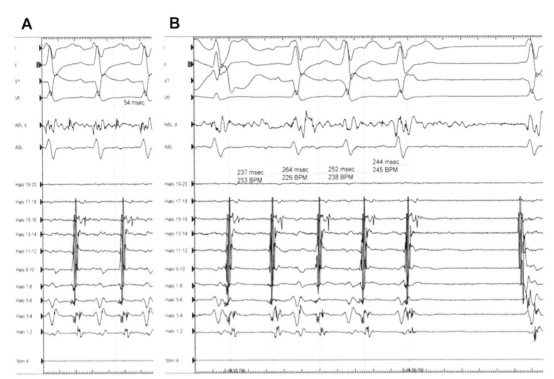

Fig. 7. The ablation catheter is in the aortomitral continuity with atrial activation 54 milliseconds pre-P wave (*A*). Ablation at this site causes slowing and termination of the tachycardia (*B*).

the evaluation of catheter position in relation to the coronaries.[4] Intracardiac echocardiography (ICE) has also been useful to assess for location of arteries, catheter contact, and relation to other cardiac structures.[5,6]

CLINICAL COURSE

Femoral arterial access was obtained and mapping was performed in the noncoronary cusp. The ICE catheter was advanced through the left femoral vein, but would not cross the azygous into the superior vena cava. The catheter was withdrawn back into the azygous where visualization of cardiac structures was possible, and the images obtained were similar to those acquired by transesophageal echocardiography (**Fig. 6**). Ablation was performed in the noncoronary cusp, where atrial signals were 30 milliseconds pre-QRS, after performing coronary angiography to ensure safe catheter position and to exclude the possibility of anomalous coronary arteries in a patient with known congenital vascular malformations (ICE was unable to identify the coronaries with accuracy). Ablation at this site did not alter the tachycardia. Using electroanatomic mapping and ICE for guidance, the ablation catheter was advanced into the aortomitral continuity. Atrial activation at

this site was 54 milliseconds pre-P wave. Ablation at this site slowed and terminated the tachycardia (**Fig. 7**) with subsequent noninducibility. The patient has not had recurrence of symptoms over a 1-year follow-up.

SUMMARY

The noncoronary cusp and aortomitral continuity should be evaluated for early atrial activation when atrial tachycardias are noted to arise near the His bundle region, especially when the activation is diffuse around the His and when the P-wave morphology predicts a left atrial focus. In patients with congenital anomalies, alternate routes for catheter position need to be explored, including retrograde access for left atrial tachycardias and positioning of ICE in the azygous vein for visualization of intracardiac structures. Consideration of remote magnetic navigation, if available, is another approach.

REFERENCES

1. Nguyen DT, Gupta R, Kay J, et al. Percutaneous transhepatic access for catheter ablation of cardiac arrhythmias. Europace 2013;15(4):494–500.
2. Kistler PM, Roberts-Thomson KC, Haqqani HM, et al. P-wave morphology in focal atrial tachycardia:

development of an algorithm to predict the anatomic site of origin. J Am Coll Cardiol 2006; 48(5):1010–7.

3. Tada H, Naito S, Miyazaki A, et al. Successful catheter ablation of atrial tachycardia originating near the atrioventricular node from the noncoronary sinus of Valsalva. Pacing Clin Electrophysiol 2004;27(10): 1440–3.

4. Sasaki T, Hachiya H, Hirao K, et al. Utility of distinctive local electrogram pattern and aortographic anatomical position in catheter manipulation at coronary cusps. J Cardiovasc Electrophysiol 2011; 22(5):521–9.

5. Mlčochová H, Wichterle D, Peichl P, et al. Catheter ablation of focal atrial tachycardia from the aortic cusp: the role of electroanatomic mapping and intracardiac echocardiography. Pacing Clin Electrophysiol 2013;36(1):e19–22.

6. Hoffmayer KS, Dewland TA, Hsia HH, et al. Safety of radiofrequency catheter ablation without coronary angiography in aortic cusp ventricular arrhythmias. Heart Rhythm 2014;11(7):1117–21.

Atrioventricular Nodal Reentrant Tachycardia with 2:1 Atrioventricular Block

Leila Larroussi, MD[a], Nitish Badhwar, MD, FHRS[a,b,*]

KEYWORDS

- AVNRT • AV block • Atrioventricular nodal reentrant tachycardia

KEY POINTS

- This report illustrates an interesting case of atrioventricular nodal reentrant tachycardia that presented with 2 different ventricular cycle lengths due to a 2:1 block in the lower common pathway.
- At the induction of the tachycardia, a long-short sequence above the His creates a phase 3 block resulting in a 2:1 conduction in the lower common pathway.
- A premature ventricular contraction, by retrograde penetration of the His, eliminates the long-short sequence and brings the conduction back to 1:1.

CLINICAL PRESENTATION

A 50-year-old woman with no known medical condition presents with a longstanding history of palpitations with abrupt onset and offset that was responsive to vagal maneuvers. **Fig. 1**A shows her baseline electrocardiogram (ECG) with a normal PR interval and right bundle branch block (RBBB).

ELECTROPHYSIOLOGY STUDY

The patient is referred to the authors' department for electrophysiology study and ablation in the setting of probable supraventricular tachycardia (SVT). During the procedure, the baseline intervals are atrial-His 58 milliseconds and His-ventricular 37 milliseconds. On isoproterenol, this tachycardia was induced with programmed atrial stimulation (see **Fig. 1**B).

The tachycardia is a wide complex tachycardia with an RBBB pattern that is similar to RBBB morphology in sinus rhythm. This finding supports the diagnosis of SVT with aberrancy. The ventricular heart rate is 200 beats per minute. Looking for P waves, there is a notch in the terminal portion of the QRS in lead II that is not present during sinus rhythm. This notch makes it an A on V tachycardia and argues against an accessory pathway (AP). The most likely diagnosis is atrioventricular nodal reentrant tachycardia (AVNRT), but atrial tachycardia (AT) cannot be excluded.

Fig. 2A shows the intracardiac electrograms during tachycardia; the authors note that the VA interval is less than 70 milliseconds, excluding again AP-mediated tachycardia.[1] Ventricular overdrive pacing consistently terminated the tachycardia by pulling in the A and, therefore, could not be used to differentiate AVNRT from AT. Atrial

Disclosures: none.
[a] Section of Cardiac Electrophysiology, Division of Cardiology, Department of Medicine, University of California, San Francisco, San Francisco, CA, USA; [b] UCSF Medical Center, 500 Parnassus Avenue, MUE-431, San Franicsco, CA 94143, USA
* Corresponding author. UCSF Medical Center, 500 Parnassus Avenue, MUE-431, San Francisco, CA 94143.
E-mail address: nitish.badhwar@ucsf.edu

A

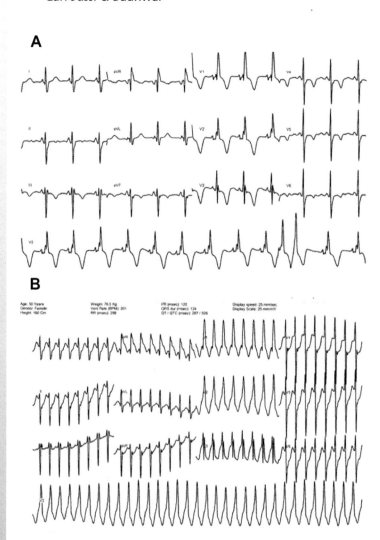

Fig. 1. (*A*) Baseline electrocardiogram (ECG) in SR. (*B*) ECG in tachycardia.

B

overdrive pacing (AOD) during tachycardia shows dissociation of the atrial electrogram (accelerated to the pacing cycle length [CL]) from the His and ventricular signals that are marching at the tachycardia CL (see **Fig. 2**B). This dissociation excludes AT. Note there is a pseudo-AHHA response after AOD that would be consistent with junctional tachycardia (JT) if the atrium had captured the His and V. **Fig. 2**C shows termination of tachycardia with a late premature atrial complex (*arrow*) that does not affect the subsequent V. This finding argues against JT.[2] Based on these findings, the most likely diagnosis is AVNRT.

QUESTION

During the pacing maneuvers, a second tachycardia was induced (**Fig. 3**). What is the most likely mechanism?

DISCUSSION

Looking at the beginning of the bottom strip, the authors note that the ventricular CL on the left is twice the CL at the end of the strip. This finding should raise the possibility of a 2:1 ventricular conduction. Looking at the P waves, the authors note

A

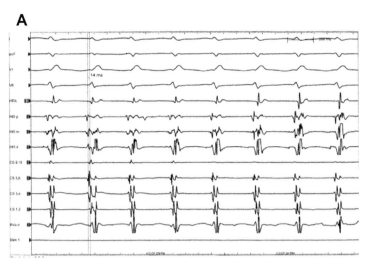

B

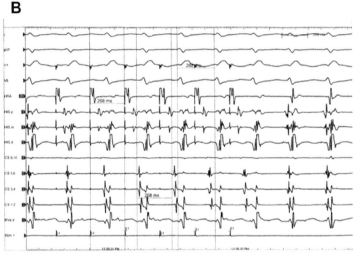

C

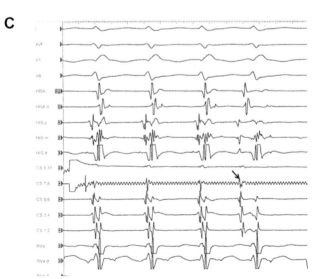

Fig. 2. (*A*) Intracardiac electrogram during tachycardia showing VA timing less than 70 milliseconds. (*B*) Intracardiac electrogram atrial overdrive pacing during tachycardia. The atrium is dissociated from the tachycardia. (*C*) Intracardiac electrograms showing tachycardia termination with late premature atrial complex (PAC) (*arrow*) that does not affect the subsequent V. This finding rules out junctional tachycardia and is consistent with AVNRT.

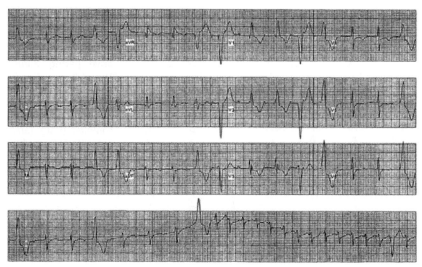

Fig. 3. ECG of tachycardia 2.

that there are indeed 2 P waves for each QRS (excluding the premature ventricular contractions [PVCs]). Also, the P-wave morphology does not change and is negative in leads II, III, and aVF, suggestive of a retrograde conduction. After the third PVC, the tachycardia conducts 1 to 1 and is similar to the initial tachycardia. This finding suggests that the tachycardia with a slower ventricular rate is also AVNRT with a 2:1 block in the lower common pathway. In the intracardiac electrogram (**Fig. 4**), the authors can see that there is no H deflection when the beat is blocked, which shows that the site of block is above the His bundle.

AVNRT with 2:1 AV block is usually present at initiation because of a long-short sequence when the jump in the slow pathway occurs. The following His depolarization is short as the patient is now in tachycardia. This tachycardia results in a functional phase 3 block in the His bundle. When a PVC occurs, it produces a retrograde depolarization of

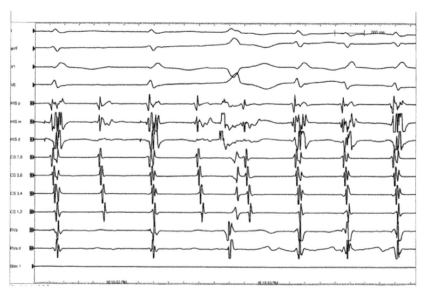

Fig. 4. Intracardiac electrograms during tachycardia 2.

the bundle of His, eliminating the long-short sequence that was perpetuating the 2:1 block.[3]

SUMMARY

This report illustrates an interesting case of AVNRT that presented with 2 different ventricular CLs because of a 2:1 block in the lower common pathway. At the induction of the tachycardia, a long-short sequence above the His creates a phase 3 block resulting in a 2:1 conduction in the lower common pathway. A PVC, by retrograde penetration of the His, eliminates the long-short sequence and brings the conduction back to 1:1.

REFERENCES

1. Knight BP, Ebinger M, Oral H, et al. Diagnostic value of tachycardia features and pacing maneuvers during paroxysmal supraventricular tachycardia. J Am Coll Cardiol 2000;36:574–782.
2. Viswanathan MN, Scheinman MM, Badhwar N. A new diagnostic maneuver to differentiate atrioventricular nodal reentrant tachycardia from junctional tachycardia: a difficult distinction [abstract]. Heart Rhythm 2007;4(5):S288.
3. Ching Man K, Brinkman K, Bogun F, et al. 2:1 atrioventricular block during atrioventricular node reentrant tachycardia. J Am Coll Cardiol 1996;28(7): 1170–4.

Implantable Cardioverter-Defibrillator Shock Caused by Uncommon Variety of Nonreentrant Atrioventricular Nodal Tachycardia

David K. Singh, MD[a],*, Nitish Badhwar, MD, FHRS[b]

KEYWORDS

- Catheter ablation • Double fire • ICD

KEY POINTS

- This article reports a typical case of incessant double-fire tachycardia resulting in implantable cardioverter-defibrillator discharge caused by the device's misdiagnosis of ventricular tachycardia.
- At electrophysiology study, the presence of double-fire physiology was confirmed, and modification of the slow pathway resulted in elimination of repetitive double fires.
- Although this is an unusual entity, it is important to recognize, because it may be misdiagnosed as atrial fibrillation, resulting in inappropriate anticoagulation and/or antiarrhythmic therapy.
- Modification of the slow pathway and elimination of double-fire physiology can result in marked improvement in quality of life and reversal of tachycardia-mediated cardiomyopathy.

CLINICAL PRESENTATION

A 56-year-old man with a history of atrial fibrillation, ischemic cardiomyopathy with an ejection fraction of 30%, and coronary artery bypass surgery was referred to our electrophysiology (EP) clinic. At the time of the referral the patient was on amiodarone for his atrial fibrillation, and reported no significant symptoms other than mild exercise intolerance. Shortly thereafter, a dual-chamber implantable cardioverter-defibrillator (ICD) was placed. His amiodarone was subsequently stopped out of concern for the long-term side effects of this therapy. Several months later the patient presented to the emergency department reporting that he had been shocked by his device. An electrocardiogram (ECG) taken around the time of his admission revealed an irregular, narrow complex tachycardia (**Fig. 1**). Device interrogation was performed. Tracings from ICD discharge revealed an irregular tachycardia with more ventricular electrograms than atrial electrograms (**Fig. 2**).

QUESTION

What is the mechanism of the tachycardia and the reason for the for the ICD discharge?

Disclosures: None.
[a] Section of Cardiac Electrophysiology, Division of Cardiology, Department of Medicine, Queens Medical Center, Honolulu, HI, USA; [b] Section of Cardiac Electrophysiology, Division of Cardiology, Department of Medicine, University of California, San Francisco, San Francisco, CA, USA
* Corresponding author. Department of Internal Medicine, Queens Medical Center, POB III, 550 South Beretania Street, Suite 601, Honolulu, HI 96814.
E-mail address: dsingh@queens.org

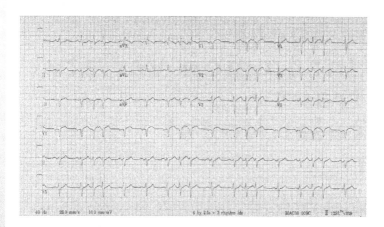

Fig. 1. Twelve-lead ECG showing regularly irregular narrow complex tachycardia with more QRS complexes than P waves.

DISCUSSION

Inspection of the ECG (see **Fig. 1**) reveals a pattern of 3 narrow complex beats followed by 1 or 2 narrow complex beats. There is a regular atrial rate at approximately 90 beats per minute. The ventricular rate alters between 90 beats per minute and approximately 150 beats per minute. The 3 narrow complex beats uniformly begin with a QRS preceded by a P wave followed by a QRS with no preceding P wave, and eventually another QRS preceded by a P wave.

The ICD interrogation reveals a similar pattern whereby 1 atrial electrogram is frequently followed by 2 ventricular electrograms with a cycle length of approximately 300 milliseconds. The far-field electrogram shows a consistent morphology. This cycle length is within the ventricular tachycardia (VT) zone of the device, resulting in a 41-J shock that seems to terminate the arrhythmia.

The differential diagnosis for a narrow complex tachycardia that manifests more ventricular beats than atrial beats is limited and includes junctional tachycardia with ventriculoatrial block, fascicular tachycardia (often associated with AV dissociation), AV nodal reentrant tachycardia with upper common pathway block, nodofascicular tachycardia with variable upper common pathway block, and paroxysmal nonreentrant supraventricular tachycardia (PNSVT) caused by repetitive double fires. The first 3 on this list would all be expected to manifest retrograde P waves. Inspection of the surface ECG clearly reveals an underlying sinus mechanism, thereby establishing PNSVT as the most likely diagnosis. This entity is seen in patients with dual atrioventricular (AV) nodal pathways. A single atrial impulse conducts first through the fast pathway followed by conduction down the slow pathway, which explains why 1 P wave can be associated with 2 QRS complexes.

ELECTROPHYSIOLOGY STUDY AND ABLATION

The patient was brought to the EP laboratory for EP study and ablation. Multipolar catheters were placed in the right atrium, His-bundle region, right

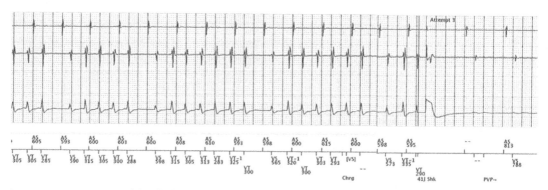

Fig. 2. ICD interrogation of the rhythm leading to shock. There are more ventricular electrograms than atrial electrograms. Often 1 atrial electrogram is followed by 2 ventricular electrograms.

ventricle (RV), and coronary sinus in standard positions. The double-fire phenomenon was observed with programmed electrical stimulation from the coronary sinus (**Fig. 3**). On cessation of pacing, a conducted beat was observed, followed by a second conducted beat with no preceding atrial depolarization.

Fig. 4 also revealed an interesting phenomenon. The first and second atrial complexes conduct to the ventricle via the fast pathway. The third ventricular complex is the result of slow pathway conduction from the prior atrial complex. The following atrial complex conducts to the ventricle via the fast pathway but the AV interval is prolonged compared with the previous fast pathway activations. The last atrial complex conducts to the ventricle via slow pathway and fast pathway activation is absent. The most likely explanation for this is slow prolongation of conduction in the fast pathway with block caused by concealed conduction from the preceding slow pathway activation (although Wenckebach periodicity in the fast pathway cannot be ruled out).

Ablation in the slow pathway region using an anatomic approach was performed. Following this, no double fires were observed either spontaneously or with programmed electrical stimulation. At 1-year follow-up, the patient has not had any ICD shocks or device-detected tachycardia.

DISCUSSION

AV reentrant tachycardia (either typical or atypical) is the most common manifestation of dual AV nodal physiology. The phenomenon of double fire, whereby a single atrial impulse is conduced down both the fast pathway and the slow pathway was first described by Csapo[1] in 1979. Since that time, there has been increasing recognition of this uncommon arrhythmia. The hallmark is a so-called 1 to 2 response, in which a single atrial impulse results in 2 QRS complexes. As with the patient described earlier, it is common for the arrhythmia to be misdiagnosed as atrial fibrillation. It is also common for patients to report palpitations and other symptoms associated with supraventricular tachycardias. Perhaps most importantly, patients with frequent and repetitive double fires can develop a tachycardia-related cardiomyopathy. Ablation of the slow pathway can eliminate the double fires and reverse the patient's cardiomyopathy.

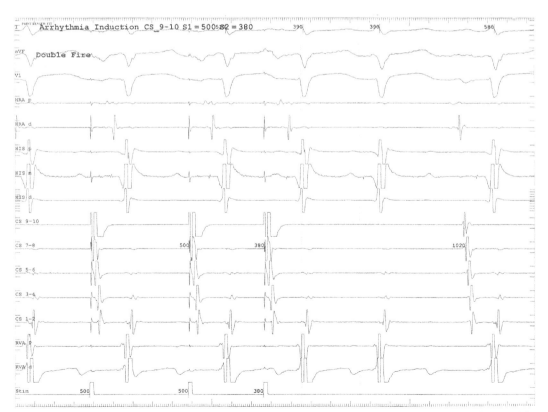

Fig. 3. Pacing from coronary sinus catheter shows double-fire response with 1 atrial paced beat followed by 2 QRS complexes each associated with His, suggesting activation through conduction system.

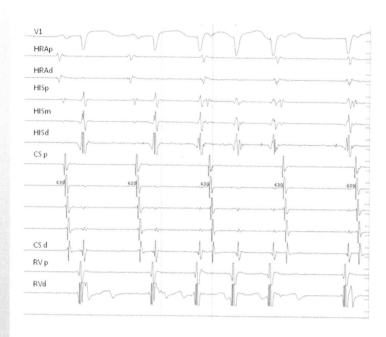

Fig. 4. The first and second atrial complexes conduct to the ventricle via the fast pathway. The third ventricular complex is the result of slow pathway conduction from the prior atrial complex. The following atrial complex conducts to the ventricle via the fast pathway but the AV interval is prolonged compared with the previous fast pathway activations. The last atrial complex conducts to the ventricle via slow pathway and fast pathway activation is absent.

Conditions that have been reported to promote double-fire physiology include[2]:

1. Sufficient antegrade dissociation of AV node
2. Absence of retrograde conduction over each AV nodal pathway following antegrade conduction over its counterpart
3. Differences between fast and slow pathway conduction times exceeding His-Purkinje refractoriness
4. Critical timing of sinus impulses relative to preceding AV nodal conduction

Although it has been reported that this arrhythmia is resistant to antiarrhythmic therapy, the patient described herein only manifested double-fire physiology following cessation of amiodarone therapy. It is possible that amiodarone altered the conduction properties of the slow pathway, fast pathway, or the His-Purkinje system, thus changing the conditions necessary for double fires to occur.

Another interesting feature of this case was the presence of an ICD. The patient had ischemic cardiomyopathy with an ejection fraction of 20% to 25%. Implantation of the ICD was probably necessary given that the double-fire physiology was not observed until after the ICD was implanted and amiodarone was withdrawn. Nonetheless, it is important to emphasize how the device may misinterpret double-fire tachycardia for VT and

deliver inappropriate therapy. Often SVT/VT discriminators rely, among other things, on more ventricular electrograms than atrial electrograms. As in this case, the patient's arrhythmia was classified as VT, resulting in a 41-J shock.

SUMMARY

This article reports a typical case of incessant double-fire tachycardia resulting in ICD discharge caused by the device's misdiagnosis of VT. At EP study, the presence of double-fire physiology was confirmed, and modification of the slow pathway resulted in elimination of repetitive double fires. Although this is an unusual entity, it is important to recognize, because it may be misdiagnosed as atrial fibrillation, resulting in inappropriate anticoagulation and/or antiarrhythmic therapy. In addition, modification of the slow pathway and elimination of double-fire physiology can result in marked improvement in quality of life and reversal of tachycardia-mediated cardiomyopathy.

REFERENCES

1. Csapo G. Paroxysmal nonreentrant tachycardias due to simultaneous conduction in dual atrioventricular nodal pathways. Am J Cardiol 1979;43(5):1033–45.
2. Gaba D, Pavri BB, Greenspon AJ, et al. Dual antegrade response tachycardia induced cardiomyopathy. Pacing Clin Electrophysiol 2004;27(4):533–6.

Incessant Palpitations and Narrow Complex Tachycardia

Frederick T. Han, MD, FHRS

KEYWORDS

- Supraventricular tachycardia • AV dissociation • Junctional tachycardia

KEY POINTS

- Junctional tachycardia (JT) is rare cause of supraventricular tachycardia.
- The intracardiac activation sequence is similar to atrioventricular nodal reentrant tachycardia (AVNRT).
- Premature atrial contractions inserted during tachycardia can help distinguish JT from AVNRT.
- As noted in this case, slow pathway ablation for JT may not always be effective for termination of JT.
- Activation mapping during JT identified a low-amplitude potential in the region of the coronary sinus ostium and the inferior margin of the triangle of Koch that marked the successful ablation site for JT.

CLINICAL PRESENTATION

A 48-year-old woman presented for evaluation and management of daily palpitations, lasting for hours. The palpitations started when the patient was in her 20s, but gradually progressed, such that in the months before presentation the palpitations occurred for up to 8 hours a day on a daily basis. The palpitations occurred irrespective of whether the patient was at rest or exercising. Physical examination, laboratory studies, and echocardiogram were normal. Ambulatory monitoring identified multiple episodes of palpitations correlating with a narrow complex tachycardia occurring throughout the day (**Fig. 1**). The patient was subsequently referred for electrophysiology study and catheter ablation.

ELECTROPHYSIOLOGY STUDY
Tachycardia Induction

Quadripolar electrode catheters were positioned in the high right atrium, right ventricular apex, and the His bundle region. A decapolar electrode catheter was placed in the coronary sinus. Normal atrial-His and His-ventricular intervals were recorded in sinus rhythm. Ventricular-atrial conduction was present with ventricular pacing; there was a concentric retrograde atrial activation pattern. A sustained A on V narrow QRS complex tachycardia at a cycle length of 386 to 573 milliseconds was induced with ventricular overdrive pacing (VOD), single ventricular extrastimulus testing, and atrial overdrive pacing from the coronary sinus on and off isoproterenol infusion up to 10 μg/min (**Fig. 2**). Significant cycle length variation was observed with variations in isoproterenol dosing. Spontaneous variations in the His-His interval preceded changes in the atrial-atrial and ventricular-ventricular intervals during tachycardia (**Fig. 3**).

QUESTION

What is the differential diagnosis for a narrow QRS complex tachycardia? How can the tachycardia mechanism be established?

Section of Cardiac Electrophysiology, Division of Cardiovascular Medicine, University of Utah Health Sciences Center, 30 North 1900 East, Room 4A-100 SOM, Salt Lake City, UT 84132, USA
E-mail address: frederick.han@hsc.utah.edu

Card Electrophysiol Clin 8 (2016) 61–65
http://dx.doi.org/10.1016/j.ccep.2015.10.005
1877-9182/16/$ – see front matter © 2016 Elsevier Inc. All rights reserved.

cardiacEP.theclinics.com

A

B

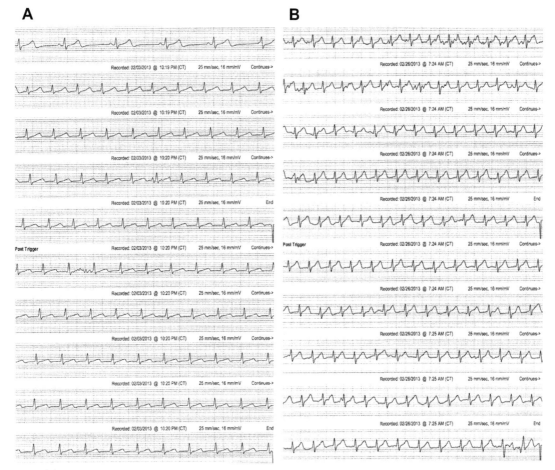

Fig. 1. (*A*) Tachycardia initiation on ambulatory monitor. (*B*) Tachycardia with atrioventricular dissociation.

MANEUVERS DURING TACHYCARDIA

The differential diagnosis of a narrow QRS complex tachycardia with a ventricular-atrial (VA) interval of 0 milliseconds includes atrioventricular nodal reentrant tachycardia (AVNRT), junctional tachycardia (JT), and circus movement tachycardia using a concealed nodofascicular (NF) accessory pathway.[1]

VOD during tachycardia entrained the tachycardia and produced a VAHV (Ventricle-Atrial-His-Ventricle) response, ruling out atrial tachycardia. His refractory premature ventricular contractions during the tachycardia did not affect the subsequent A within the confines of wobble noted in tachycardia.[2] This finding argues against concealed NF accessory pathway–mediated tachycardia.

Single early programmed atrial extrastimuli advanced the subsequent QRS via conduction down the fast atrioventricular nodal pathway with continuation of tachycardia (**Fig. 4**). Late premature atrial contractions (PACs) did not delay or terminate the tachycardia via the slow pathway.[3,4] With AVNRT, late premature atrial contractions are expected to advance the tachycardia via conduction down the slow pathway; early premature atrial contractions that conduct down the fast pathway should terminate tachycardia.

MAPPING AND ABLATION

A 4-mm quadripolar radiofrequency ablation catheter was used for mapping and ablation. All lesions were delivered in the temperature-controlled mode at 50 W with a 60°C temperature limit for up to 60 seconds. For ablation of the JT, we decided to proceed with a stepwise approach with inducibility testing after each series of ablations. First, we targeted the slow pathway during sinus rhythm. Two radiofrequency lesions were in the slow pathway region with junctional beats observed during ablation. The JT remained inducible (the 2 red lesions in **Fig. 5**).

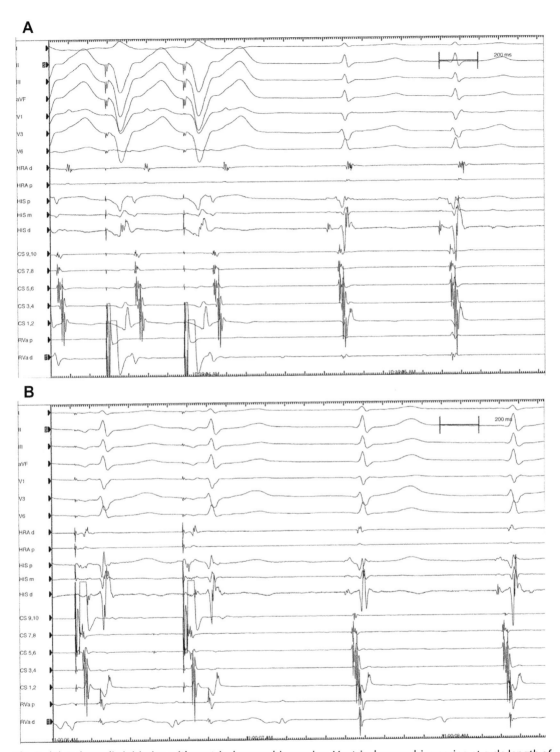

Fig. 2. (*A*) Tachycardia initiation with ventricular overdrive pacing. Ventricular overdrive pacing at cycle length of 400 milliseconds induced a narrow QRS complex tachycardia with a VAHV initiation. (*B*) Tachycardia initiation with atrial overdrive pacing. Atrial overdrive pacing the proximal coronary sinus (CS 9,10) at 550 milliseconds induced a narrow QRS complex tachycardia with a AHHA (atrial-His-His-atrial) initiation pattern.

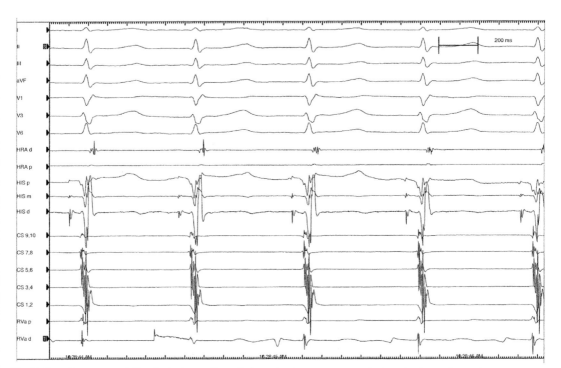

Fig. 3. Spontaneous variation in tachycardia cycle length. Spontaneous variations in the tachycardia cycle length were noted with variations in the His-His interval preceding changes in the atrial-atrial and ventricular-ventricular intervals.

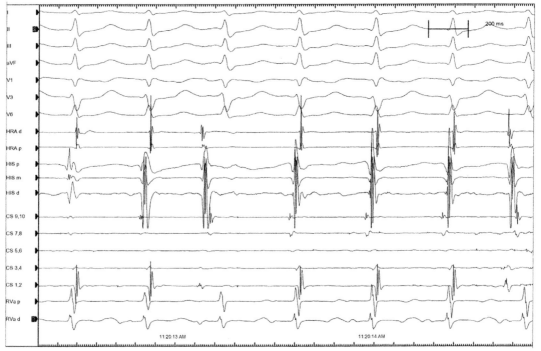

Fig. 4. Spontaneous right atrial premature atrial contraction during tachycardia. A spontaneous late right atrial premature atrial contraction advances the next QRS via conduction down the fast atrioventricular nodal pathway with continuation of tachycardia that rules out AVNRT.

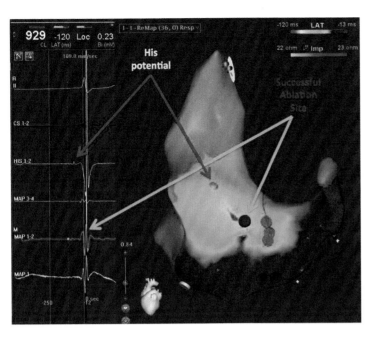

Fig. 5. CARTO activation map of JT in left anterior oblique cranial view. Activation mapping of JT after 2 slow pathway ablations and 3 ablations on the roof of the proximal coronary sinus failed to terminate the JT. The lesion at the successful ablation site identified a low-amplitude potential that preceded the His potential during tachycardia. Ablation at this site rendered the tachycardia noninducible.

Next, during tachycardia we mapped the earliest atrial activation and delivered 3 lesions at the roof of the proximal coronary sinus.[5] The tachycardia remained inducible at this point. During tachycardia, we performed mapping to identify a prepotential during the tachycardia. As noted in **Fig. 5**, we identified a low-amplitude potential at the roof of the coronary sinus ostium that preceded the His potential during tachycardia. A single radiofrequency lesion delivered at this site terminated the tachycardia and rendered it noninducible.

SUMMARY

JT is rare cause of supraventricular tachycardia. The intracardiac activation sequence is similar to AVNRT. Premature atrial contractions inserted during tachycardia can help distinguish JT from AVNRT. As noted in this case, slow pathway ablation for JT may not always be effective for termination of JT. Activation mapping during JT identified a low-amplitude potential in the region of the coronary sinus ostium and the inferior margin of the triangle of Koch that marked the successful ablation site for JT.

REFERENCES

1. Hamdan MH, Page RL, Scheinman MM. Diagnostic approach to narrow complex tachycardia with VA block. Pacing Clin Electrophysiol 1997;20:2984–8.

2. Knight BP, Ebinger M, Oral H, et al. Diagnostic value of tachycardia features and pacing maneuvers during paroxysmal supraventricular tachycardia. J Am Coll Cardiol 2000;36:574–82.

3. Viswanathan MN, Scheinman MM, Badhwar N. A new diagnostic maneuver to differentiate atrioventricular nodal reentrant tachycardia from junctional tachycardia: a difficult distinction [abstract]. Heart Rhythm 2007;4(5):S288.

4. Padanilam BJ, Manfredi JA, Steinberg LA, et al. Differentiating junctional tachycardia and atrioventricular node re-entry tachycardia based on response to atrial extrastimulus pacing. J Am Coll Cardiol 2008; 52:1711–7.

5. Hamdan MH, Badhwar N, Scheinman MM. Role of invasive electrophysiologic testing in the evaluation and management of adult patients with focal junctional tachycardia. Card Electrophysiol Rev 2002; 6(4):431–5.

Narrow Complex Tachycardia
What is the Mechanism?

Marwan M. Refaat, MD, FHRS, FESC[a],*,
Melvin Scheinman, MD[b], Nitish Badhwar, MD, FHRS[b]

KEYWORDS

- Catheter ablation • Junctional tachycardia • Atrioventricular nodal reentrant tachycardia

KEY POINTS

- This article presents a diagnostic dilemma in which atrioventricular nodal reentrant tachycardia (AVNRT) and junctional tachycardia (JT) were differentiated based on tachycardia initiation with atrial extrastimulus as well as on the response to progressive decremental atrial extrastimuli.
- The progressive increase in A2H2′ (Atrial His interval) and H2H2′ (His-His interval) in response to atrial extrastimuli favors reentry as the mechanism of the tachycardia.
- This is a novel mechanistic differentiation of AVNRT from focal JT.

CLINICAL PRESENTATION

A 51-year-old man presented with incessant supraventricular tachycardia (SVT) despite treatment with β-blockers. He was referred for electrophysiology study and catheter ablation. SVT initiation was characterized by dual ventricular response to the programmed premature atrial complex (PAC) and the atrial depolarization was linked to the second ventricular response (**Fig. 1**). His-refractory premature ventricular contraction (PVC) had no effect on the SVT and ventricular overdrive pacing during SVT did not preexcite or postexcite the first fused beat. Atrial overdrive pacing (AOD) during SVT led to an AHHA response. As shown in **Fig. 2**, with AOD from the proximal coronary sinus at 600 milliseconds, progressively tighter extrastimuli (360 milliseconds in **Fig. 2**A, 340 milliseconds in **Fig. 2**B,

320 milliseconds in **Fig. 2**C) lead to longer A2H2′ and H2H2′.

QUESTION

What is the diagnosis of the narrow complex tachycardia?

DISCUSSION

An A-on-V SVT with septal VA timing less than 70 milliseconds rules out extranodal accessory pathway–mediated SVT. The differential diagnosis of an A-on-V SVT is typical slow-fast atrioventricular (AV) nodal reentrant tachycardia (AVNRT), atrial tachycardia, focal junctional tachycardia (JT), concealed nodofascicular/nodoventricular tachycardia, as well as intrahisian reentrant tachycardia. Because His-refractory PVC had no effect

Disclosures: None.
[a] Section of Cardiac Electrophysiology, Division of Cardiology, Department of Medicine, Faculty of Medicine and Medical Center, American University of Beirut, PO Box 11-0236, Riad El-Solh, Beirut 1107 2020, Lebanon;
[b] Section of Cardiac Electrophysiology, Division of Cardiology, Department of Medicine, University of California, 500 Parnassus Avenue, San Francisco, CA 94143, USA
* Corresponding author. Cardiology/Cardiac Electrophysiology, Departments of Internal Medicine and Biochemistry and Molecular Genetics, Faculty of Medicine and Medical Center, American University of Beirut, PO Box 11-0236, Riad El-Solh, Beirut 1107 2020, Lebanon.
E-mail address: mr48@aub.edu.lb

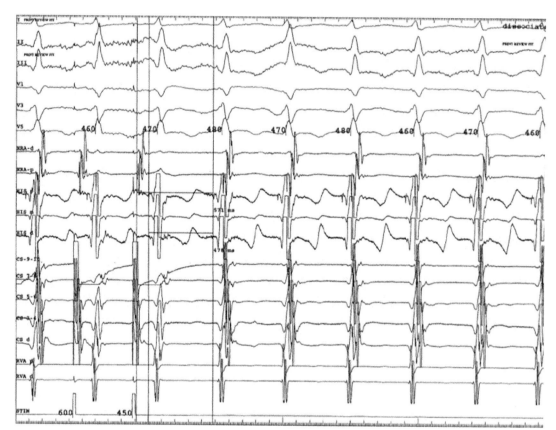

Fig. 1. SVT initiation with atrial extrastimulus that leads to AHHA response. This finding is consistent with junctional tachycardia as well as atrioventricular nodal reentrant tachycardia initiating with double fire.

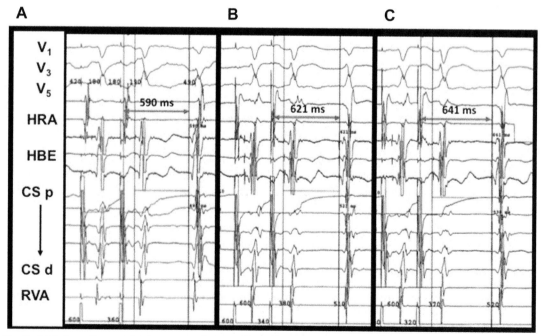

Fig. 2. AOD from the proximal coronary sinus at 600 milliseconds, progressive tighter extrastimuli (360 milliseconds in [A], 340 milliseconds in [B], 320 milliseconds in [C]) lead to longer A2H2' and H2H2'. CSd, distal coronary sinus electrogram; CSp, proximal coronary sinus electrogram; HBE, His Bundle electrogram; HRA, high right atrium; RVA, right ventricular apex electrogram.

on the SVT, and ventricular overdrive pacing during SVT did not preexcite or postexcite the first fused beat, a concealed nodofascicular or nodoventricular reentrant tachycardia is less likely. VA linking argues against atrial tachycardia. An extranodal accessory pathway is excluded by the short VA interval (<70 milliseconds). AOD during SVT led to an AHHA response, which could be caused by JT or AVNRT termination with AOD and reinduction with a 2:1 response to atrial pacing.[1] Thus, the main differential diagnosis was between JT and AVNRT initiating with double fire. AVNRT involves a reentrant circuit within the AV node, whereas the mechanism of JT in adults is enhanced automaticity or triggered activity.

As shown in **Fig. 2**, progressively tighter extrastimuli (360 milliseconds in [A] to 320 milliseconds in [C]) lead to longer A2H2′ and H2H2′ that favors a reentrant mechanism (AVNRT). A focus with triggered activity (JT) would have yielded a shorter A2H2′ and H2H2′ with tighter extrastimuli. A late PAC induced during His bundle refractoriness delayed the next His and A. These findings exclude focal JT and favor AVNRT as the diagnosis.[2,3]

Following determination of the SVT mechanism, a deflectable-tip mapping/ablation catheter was maneuvered into position along the medial tricuspid annulus at the traditional slow pathway region, to about one-third of the way between the coronary sinus os and the His recording position; this latter distance comprised about 5 mm fluoroscopically. The patient had a small circuit with a narrow distance from the coronary sinus to the His catheter. At this location, the local electrogram showed a configuration consistent with an AV nodal slow-pathway potential. The bipolar signal in sinus rhythm had a small atrial component ending in a small upward deflection, and a larger ventricular component. Catheter ablation at this site led to junctional beats and made SVT noninducible. The patient has been symptom free for 18 months.

This article presents a diagnostic dilemma in that AVNRT and JT were differentiated based on tachycardia initiation with atrial extrastimulus as well as on the response to progressive decremental atrial extrastimuli. The progressive increase in A2H2′ and H2H2′ in response to atrial extrastimuli favors reentry as the mechanism of the tachycardia, which is a novel mechanistic differentiation of AVNRT from focal JT.

REFERENCES

1. Fan R, Tardos JG, Almasry I, et al. Novel use of atrial overdrive pacing to rapidly differentiate junctional tachycardia from atrioventricular nodal reentrant tachycardia. Heart Rhythm 2011;8:840–4.
2. Viswanatham MN, Scheinman MM, Badhwar N. A new diagnostic maneuver to differentiate atrioventricular nodal reentrant tachycardia from junctional tachycardia: a difficult distinction. Heart Rhythm 2007;4(5):S288.
3. Padanilam BJ, Manfredi JA, Steinberg LA, et al. Differentiating junctional tachycardia and atrioventricular node re-entry tachycardia based on response to atrial extrastimulus pacing. J Am Coll Cardiol 2008; 52(21):1711–7.

Incessant Long R-P Tachycardia

Bernard Abi-Saleh, MD, FHRS[a,b,1], Marwan M. Refaat, MD, FHRS, FESC[a,b,c,*,1],
Fadi F. Bitar, MD[d], Maurice Khoury, MD[a,b], Mariam Arabi, MD[d]

KEYWORDS

- Catheter ablation • Atrial tachycardia • Left atrial appendage

KEY POINTS

- A 13-year-old boy had a positive P wave in V1 with a negative P wave in lead I, aVL, and aVR, as well as a positive P wave in the inferior leads, which correlated with a left atrial appendage (LAA) atrial tachycardia (AT) focus.
- Many features of this case are helpful to the diagnosis and treatment of LAA AT.
- P-wave morphologies can provide clues regarding an AT's origin, and our case with a P-wave negative in lead I favored LAA AT.
- The atrial activation sequence was earliest in the LAA.
- Careful mapping along the atria and coronary sinus to determine the earliest site of activation for the surface P-wave is a reliable method for precisely localizing the AT origin as a target for catheter ablation.

CLINICAL PRESENTATION

A 13-year-old boy presented to the hospital for acute appendicitis and was noted to be in tachycardia with a heart rate of 220 beats per minute (bpm). An electrocardiogram was performed and it showed a narrow complex tachycardia at 220 bpm. The patient reported occasional palpitations, especially on heavy exercise, but denies any dizziness or syncope. His transthoracic echocardiogram showed a severely depressed left ventricular systolic function with ejection fraction (EF) at 20% to 24%.

He was started on propranolol 40 mg 3 times a day then loaded with amiodarone and followed by a maintenance dose of 200 mg a day. Six months later, the amiodarone was switched to flecainide 100 mg twice a day. The patient continued to have intermittent palpitations. His follow-up electrocardiogram revealed the same narrow complex tachycardia but slower, at 110 to 130 bpm, with only occasional sinus beats. He was referred for an electrophysiology (EP) study and ablation.

ELECTROPHYSIOLOGY STUDY

In the EP laboratory, an octapolar coronary sinus was introduced percutaneously from the right femoral vein and positioned into the coronary

Disclosures: None.
[a] Cardiac Electrophysiology Section, Cardiology Division, American University of Beirut Medical Center, Beirut, Lebanon; [b] Cardiac Electrophysiology Section, Cardiology Division, Department of Internal Medicine, American University of Beirut Faculty of Medicine and Medical Center, PO Box 11-0236, Riad El-Solh, Beirut 1107 2020, Lebanon; [c] Department of Biochemistry and Molecular Genetics, American University of Beirut Faculty of Medicine and Medical Center, PO Box 11-0236, Riad El-Solh, Beirut 1107 2020, Lebanon; [d] Department of Pediatrics and Adolescent Medicine, American University of Beirut Medical Center, Beirut, Lebanon
[1] The authors contributed equally to this article.
* Corresponding author. Department of Biochemistry and Molecular Genetics, American University of Beirut Faculty of Medicine and Medical Center, PO Box 11-0236, Riad El-Solh, Beirut 1107 2020, Lebanon.
E-mail address: mr48@aub.edu.lb

cardiacEP.theclinics.com

sinus. A detailed mapping of the tachycardia was performed using the 8-Fr Thermocool open irrigated mapping/ablation catheter with a 3.5-mm tip. Bipolar electrograms (30–500 Hz) were displayed and stored using a digital recording system (EP MedSystems, West Berlin, NJ). Three-dimensional electroanatomic mapping was performed with Ensite NavX (St Jude Medical, St Paul, MN) as well as the triggered sweep for detailed determination of the site of origin of the tachycardia. There was evidence of wobbling of the tachycardia cycle length with a change in atrial rate driving the change in the ventricular rate that favored a diagnosis of atrial tachycardia (AT).

QUESTION: WHERE IS THE SITE OF ORIGIN OF THE FOCAL ATRIAL TACHYCARDIA?

Analysis of P-wave morphology during tachycardia revealed a positive P wave in lead V1, positive in inferior leads, negative in lead I, and flat in V5 and V6 (**Fig. 1**), indicating that the tachycardia is originating from the left atrium.

Mapping of the left atrial (LA) cavity, the pulmonary veins, the mitral annulus, and the LA appendage (LAA) showed that the earliest atrial activation was located in the apex of the LAA (**Fig. 2**). A lesion was delivered with an irrigated ablation catheter with 30 W for 60 seconds, causing

intermittent interruption of the tachycardia (**Fig. 3**). Five additional lesions received 35 W for 60 seconds each at and around the site of earliest activation in the LAA (**Fig. 4**). The tachycardia never recurred, even after a waiting period of 90 minutes on and off isoproterenol as well as after 24 hours of telemetry monitoring. His EF normalized to 60% and he has remained symptom free over the last 2 years.

DISCUSSION

Focal ATs are uncommon causes of supraventricular tachycardia (SVT) in adults, accounting for 5% to 10% of cases. They usually occur along the crista terminalis in the right atrium and near the pulmonary veins in the left atrium. Less frequently, they can arise from the aortic cusps, coronary sinus ostium and musculature, the para-Hisian region, the right atrial appendage and LAA, or along the tricuspid or mitral annulus.[1,2] This case involves an AT originating from the LAA, which is a rare focus and accounts to 0.6% of focal AT.[1]

Analysis of P-wave morphology during SVT and/or ectopic atrial impulses is useful in localizing the site of focal ATs. Several P-wave algorithms have been developed to help determine the AT site of origin.[1,3,4] In a recent algorithm, Kistler and colleagues[1] reported that a positive P wave in leads V1 to V3 with isoelectric P wave in lead V6, a

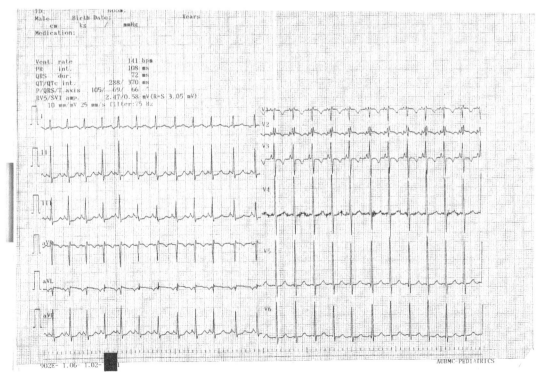

Fig. 1. Long R-P tachycardia with P-wave morphology in supraventricular tachycardia.

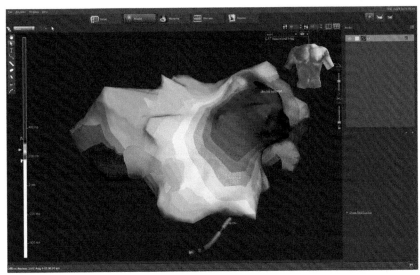

Fig. 2. Electroanatomic map in the right anterior oblique view showing the site of earliest atrial activation in the LAA.

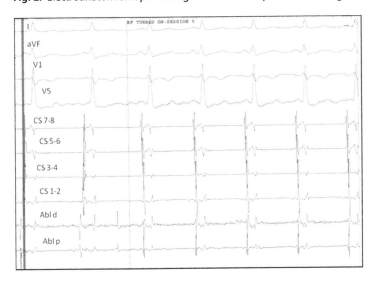

Fig. 3. Termination of the AT and change in atrial activation sequence with successful ablation of the LAA AT.

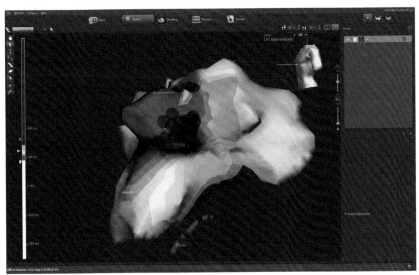

Fig. 4. Electroanatomic map in left anterior oblique view showing the ablation lesions delivered at the site with earliest atrial activation in the LAA.

negative P wave in aVL, a negative P wave in lead I, with positive P wave in the inferior leads favored an LAA focus. In the 2 cases of LAA AT out of the 196 focal AT, 1 patient had an isoelectric P wave in aVR and 1 patient had a negative P wave in aVR.[1] Our case had a positive P wave in V1 with a negative P wave in lead I, aVL, and aVR, as well as a positive P wave in the inferior leads, which correlated with an LAA AT focus.

Many features of this case are helpful to the diagnosis and treatment of LAA AT. P-wave morphologies can provide clues regarding an AT's origin and this case with a P-wave negative in lead I favored LAA AT. The atrial activation sequence was earliest in the LAA. Careful mapping along the atria and coronary sinus to determine the earliest site of activation for the surface P wave is a reliable method for precisely localizing the AT origin as a target for catheter ablation.

REFERENCES

1. Kistler PM, Roberts-Thomson KC, Haqqani HM, et al. P-wave morphology in focal atrial tachycardia: development of an algorithm to predict the anatomic site of origin. J Am Coll Cardiol 2006; 48(5):1010–7.
2. Gonzalez MD, Contreras LJ, Jongbloed MR, et al. Left atrial tachycardia originating from the mitral annulus-aorta junction. Circulation 2004;110(20): 3187–92.
3. Tang CW, Scheinman MM, Van Hare GF, et al. Use of P wave configuration during atrial tachycardia to predict site of origin. J Am Coll Cardiol 1995;26(5): 1315–24.
4. Ellenbogen KA, Wood MA. Atrial tachycardia. In: Zipes DP, Jalife J, editors. Cardiac electrophysiology: from cell to bedside. 4th edition. Philadelphia: Saunders; 2004. p. 500–11.

Section 2: Ventricular Tachycardia

Editor: Henry H. Hsia

Ventricular Tachycardias

Henry H. Hsia, MD, FHRS

KEYWORDS

- Ventricular tachycardia • Electrocardiographic localization and anatomy
- Electrophysiology mapping • Electroanatomical substrate

KEY POINTS

- Understanding the underlying substrate is critical for preprocedural planning to optimize ablation outcomes and minimize procedural risk.
- Careful analysis of the electrocardiogram pattern is useful for localization of the ventricular tachyarrhythmia site of origin.
- Detailed knowledge of the anatomy is essential for developing mapping and ablation strategies.
- A hybrid approach of both conventional activation-entrainment mapping and substrate characterization is needed for successful ablation.

Ventricular tachyarrhythmia (VT) is an important cause of morbidity and sudden death in patients with structural heart disease. Although implantable cardioverter-defibrillator (ICD) reduces the risk of sudden arrhythmic death,[1,2] ICD therapies have been associated with increased mortality[3,4] as well as a significant negative impact on patients' quality of life.[5,6] Antiarrhythmic drugs, including amiodarone, may be effective in preventing arrhythmia recurrences and ICD therapies but have an increased risk of drug-related adverse effects and noncardiac mortality.[7,8]

In recent years, utilization of VT catheter ablation has increased and evolved.[9,10] This section of the monograph is devoted entirely on ventricular arrhythmias. These cases are uniquely thought provoking, with emphasis on important electrocardiographic and anatomic features, illustrating crucial points in the use of diagnostic maneuvers, mapping techniques, imaging integration, as well as formulating the appropriate ablation strategies.

The right ventricular (RV) and left ventricular (LV) outflow tracts share many similar characteristics because of the common embryonic origin.[11] Identifying the precise arrhythmia location and achieving successful ablation may be challenging because of the complex anatomic relationship and close proximity of various structures. However, several electrocardiographic features can provide clues.[12–16] The utility of 12-lead electrocardiogram (ECG), coupled with a detailed understanding of the anatomy, remains invaluable in localizing such arrhythmia foci. A systematic approach to mapping of outflow tract arrhythmias, along with real-time image guidance, such as intracardiac echocardiography, helps to improve procedural outcome and minimize complications.

Ventricular arrhythmias originating from the aortic noncoronary cusp is rare and usually occurs in young patients. The ECG morphology is often similar to those that arise from the right coronary cusp or para-Hisian locations.[17] Motonaga and colleagues presented such an unusual case and provided an excellent discussion on the complex anatomic relationship between the RV and LV outflow tracts (see: Motonaga K, Ceresnak S, Hsia H. Unusual outflow tract ventricular tachycardia, in this issue).

Ventricular arrhythmias arising from the LV summit may account for up to 18% of the idiopathic arrhythmias from the LV outflow tract.[18] The LV summit represents the most superior portion of the LV, including the epicardial surface bisected by the coronary vasculature. Ablation is often

Arrhythmia Service, VA San Francisco, Building 203, Room 2A-52A, MC 111C-6, 4150 Clement Street, San Francisco, CA 94121, USA
E-mail address: henry.hsia@ucsf.edu

Card Electrophysiol Clin 8 (2016) 75–78
http://dx.doi.org/10.1016/j.ccep.2015.10.008
1877-9182/16/$ – see front matter Published by Elsevier Inc.

limited by the proximity to the coronary arteries and the presence of epicardial fat. Intraoperative imaging is essential to avoid coronary arterial damage,[19] and effective ablation may be achieved from anatomically adjacent sites as an alternative target. Groups from both the University of Pennsylvania and the Brigham and Women's Hospital provided illustrative case studies of such challenging arrhythmia (see: Santangeli P, Lin D, Marchlinski F. Catheter ablation of ventricular arrhythmias arising from the left ventricular summit and Kumar S, Tedrow U, Stevenson W. Ventricular arrhythmias from the left ventricular summit: critical importance of anatomy, imaging and detailed mapping to allow safe and effective ablation, in this issue). Recently, specific electrocardiographic indices have been described that predict ablation success.[20] ECG analysis is, therefore, crucial for planning of the most appropriate mapping approach for LV summit arrhythmias.

Ventricular arrhythmias originating from the cardiac crux represents another unusual arrhythmia that has also been increasingly recognized.[21,22] Laroussi and colleagues presented an idiopathic ventricular tachycardia originating from the LV apical crux region that was mapped and successfully ablated via an epicardial approach (see: Larroussi L, Badhwar N. Ventricular tachycardia arising from cardiac crux: ECG recognition and site of ablation, in this issue). This case highlighted again the importance of ECG analysis in predicting the potential location of the target site.

Nogami and colleagues presented an excellent review of the anatomy and mechanism of fascicular VT. Patients with fascicular VT may not be easily inducible, perhaps because of the subendocardial location of the Purkinje fibers that is vulnerable to catheter trauma during mapping. This case report provided an effective strategy for anatomically based ablation when fascicular VT is noninducible or if diastolic Purkinje potential cannot be recorded during mapping (see: Talib A, Nogami A. Anatomical ablation strategy for non-inducible fascicular tachycardia, in this issue). Pace mapping at the successful ablation site is often not perfect because selective capture of the orthodromic limb of the circuit is difficult and there may be a "lower common pathway" in some patients.

Postinfarction VTs are mostly due to scar-based reentry with nonuniform anisotropic conduction, multiple potential circuits with interconnecting channels. Such scar substrate may be identified by low-voltage recordings as well as the presence of local abnormal ventricular activities (LAVA) or late potentials. Most of the VTs in patients with ischemic heart disease and prior myocardial infarctions can be successfully ablated by an endocardial

approach targeting the late potentials/LAVA, which are surrogates for the surviving myocardial bundles. A combination of activation mapping, entrainment, electroanatomical substrate characterization, and pace mapping is required. As illustrated by the case from University of Oklahoma, a systematic approach is essential to improve ablation success and safety (see: Garabelli P, Stavrakis S, Po S. Ablation of ventricular tachycardia in patients with ischemic cardiomyopathy, in this issue).

By contrast, scar in nonischemic cardiomyopathy is commonly located in the midmyocardium or epicardium, associated with smaller areas of endocardial low-voltage abnormalities.[23–26] The subset of patients with predominantly intramural septal scar poses particularly challenges, with high long-term arrhythmia recurrence despite multiple ablations.[27] Nazer and colleagues presented an interesting case of pleomorphic ventricular tachycardia, reflecting variable fusions from multiple exits of a septal VT (see: Nazer B, Hsia H. Pleomorphic ventricular tachycardias in nonischemic cardiomyopathy, in this issue). With careful analysis and patience, an isthmus site of the reentrant circuit was ultimately identified and successfully ablated. The group from University of Colorado presented an unusual patient with biventricular noncompaction with both endocardial and epicardial VTs (see: Gonzalez J, Tzou W, Sauer W, et al. Ventricular tachycardia in a patient with bi-ventricular non-compaction, in this issue). A hybrid approach of conventional mapping techniques coupled with substrate analysis was again required for a successful result. This case highlighted the potential epicardial substrate in patients with uncommon forms of nonischemic cardiomyopathies.

This collection of challenging real-life cases emphasizes several important points about mapping and ablation of ventricular arrhythmias: (1) Careful preprocedural planning based on patients' history and clinical data is essential. Analysis of ECG is critical for localizing the potential arrhythmia foci/substrate and helps to formulate mapping approaches. (2) A detailed understanding of anatomy is important. A strategy of mapping all potential target sites in proximity and the use of an alternative location for ablation energy delivery may be required, particularly for ventricular arrhythmias originating from the LV summit or crux. (3) For scar-based VTs, a systematic approach with a combination of activation mapping, entrainment, and pace mapping as well as detailed substrate characterization are required for a successful outcome. (4) The use of imaging guidance is important to facilitate mapping and to minimize risk/complications.

REFERENCES

1. A comparison of antiarrhythmic-drug therapy with implantable defibrillators in patients resuscitated from near-fatal ventricular arrhythmias. The Antiarrhythmics versus Implantable Defibrillators (AVID) Investigators. N Engl J Med 1997;337:1576–83.
2. Bardy G, Lee K, Mark D, et al. Sudden Cardiac Death in Heart Failure Trial (SCD-HeFT) Investigators. Amiodarone or an implantable cardioverter-defibrillator for congestive heart failure. N Engl J Med 2005;352(3):225–37.
3. Poole J, Johnson G, Hellkamp A, et al. Prognostic importance of defibrillator shocks in patients with heart failure. N Engl J Med 2008;359:1009–17.
4. Sweeney M, Sherfesee L, DeGroot P, et al. Differences in effects of electrical therapy type for ventricular arrhythmias on mortality in implantable cardioverter-defibrillator patients. Heart Rhythm 2010;7:353–60.
5. Wathen M, Sweeney M, DeGroot P, et al, PainFREE Investigators. Shock reduction using antitachycardia pacing for spontaneous rapid ventricular tachycardia in patients with coronary artery disease. Circulation 2001;104:796–801.
6. Sears S, Conti J. Quality of life and psychological functioning of ICD patients. Heart 2002;87(5):488–93.
7. Connolly S, Dorian P, Roberts R, et al, Optimal Pharmacological Therapy in Cardioverter Defibrillator Patients (OPTIC) Investigators. Comparison of beta-blockers, amiodarone plus beta-blockers, or sotalol for prevention of shocks from implantable cardioverter defibrillators: the OPTIC Study: a randomized trial. JAMA 2006;295(2):165–71.
8. Packer D, Prutkin J, Hellkamp A, et al. Impact of implantable cardioverter-defibrillator, amiodarone, and placebo on the mode of death in stable patients with heart failure: analysis from the sudden cardiac death in heart failure trial. Circulation 2009;120(22):2170–6.
9. Sacher F, Tedrow U, Field M, et al. Ventricular tachycardia ablation: evolution of patients and procedures over 8 years. Circ Arrhythm Electrophysiol 2008;1:153–61.
10. Palaniswamy C, Kolte D, Harikrishnan P, et al. Catheter ablation of post infarction ventricular tachycardia: ten-year trends in utilization, in-hospital complications, and in-hospital mortality in the United States. Heart Rhythm 2014;11(11):2056–63.
11. Kramer T. The partition of the truncus and conus and the formation of the membraneous portion of the interventricular septum in human heart. Am J Anat 1942;71(3):343–70.
12. Jadonath R, Schwartzman D, Preminger M, et al. Utility of the 12-lead electrocardiogram in localizing the origin of right ventricular outflow tract tachycardia. Am Heart J 1995;130:1107–13.
13. Yamauchi Y, Aonuma K, Takahashi A, et al. Electrocardiographic characteristics of repetitive monomorphic right ventricular tachycardia originating near the His-bundle. J Cardiovasc Electrophysiol 2005;16(10):1041–8.
14. Yoshida N, Inden Y, Uchikawa T, et al. Novel transitional zone index allows more accurate differentiation between idiopathic right ventricular outflow tract and aortic sinus cusp ventricular arrhythmias. Heart Rhythm 2011;8(3):349–56.
15. Hutchinson M, Garcia F. An organized approach to the localization, mapping, and ablation of outflow tract ventricular arrhythmias. J Cardiovasc Electrophysiol 2013;24(10):1189–97.
16. Yoshida N, Yamada T, McElderry H, et al. A novel electrocardiographic criterion for differentiating a left from right ventricular outflow tract tachycardia origin: the V2S/V3R index. J Cardiovasc Electrophysiol 2014;25(7):747–53.
17. Yamada T, Lau Y, Litovsky S, et al. Prevalence and clinical, electrocardiographic, and electrophysiologic characteristics of ventricular arrhythmias originating from the noncoronary sinus of Valsalva. Heart Rhythm 2013;10(11):1605–12.
18. Yamada T, McElderry H, Doppalapudi H, et al. Idiopathic ventricular arrhythmias originating from the left ventricular summit: anatomic concepts relevant to ablation. Circ Arrhythm Electrophysiol 2010;3(6):616–23.
19. Roberts-Thomson K, Steven D, Seiler J, et al. Coronary artery injury due to catheter ablation in adults: presentations and outcomes. Circulation 2009;120:1465–73.
20. Jauregui Abularach M, Campos B, Park K, et al. Ablation of ventricular arrhythmias arising near the anterior epicardial veins from the left sinus of Valsalva region: ECG features, anatomic distance, and outcome. Heart Rhythm 2012;9(6):865–73.
21. Doppalapudi H, Yamada T, Ramaswamy K, et al. Idiopathic focal epicardial ventricular tachycardia originating from the crux of the heart. Heart Rhythm 2009;6(1):44–50.
22. Kawamura M, Gerstenfeld E, Vedantham V, et al. Idiopathic ventricular arrhythmia originating from the cardiac crux or inferior septum: an epicardial idiopathic ventricular arrhythmia. Circ Arrhythm Electrophysiol 2014;7(6):1152–8.
23. Soejima K, Stevenson W, Sapp J, et al. Endocardial and epicardial radiofrequency ablation of ventricular tachycardia associated with dilated cardiomyopathy: the importance of low-voltage scars. J Am Coll Cardiol 2004;43:1834–42.
24. Cesario D, Vaseghi M, Boyle N, et al. Value of high-density endocardial and epicardial mapping for catheter ablation of hemodynamically unstable ventricular tachycardia. Heart Rhythm 2006;3(1):1–10.

25. Nakahara S, Tung R, Ramirez R, et al. Characterization of the arrhythmogenic substrate in ischemic and nonischemic cardiomyopathy implications for catheter ablation of hemodynamically unstable ventricular tachycardia. J Am Coll Cardiol 2010;55(21): 2355–65.

26. Cano O, Hutchinson M, Lin D, et al. Electroanatomic substrate and ablation outcome for suspected epicardial ventricular tachycardia in left ventricular nonischemic cardiomyopathy. J Am Coll Cardiol 2009;54(9):799–808.

27. Haqqani H, Tschabrunn C, Tzou W, et al. Isolated septal substrate for ventricular tachycardia in nonischemic dilated cardiomyopathy: incidence, characterization, and implications. Heart Rhythm 2011; 8(8):1169–76.

Unusual Outflow Tract Ventricular Tachycardia

Kara S. Motonaga, MD[a],*, Scott R. Ceresnak, MD[a], Henry H. Hsia, MD, FHRS[b]

KEYWORDS

- Ventricular tachycardia • Outflow tract • Ventricular arrhythmia • Heart

KEY POINTS

- Distinguishing premature ventricular contractions/ventricular tachycardia from the right ventricular outflow tract (RVOT) versus the left ventricular outflow tract (LVOT) can be difficult by electrocardiogram (ECG) findings alone, particularly when the origin is above the aortic valve, because of their close anatomic relationships.
- When the ECG shows a left bundle branch block morphology with an inferior axis and an R-wave transition at or later than V3 to V4, mapping first in the RVOT is reasonable.
- When ablation in the RVOT is unsuccessful despite early activation signals, mapping of the LVOT in the aortic cusps should be considered.
- A thorough understanding of the outflow tract anatomy as well as a systematic and meticulous approach to mapping of the ventricular outflow regions and great vessels increases the success rate and decreases the risk of damage to adjacent structures and the conduction system.
- The use of multimodality imaging, particularly real-time intracardiac echocardiographic guidance, is essential for defining anatomy, ensuring adequate catheter contact, and minimizing risks.

INTRODUCTION

The right ventricular outflow tract (RVOT) and left ventricular outflow tract (LVOT) are the most common sites of origin for ventricular arrhythmias in structurally normal hearts. These arrhythmias often arise from endocardial sites in the ventricles and can be successfully treated with radiofrequency catheter ablation.[1] They are generally focal with automatic/triggered activity and not related to scar-based reentry mechanisms.[2] However, ventricular outflow tract arrhythmias can arise from adjacent structures such as the proximal pulmonary artery and coronary cusps. It is important to understand the relationship between the relevant cardiac structures in this area for successful mapping and ablation. This article discusses unusual outflow tract ventricular tachycardias (VTs) using a clinical case presentation to highlight the key anatomic features as well as mapping and ablation techniques for this region.

ANATOMY OF THE OUTFLOW TRACTS

In a structurally normal heart, the RVOT and LVOT cross over each other with the RVOT located anteriorly and leftward relative to the aortic root and ventricular septum, whereas the LVOT is posterior and rightward. The RVOT wraps anteriorly around the aortic root and is in close proximity to the right coronary cusp (RCC) (**Fig. 1**). The pulmonary valve is anterior and superior to the aortic valve with a 90° orientation to the aortic valve in the horizontal plane (see **Fig. 1**). The pulmonary trunk is adjacent to the left coronary cusp (LCC). The noncoronary cusp (NCC) is located over the anterior atrial

[a] Department of Pediatrics, Division of Pediatric Cardiology, Stanford University, Palo Alto, CA, USA;
[b] Department of Medicine, Division of Cardiology, University of California, San Francisco, San Francisco, CA, USA
* Corresponding author. Department of Pediatrics, Division of Pediatric Cardiology, Stanford University, 750 Welch Road, Suite 321, Palo Alto, CA 94304.
E-mail address: sachie@stanford.edu

Card Electrophysiol Clin 8 (2016) 79–88
http://dx.doi.org/10.1016/j.ccep.2015.10.032
1877-9182/16/$ – see front matter © 2016 Elsevier Inc. All rights reserved.

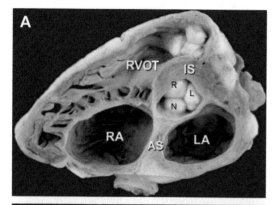

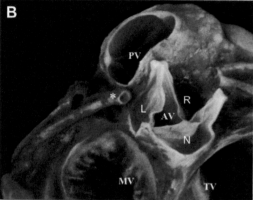

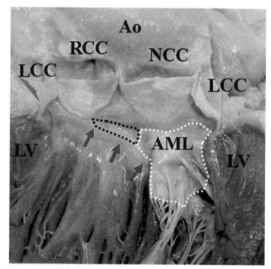

Fig. 1. Anatomic specimens demonstrating the outflow tract anatomy. (*A*) Cross section at the base of the heart showing the relationship of the aortic cusps to the atria and right ventricular outflow tract (RVOT). The RVOT wraps anteriorly around the aortic root with the right coronary cusp (R) adjacent to the thick interventricular septum (IS) in the posterior RVOT. The left coronary cusp (L) lies adjacent to the left atrium (LA) and the proximal pulmonary trunk. The noncoronary cusp (N) lies adjacent to the interatrial septum (AS) and the LA and right atria (LA). (*B*) The pulmonary valve (PV) is anterior and approximately 1-2 cm superior to the aortic valve (AV) with a 90° orientation in the horizontal plane. The posterior PV cusp is adjacent to the left main coronary artery in the epicardial space (*asterisk*) and the L cusp. The N cusp is the most inferior and posterior of all three cusps with its position adjacent to the AS. MV, mitral valve; TV, tricuspid valve. ([*A*] *From* Madhavan M, Asirvatham SJ. What are we ablating above the semilunar valves? Insights from electrical navigation. J Cardiovasc Electrophysiol 2011;22:530–33, with permission and [*B, C*] *From* Gami AS, Noheria A, Lachman N, et al. Anatomical correlates relevant to ablation above the semilunar valves for the cardiac electrophysiologist: a study of 603 hearts. J Interv Card Electrophysiol 2011;30:5–15; with permission).

septum in continuity with the anterior leaflet of the mitral valve (MV) (**Fig. 2**). The His bundle is a right atrial structure that goes across to the left ventricle (LV) via the membranous septum just under RCC-NCC commissure.

The superior RVOT is considered an epicardial structure because it is located above the LV with the pulmonary valve cusps adjacent to the epicardial coronary vasculature within the LV summit (see **Fig. 1**B). The pulmonary trunk is a completely infundibular muscular structure. The muscular fibers can extend into the interleaflet triangles and even above the sinotubular junction of the pulmonary valve along the entire circumference of the pulmonary trunk[3] (**Fig. 3**).

The LVOT is located posteriorly and rightward to the RVOT with the RCC positioned above the ventricular septum. Unlike the RVOT, the LVOT only has ventricular muscular extensions into the aortic valves under the RCC and LCC[3,4] (see **Fig. 2**). The NCC usually does not have any muscular connections because it has fibrous connections to the anterior leaflet of the MV and the membranous septum.

Fig. 2. Heart specimen demonstrating anatomy of the non-coronary cusp (NCC) which is in fibrous continuity with the anterior mitral valve leaflet (AML, *white dotted circle*) and the membranous septum (*black dotted circle*) which sits beneath the NCC-right coronary cusp (RCC) commissure. Therefore, the NCC is usually separated from the left ventricular (LV) myocardium by fibrous tissue (*red arrows*). (*From* Yamada T, Lau YR, Litovsky SH, et al. Prevalence and clinical, electrocardiographic, and electrophysiologic characteristics of ventricular arrhythmias originating from the noncoronary sinus of Valsalva. Heart Rhythm 2013;10:1605–12; with permission.)

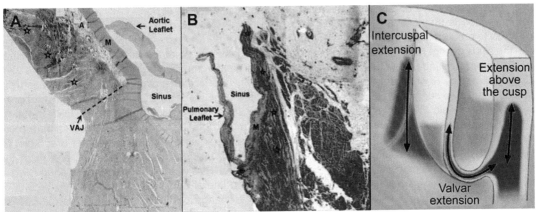

Fig. 3. Histologic specimen stained with Gomori's trichrome demonstrating myocardial extensions above the ventriculo-arterial junctions (VAJ). (*A*) Long axis view of the aortic root showing continuous, epicardial ventricular muscle extensions above the VAJ denoted by stars. (*B*) Long axis view of the pulmonary root demonstrating continuous, adventitial ventricular muscle extension beyond the VAJ of the pulmonic valves denoted by stars. (*C*) Illustration showing sites of myocardial extensions above the cusp, into the valve, and into the inter-cusp triangle. A, adventitia; M, media. (*From* Hasdemir C, Aktas S, Govsa F, et al. Demonstration of ventricular myocardial extensions into the pulmonary artery and aorta beyond the ventriculo-arterial junction. Pacing Clin Electrophysiol 2007;30:534–9; with permission.)

These anatomic relationships are important when mapping and ablating ventricular arrhythmias in the outflow tracts, as shown in the following case.

CASE PRESENTATION

A previously healthy 18-year-old woman presented with symptomatic premature ventricular contractions (PVCs) and nonsustained VT (NSVT). She had a structurally normal heart with normal cardiac function by echocardiography with no evidence of wall motion abnormalities or hypertrophy. Cardiopulmonary exercise testing showed a normal functional capacity with frequent PVCs and VT that was present throughout the exercise test. Serial 24-hour Holter monitors showed a ventricular ectopy burden between 30% and 40%. She was initially treated with atenolol and then changed to high-dose diltiazem with no improvement in her symptoms or ventricular ectopy burden. A prior attempt of catheter ablation at the RVOT was unsuccessful. She was therefore referred for a repeat electrophysiology (EP) study and catheter ablation.

The baseline 12-lead electrocardiogram (ECG) with NSVT is shown in **Fig. 4**. The left bundle branch block (LBBB) morphology with an inferior QRS axis is consistent with an outflow tract origin. The precordial R-wave transition zone is between

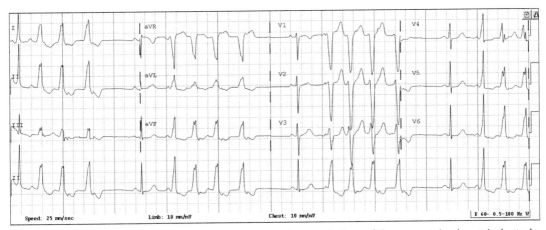

Fig. 4. Baseline 12-lead electrocardiogram demonstrating the morphology of the nonsustained ventricular tachycardia with a left bundle branch block morphology and inferior QRS axis. The R wave transition is relatively late (V3-V4), but similar to that of sinus rhythm.

V3 and V4 for the NSVT and is the same for sinus rhythm, which is suggestive of an RVOT origin. A PVC/VT precordial R-wave transition earlier than the sinus rhythm would favor an LVOT origin.[5] The R/S amplitude index less than 30% in V1 and V2 as well as the R-wave duration index of less than 50% are also suggestive of an RVOT origin.[6] The tall monophasic R wave in lead I, the smaller R-wave amplitude in III compared with II, the R wave in aVL, and the PVC QRS duration/sinus rhythm QRS duration ratio of less than 1.9 are suggestive of a site of origin near the septal RVOT para-Hisian region based on predictive ECG algorithms (**Fig. 5**).[7,8]

At the beginning of the EP study, mapping was first performed in the right ventricle (RV) based on the ECG findings. The earliest activation (far-field signal) during a spontaneous PVC was at the proximal His (His$_p$), which was 35 milliseconds earlier than the surface QRS and earlier than the distal His recordings (**Fig. 6**). The earliest signals in the para-Hisian region were near the tricuspid annulus (with a large atrial electrogram and a small far-field ventricular signal) (**Fig. 7**). Two cryoablation lesions were placed at this site, which did not eliminate the PVCs but resulted in a change in QRS morphology with a longer QRS duration, a more notched appearance of the QRS, a more positive R wave in aVL, and a later precordial R-wave transition (now V4–V5) compared with the original PVC (**Fig. 8**). This finding suggested a more lateral and inferior activation in the RVOT. This change in QRS morphology was likely caused by the altering of the exit of the PVC with the cryoablation. Mapping after the cryoablation showed late activation in the para-Hisian region and no other sites in the RV were early compared with surface QRS.

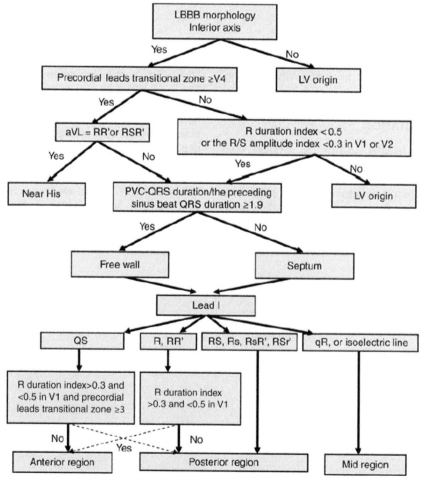

Fig. 5. An algorithm for predicting the location of the ventricular tachycardia within the right ventricle with sensitivity 78.1%, specificity 88.9% and positive predictive value 84.2%. (*From* Zhang F, Chen M, Yang B, et al. Electrocardiographic algorithm to identify the optimal target ablation site for idiopathic right ventricular outflow tract ventricular premature contraction. Europace 2009;11:1214–20; with permission.)

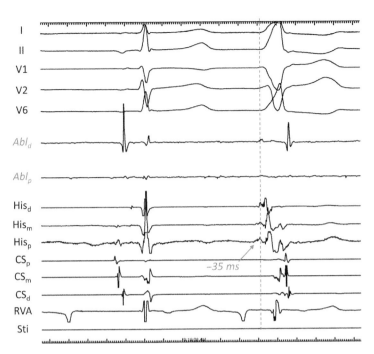

Fig. 6. Baseline intracardiac electrograms showing a far-field signal on the proximal His that is 35 msec ahead of the PVC onset, and is earlier than distal His.

Subsequent mapping of the LVOT was performed with delineation of the aortic cusps by three-dimensional (3D) electroanatomic mapping and Cartosound intracardiac echocardiography (ICE) (Biosense Webster, Diamond Bar, CA). Mapping was performed in the RCC and the LCC but did not show any early activation signals. The earliest intracardiac signal during PVCs was recorded in the NCC, which was 54 milliseconds earlier than QRS (**Fig. 9**). The large atrial electrogram during a sinus beat at this earliest location also confirms the catheter position in the NCC adjacent to the interatrial septum. Radiofrequency ablation using a Thermocool irrigated-tip catheter resulted in immediate termination of ventricular ectopy (**Fig. 10**). There was no further ventricular

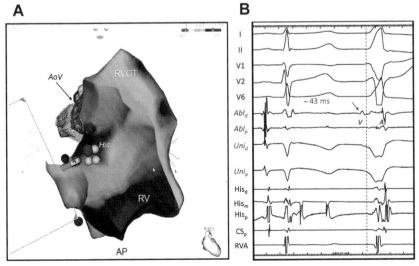

Fig. 7. (*A*) Three-dimensional activation map demonstrating the site of earliest activation (*red*) in a para-Hisian location near the tricuspid valve. The yellow dots represent the "His cloud" and the pink dots represent the sites of earliest activation where two cryoablation lesions were placed. (*B*) Intracardiac electrograms at the site of earliest para-Hisian activation (43 msec earlier than surface QRS) near the tricuspid valve with a large atrial electrogram recording and small, far-field ventricular signals. The unipolar recordings showed a slurred QS pattern.

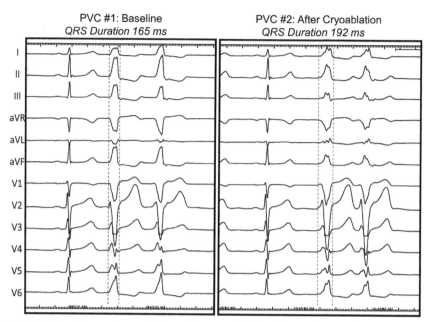

PVC #1: Baseline
QRS Duration 165 ms

PVC #2: After Cryoablation
QRS Duration 192 ms

Fig. 8. Change in QRS duration and morphology after cryoablation lesions. The QRS became wider with a more positive R in lead aVL, and an even later R wave transition between V4-V5. This is suggestive of a more lateral, inferior RV activation.

ectopy seen after ablation and no inducible ventricular ectopy with or without isoproterenol. Selective coronary angiography following ablation confirmed normal coronaries with no evidence of ostial or coronary damage. At 1-year follow-up, the ECG was normal, with no significant ventricular ectopy on Holter monitoring.

UNUSUAL OUTFLOW TRACT VENTRICULAR TACHYCARDIA

The RVOT is the classic site for idiopathic ventricular arrhythmias in patients with structurally normal hearts. However, it is increasingly recognized that PVCs/VT originating from other outflow tract locations can produce similar ECG characteristics of an LBBB QRS morphology and an inferior axis. Numerous ECG algorithms have been developed to distinguish RVOT versus LVOT arrhythmias; however, significant limitations remain.[5,8–17]

The similarity in ECG findings between PVCs/VT originating from the His bundle region of the RVOT versus the aortic cusps is likely related to their close anatomic relationship and rapid transseptal conduction.[6,12,18,19] Yamada and colleagues[20] showed that 20% of arrhythmias with an origin in the aortic cusps showed a late QRS transition after V3, which is suggestive of an RVOT origin. In addition, approximately 25% of the ventricular arrhythmias with an aortic cusp origin had a preferential localized breakout site in the RVOT, which may

also explain the difficulty in using ECG algorithms for accurate localization of VT arising in the aortic cusps. Successful ablation was more accurately guided by targeting the earliest ventricular activation site, whereas pace mapping identified a preferential breakout site. Therefore the utility of pace mapping for PVC/VT ablation in the outflow tracts may be limited.

Most VTs originating in the aortic cusps arise from the LCC, RCC, or the LCC-RCC commissure because of their relationship with the LV myocardium. These cusps are in direct contact with the most superior segment of the LV, with myocardial extensions reaching the interleaflet triangles and the sinotubular junction[3] (see **Fig. 5**). Gami and colleagues[21] found myocardial extensions into the aortic sinuses in 57% of patients, with 55% of those in the RCC and 24% in the LCC.

VT originating in the NCC is extremely rare with successful ablation reported in only a small number of cases.[18,22–24] Yamada and colleagues[24] studied 90 patients with PVCs/VT arising from the aortic root and found that only 6 (7%) were located in the NCC compared with 33 (37%) in the LCC, 32 (36%) in the RCC, and 19 (21%) at the LCC-RCC junction. Patients with PVCs/VT arising from the NCC were young (all <35 years old). The ECG and electrophysiologic findings of NCC arrhythmias were similar to those of RCC but were characterized by a narrower QRS duration (<150 milliseconds), smaller lead III/II R-wave amplitude ratio (<0.65), with an earlier local

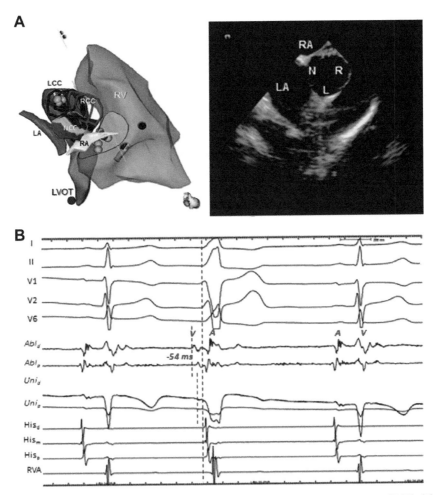

Fig. 9. (A) Activation map demonstrating the earliest signal (*red*) in the non-coronary cusp (NCC). (B) Recordings from the NCC showed a large atrial electrogram and a far-field ventricular signal in sinus rhythm. It registered the earliest intracardiac activation during PVC which was 54 msec earlier than QRS. The unipolar recording shows a QS pattern. Note the relationship of the NCC adjacent to the left (LA) and right atria (RA). L, left coronary cusp; LCC, left coronary cusp; LVOT, left ventricular outflow tract; N, non-coronary cusp; R, right coronary cusp; RCC, right coronary cusp; RV, right ventricle.

activation in the His bundle region (preceded QRS onset by >25 milliseconds) and a larger atrial/ventricular electrogram amplitude ratio (>1) at the successful ablation site.[24]

These ECG characteristics are consistent with the anatomic location of the NCC in the most inferior, posterior, and medial position among the aortic cusps. The most inferior portion of the NCC and RCC are in contact with the membranous portion of the interventricular septum where it comes in close apposition to the penetrating His bundle.[25] Because of this close proximity, early activation can be recorded from a catheter in the para-Hisian position across the tricuspid annulus and likely represents a breakout point into the RV myocardium. Therefore, ablation of the connection from the cusp to the ventricular

myocardium may change the activation pattern and thus the morphology of the QRS complex. Special attention should be paid to changes in VT QRS morphology following attempted ablation in the RV His region because this may be a clue for a focus in the aortic cusps with breakout points in the RV.

Although the proximity of the NCC to the atrial septum has been well appreciated, the relation of this structure to the ventricular myocardium has not been well described.[19,26] The NCC is usually separated from the ventricular myocardium by the membranous septum and the fibrous aortomitral continuity. However, ventricular myocardial extensions into the NCC have been found in up to 4% of autopsied hearts, which is the most likely explanation for the rare cases of PVCs/VT

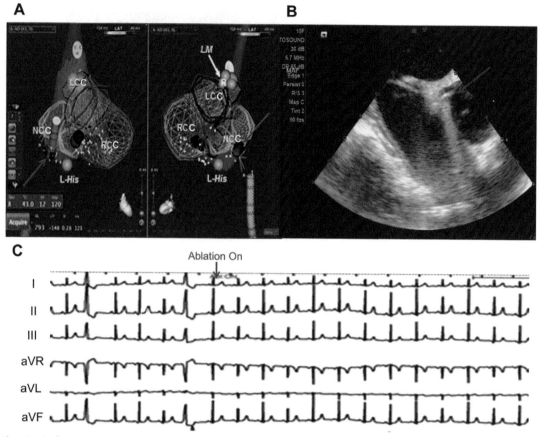

Fig. 10. Catheter position (*red arrows*) at successful ablation site in the non-coronary cusp (NCC) by three-dimensional mapping (*A*) and intracardiac echocardiography (*B*). The catheter position in the NCC is adjacent to the inter-atrial septum. The His Bundle (*yellow dot*) penetrates the membranous septum beneath the NCC-right coronary cusp (RCC) commissure. (*C*) Radiofrequency ablation in the NCC results in immediate termination of ventricular ectopy. LA, left atrium; LM, left main coronary artery; RA, right atrium.

successfully ablated in the NCC.[3,21–24] Ya and colleagues[27] showed that, during embryogenesis in animal hearts, the distal part of the outflow tract loses its myocardial phenotype to form the proximal part of the ascending aorta and pulmonary trunk. Incomplete myocardial regression could explain the presence of myocardial extensions into the aortic sinuses and the pulmonary artery thus providing substrate for ventricular arrhythmias.

During ablation in the aortic root, extra precaution should to be taken to avoid the small but real risk of coronary artery or aortic valve injury. The use of 3D electroanatomic mapping systems combined with ICE imaging is critical for detailed delineation and mapping of the aortic sinuses and commissures. ICE also permits real-time visualization of the aortic root to avoid catheter manipulation and energy delivery near the ostia of the right and left coronary arteries.[28] Selective coronary angiography is also helpful before ablation

in the aortic cusp to show the relationship of the ablation site to the ostia, as well as after ablation to document that there was no coronary or ostial damage following ablation.[29,30]

GENERAL APPROACH TO OUTFLOW TRACT VENTRICULAR ARRHYTHMIAS

Distinguishing PVCs/VT from the RVOT versus the LVOT can be difficult by ECG findings alone, particularly when the origin is above the aortic valve, because of their close anatomic relationships. Therefore, when the ECG shows an LBBB morphology with an inferior axis and an R-wave transition at or later than V3 to V4, mapping first in the RVOT is reasonable. However, when ablation in the RVOT is unsuccessful despite early activation signals, mapping of the LVOT in the aortic cusps should be considered. A thorough understanding of the outflow tract anatomy as well as a systematic and meticulous approach to mapping of the ventricular outflow regions and great vessels increases the success rate and decreases the risk of damage to adjacent structures and the conduction system. The use of multimodality imaging, particularly real-time intracardiac echocardiographic guidance, is essential for defining anatomy, ensuring adequate catheter contact, and minimizing risks.

REFERENCES

1. Samore NA, Imran Majeed SM, Kayani AM, et al. Outcome of radiofrequency catheter ablation as a non-pharmacological therapy for idiopathic ventricular tachycardia. J Coll Physicians Surg Pak 2009; 19:548–52.

2. Lerman BB. Response of nonreentrant catecholamine-mediated ventricular tachycardia to endogenous adenosine and acetylcholine. Evidence for myocardial receptor-mediated effects. Circulation 1993;87:382–90.

3. Hasdemir C, Aktas S, Govsa F, et al. Demonstration of ventricular myocardial extensions into the pulmonary artery and aorta beyond the ventriculo-arterial junction. Pacing Clin Electrophysiol 2007;30:534–9.

4. Sutton JP 3rd, Ho SY, Anderson RH. The forgotten interleaflet triangles: a review of the surgical anatomy of the aortic valve. Ann Thorac Surg 1995;59:419–27.

5. Yoshida N, Inden Y, Uchikawa T, et al. Novel transitional zone index allows more accurate differentiation between idiopathic right ventricular outflow tract and aortic sinus cusp ventricular arrhythmias. Heart Rhythm 2011;8:349–56.

6. Ouyang F, Fotuhi P, Ho SY, et al. Repetitive monomorphic ventricular tachycardia originating from the aortic sinus cusp: electrocardiographic characterization for guiding catheter ablation. J Am Coll Cardiol 2002;39:500–8.

7. Yamauchi Y, Aonuma K, Takahashi A, et al. Electrocardiographic characteristics of repetitive monomorphic right ventricular tachycardia originating near the His-bundle. J Cardiovasc Electrophysiol 2005; 16:1041–8.

8. Zhang F, Chen M, Yang B, et al. Electrocardiographic algorithm to identify the optimal target ablation site for idiopathic right ventricular outflow tract ventricular premature contraction. Europace 2009; 11:1214–20.

9. Callans DJ, Menz V, Schwartzman D, et al. Repetitive monomorphic tachycardia from the left ventricular outflow tract: electrocardiographic patterns consistent with a left ventricular site of origin. J Am Coll Cardiol 1997;29:1023–7.

10. Cheng Z, Cheng K, Deng H, et al. The R-wave deflection interval in lead V3 combining with R-wave amplitude index in lead V1: a new surface ECG algorithm for distinguishing left from right ventricular outflow tract tachycardia origin in patients with transitional lead at V3. Int J Cardiol 2013;168: 1342–8.

11. Hachiya H, Aonuma K, Yamauchi Y, et al. Electrocardiographic characteristics of left ventricular outflow tract tachycardia. Pacing Clin Electrophysiol 2000; 23:1930–4.

12. Ito S, Tada H, Naito S, et al. Development and validation of an ECG algorithm for identifying the optimal ablation site for idiopathic ventricular outflow tract tachycardia. J Cardiovasc Electrophysiol 2003; 14:1280–6.

13. Jadonath RL, Schwartzman DS, Preminger MW, et al. Utility of the 12-lead electrocardiogram in localizing the origin of right ventricular outflow tract tachycardia. Am Heart J 1995;130:1107–13.

14. Kamakura S, Shimizu W, Matsuo K, et al. Localization of optimal ablation site of idiopathic ventricular tachycardia from right and left ventricular outflow tract by body surface ECG. Circulation 1998;98: 1525–33.

15. Kanagaratnam L, Tomassoni G, Schweikert R, et al. Ventricular tachycardias arising from the aortic sinus of Valsalva: an under-recognized variant of left outflow tract ventricular tachycardia. J Am Coll Cardiol 2001;37:1408–14.

16. Krebs ME, Krause PC, Engelstein ED, et al. Ventricular tachycardias mimicking those arising from the right ventricular outflow tract. J Cardiovasc Electrophysiol 2000;11:45–51.

17. Lin D, Ilkhanoff L, Gerstenfeld E, et al. Twelve-lead electrocardiographic characteristics of the aortic cusp region guided by intracardiac echocardiography and electroanatomic mapping. Heart Rhythm 2008;5:663–9.

18. Yamada T, McElderry HT, Doppalapudi H, et al. Catheter ablation of ventricular arrhythmias originating in the vicinity of the His bundle: significance of mapping the aortic sinus cusp. Heart Rhythm 2008;5:37–42.

19. Ouyang F, Ma J, Ho SY, et al. Focal atrial tachycardia originating from the non-coronary aortic sinus: electrophysiological characteristics and catheter ablation. J Am Coll Cardiol 2006;48:122–31.

20. Yamada T, Murakami Y, Yoshida N, et al. Preferential conduction across the ventricular outflow septum in ventricular arrhythmias originating from the aortic sinus cusp. J Am Coll Cardiol 2007;50:884–91.

21. Gami AS, Noheria A, Lachman N, et al. Anatomical correlates relevant to ablation above the semilunar valves for the cardiac electrophysiologist: a study of 603 hearts. J Interv Card Electrophysiol 2011; 30:5–15.

22. Hlivak P, Peichl P, Cihak R, et al. Catheter ablation of idiopathic ventricular tachycardia originating from myocardial extensions into a noncoronary

aortic cusp. J Cardiovasc Electrophysiol 2012;23:98–101.

23. Sayah S, Shahrzad S, Moradi M, et al. Electrocardiographic, electrophysiologic, and anatomical features of ventricular tachycardia originating from noncoronary cusp. J Electrocardiol 2012;45:170–5.

24. Yamada T, Lau YR, Litovsky SH, et al. Prevalence and clinical, electrocardiographic, and electrophysiologic characteristics of ventricular arrhythmias originating from the noncoronary sinus of Valsalva. Heart Rhythm 2013;10:1605–12.

25. Yamada T, Litovsky SH, Kay GN. The left ventricular ostium: an anatomic concept relevant to idiopathic ventricular arrhythmias. Circ Arrhythm Electrophysiol 2008;1:396–404.

26. Beukema RJ, Smit JJ, Adiyaman A, et al. Ablation of focal atrial tachycardia from the non-coronary aortic cusp: case series and review of the literature. Europace 2014;17(6):953–61.

27. Ya J, van den Hoff MJ, de Boer PA, et al. Normal development of the outflow tract in the rat. Circ Res 1998;82:464–72.

28. Hoffmayer KS, Dewland TA, Hsia HH, et al. Safety of radiofrequency catheter ablation without coronary angiography in aortic cusp ventricular arrhythmias. Heart Rhythm 2014;11:1117–21.

29. Kumagai K. Idiopathic ventricular arrhythmias arising from the left ventricular outflow tract: tips and tricks. J Arrhythm 2014;30:211–21.

30. Hachiya H, Aonuma K, Yamauchi Y, et al. How to diagnose, locate, and ablate coronary cusp ventricular tachycardia. J Cardiovasc Electrophysiol 2002;13:551–6.

Ventricular Arrhythmias from the Left Ventricular Summit
Critical Importance of Anatomy, Imaging, and Detailed Mapping to Allow Safe and Effective Ablation

 CrossMark

Saurabh Kumar, BSc(Med), MBBS, PhD, Usha B. Tedrow, MD,
William G. Stevenson, MD*

KEYWORDS

- Ventricular arrhythmias • Left ventricular summit • Ablation • Imaging • Mapping
- Percutaneous catheter ablation

KEY POINTS

- These two cases illustrate important technical challenges posed by ventricular arrhythmias originating from structures surrounding the left ventricular summit.
- The electrocardiogram with various electrocardiographic indices may give clues to the likely site of origin, but significant limitations exist.
- Systematic and comprehensive mapping of the septal right ventricular outflow tract, coronary venous system, and aortic sinuses is critical.
- Detailed understanding and imaging of the anatomy of this region, including the location of coronaries, are important.
- Activation mapping may reveal a site of origin within close proximity to the coronaries or the phrenic nerve.

INTRODUCTION

Ventricular arrhythmias (VA) arising from the region of the left ventricular (LV) summit can be challenging for catheter-based percutaneous ablation. A detailed knowledge of the anatomy of this region and the need of high-density mapping of surrounding structures are critical in ensuring safe and effective ablation. This case-based review focuses on the particular challenges with ablation in this region.

CASE 1

A 55-year-old man with a history of hypertension was referred for catheter ablation of highly symptomatic premature ventricular contractions (PVCs; burden 19% over 24 hours, **Fig. 1**) refractory to metoprolol, amiodarone, and dofetilide associated with progressive decline in LV function over 4 years. Ablation of the septal right ventricular outflow tract (RVOT) 2 years before referral failed. Echocardiography showed an LV ejection fraction

Arrhythmia Service, Cardiovascular Division, Brigham and Women's Hospital, 75 Francis Street, Boston, MA 02115, USA
* Corresponding author.
E-mail address: wstevenson@partners.org

cardiacEP.theclinics.com

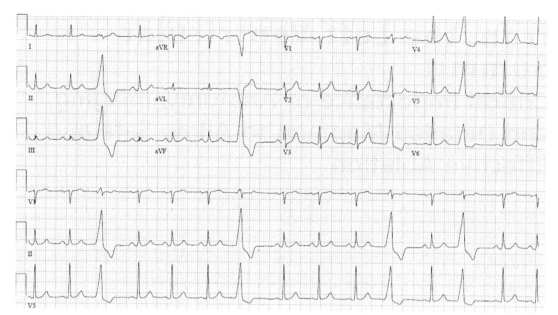

Fig. 1. PVC of patient 1.

of 35% to 40% with an LV end diastolic diameter of 60 mm.

Other than spontaneous PVCs, the baseline electrocardiogram (EKG) was normal (see **Fig. 1**). The PVC coupling interval varied from 585 milliseconds to 652 milliseconds (Δ coupling interval: maximum–minimum coupling interval = 67 milliseconds; **Fig. 2**). PVCs were right bundle (RB) lead V1 with a frontal plane axis of +100°, QRS duration of 135 milliseconds and monomorphic R waves throughout the precordium, absence of S waves in leads V5/V6 with an initial r wave in I (**Fig. 3**). The maximum deflection index (MDI) was 0.58; the R-wave amplitude ratio of leads III/II was 0.94; the QS wave ratio of aVL/ aVR was 0.89; and the peak deflection index (PDI) in the inferior leads (latest peak in the inferior leads/total QRS duration) was 0.7, respectively (see **Fig. 3**). These findings also suggested origin in the LV summit/outflow region, possibly from an epicardial site given the long MDI (discussed later).

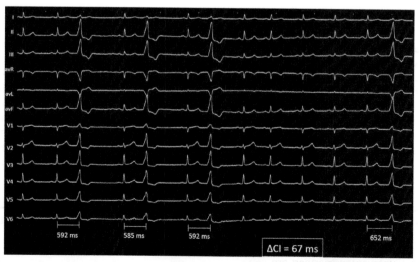

Fig. 2. Varying coupling intervals of PVC; Δ-coupling interval (CI) (maximum–minimum coupling interval) was greater than 60 milliseconds.

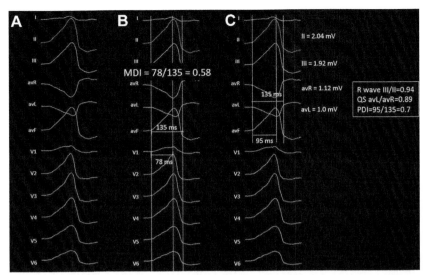

Fig. 3. (A) PVC and (B, C) calculations of maximum deflection index (MDI) and peak deflection index (PDI) calculated as the latest peak in the inferior leads/total QRS duration as described in the text.

The authors follow a systematic approach to the mapping and ablation of these arrhythmias. To avoid PVC suppression, mapping is performed initially with local anesthesia with minimal sedation. Multipolar electrode catheters were positioned in the RV apex and the His bundle region. Intracardiac echo (ICE) is used for the creation of an anatomic shell of the LV and right ventricles and the outflow tracts with particular attention to defining cusp anatomy and origin of the left and right coronary ostia. Mapping and ablation is performed using a 3.5-mm tip irrigated catheter (ThermoCool SF; Biosense Webster, Diamond Bar, California) facilitated by an electroanatomic mapping system (CARTO 3; Biosense Webster). Bipolar electrograms (EGMs) are high-pass filtered at 30 to 500 Hz; unipolar EGM from the distal electrode was filtered at 0.05 to 500 Hz and digitally recorded along with a 12-lead surface ECG (Cardiolab EP system; General Electric Healthcare, Buckinghamshire, United Kingdom). Pace mapping was performed, when necessary, using unipolar stimuli at 10 mA and a pulse width of 2 milliseconds.

In this case, the ablation catheter was first inserted out to the great cardiac vein (GCV); activation mapping at this site revealed a multicomponent ventricular signal of 27 milliseconds pre-QRS. A venogram created by injecting contrast through the open irrigation catheter showed that this site was at the origin of the anterior interventricular vein (AIV) (**Fig. 4**). Pace mapping at this site produced an excellent QRS morphology match to the PVCs (96% using the PaSo algorithm, CARTO-3, Biosense Webster;

see **Fig. 4**), but the R-wave amplitude in the inferior leads was lower with pacing compared with the spontaneous PVC (see **Fig. 4**). The authors next assess proximity of the site to the coronary arteries either with angiography or ICE. In this case, ICE imaging showed that this site was within 10 mm of the left main coronary artery (see **Fig. 4**) and within 5 mm at some points in the cardiac cycle. The authors then mapped adjacent anatomic sites. Mapping of the septal RVOT, pulmonary artery, left coronary cusp (LCC), right coronary cusp (RCC), and LCC-RCC junction showed late activation without discrete early potentials (see **Fig. 4**). The aortic-mitral continuity (AMC) directly opposite the GCV site showed a rounded, far field signal that was 21 milliseconds pre-QRS, 6 milliseconds later than in the GCV. Pace mapping showed a moderate pace-map match (88% by PaSo software, Biosense Webster, **Fig. 5**). The AMC site was greater than 10 mm away from the left main coronary by ICE imaging, and the distance between the endocardial AMC site and the GCV site was 9 mm.

Given the proximity of the arrhythmia origin in the GCV to the left main coronary artery, empirical ablation was performed in the endocardial AMC region directly opposite to the site of earliest activation in the GCV (see **Fig. 5**). Power was set to 30 W with a maximum temperature of 45°C, aiming for a minimum of 10 Ω impedance drop; power was increased in 5-W increments up to 50 W if impedance did not decrease less than 5 Ω in the first 10 seconds. With ablation via the retrograde aortic approach, there was transient PVC suppression; however, impedance decreases were less

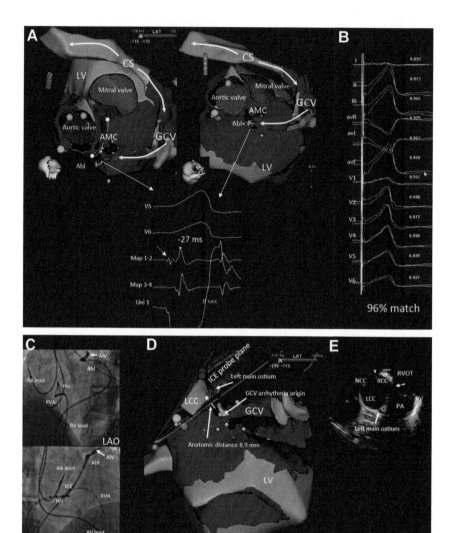

Fig. 4. (*A*) Superior and anterior view of the LV, coronary sinus (CS), GCV, and aortic-mitral continuity (AMC). Note the intimate anatomic proximity of these structures. The site of earliest activation was in the distal GCV, which was 27 milliseconds pre-QRS with a ventricular prepotential (*dotted arrow*) on the distal ablation electrode (Map 1-2) and QS signals on the unipolar distal electrode (Uni 1). Pace map (*B*) was excellent showing a 96% match. The R-wave amplitude in the inferior leads during spontaneous PVCs (*green* QRS complexes, amplitude in leads II, III, avF of 2.04, 1.92, and 2.2 mV, respectively) was greater than the paced R waves (*yellow* QRS complexes; amplitude in leads II, III, avF of 1.9, 1.6, 1.6 mV, respectively), suggesting the site of origin may have been even higher in the LV summit in the inaccessible area. (*C*) Fluoroscopic left anterior oblique (LAO) and right anterior oblique (RAO) projections of the ablation catheter (Abl) at the site of earliest activation in the GCV. Hand contrast injection was performed showing that site of origin was the AIV (*arrow*). (*D*) ICE superimposed on the electroanatomic map was used to identify the origin and course of the left main coronary, which was located within 10 mm of the arrhythmia origin. (*E*) ICE loop showing the intimate anatomic relationship of the left coronary cusp (LCC) to the anteroseptal RVOT and the left-right coronary cusp (RCC) junction and RCC to the posteroseptal RVOT (*dotted arrow*); (*F–H*) activation mapping in the posteroseptal RVOT, RCC, and LCC showed late activation. LM, left main coronary artery; NCC, noncoronary cusp; PA, pulmonary artery; RV, right ventricle.

than 10 Ω, suggesting insufficient contact. A transseptal approach to the AMC area was then undertaken, which resulted in satisfactory impedance decreases during ablation. A total of 11, long-duration RF applications (60–90 seconds each) were given; PVC suppression was ultimately observed after 4 to 5 applications. During a 30-minute waiting period, rare isolated single PVCs were seen. Unfortunately, PVCs recurred in follow-up.

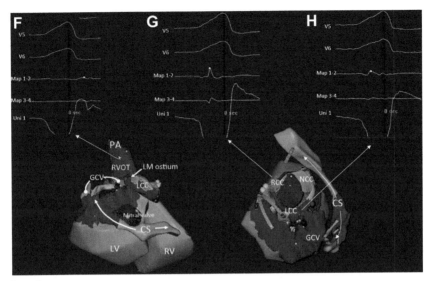

Fig. 4. (*continued*)

CASE 2

A 60-year-old man with hypertension and obstructive sleep apnea was referred for ablation of symptomatic frequent PVCs (burden 22% over 24 hours) associated with an LV ejection fraction of 40%. Metoprolol had failed to suppress PVCs.

At a prior ablation attempt, earliest activation was identified in the GCV adjacent to the left anterior descending (LAD) coronary artery; hence, no ablation was performed.

Spontaneous PVCs in electrophysiology laboratory showed a PVC Δ coupling interval of

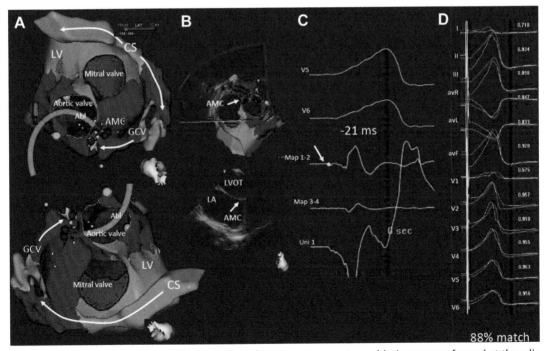

Fig. 5. Given the proximity of the GCV site to the left main coronary artery, ablation was performed at the adjacent LV endocardial site in the aortic-mitral continuity (AMC) (*red dots, A*). ICE loop through the AMC (*arrow, B*). At this site, activation was 6 milliseconds later but pre-QRS with a far field rounded signal (*C, arrow*). Pace map was not perfect (*D*). Abl, ablation catheter; CS, coronary sinus; LA, left atrium; LVOT, LV outflow tract.

75 milliseconds with an RB morphology in V1 with a frontal plane axis of +110°, QRS duration of 161 milliseconds, and monophasic R waves throughout the precordium, absence of S waves in leads V5/V6 and rs configuration in lead I (**Fig. 6**A). The MDI was 0.55; the R-wave amplitude ratio of leads III/II was 0.97; the QS wave ratio of aVL/aVR was 1; PDI in the inferior leads was 0.7, respectively. These findings also suggested origin in the LV summit/outflow region, possibly from an epicardial site given the long MDI (discussed later).

Activation mapping showed late activation of the septal RVOT with less than 10/12 pace-map match (54% match by PaSo). The GCV activation was 30 milliseconds pre-QRS with a good pace-map match (89% match by PaSo; see **Fig. 6**B, C); however, coronary angiography showed a distance of less than 5 mm from the LAD. Retrograde aortic mapping of the aortic cusps showed an even earlier presystolic signal that was 56 milliseconds pre-QRS at the LCC-RCC cusp junction with a near perfect pace-map match (95% by PaSo; see **Fig. 6**D, E). This site was 11 mm away from the earliest GCV site and 15 mm from the left main coronary ostium (see **Fig. 6**F). RF was applied at 25 to 30 W aiming for a minimum 10-Ω impedance drop this site, which promptly terminated the PVCs; additional lesions were applied immediately adjacent to this site in the cusp and just below the valve (see **Fig. 6**G). An LV voltage map showed no evidence of endocardial low-voltage scar. Programmed ventricular stimulation failed to induce sustained ventricular tachycardia. During follow-up, he has remained free of arrhythmia.

DISCUSSION

The LV summit is a triangular region of the epicardial LV outflow tract bounded by the bifurcation of the LAD and the left circumflex coronary arteries and transected laterally by the GCV at its junction with the AIV (**Fig. 7**A).[1] Approximately 12% of VAs from the LV are estimated to occur from the LV summit.[1]

The LV summit is in close proximity to outflow tracts structures, such as LCC, RCC, LCC-RCC junction, the septal RVOT, and the AMC, GCV, AIV or the perivascular epicardium, all of which can give rise to VAs (**Fig. 7**B).[1–7] Because of the anatomic contiguity of these structures, although recordings from one particular site (eg, the GCV/AIV) may be early, it may represent activation from an adjacent source.[8] This point is particularly relevant to the authors' second case when early activation was seen in the GCV; however, an even earlier signal was seen at the LCC-RCC

junction, which was ultimately the site of successful ablation.

Activation time rather than pace mapping is more reliable for identifying ablation targets in outflow tract arrhythmias, particularly in the LV outflow tract and aortic cusp. Pace mapping is less reliable due to preferential paths for conduction between the aortic root origin and breakout site, which may be in the RVOT, or to adjacent endocardial sites, such as the AMC or the epicardial surface.[9] However, in the authors' patients it did agree reasonably with the best target site identified by activation mapping.

Success of catheter ablation of VA originating from within the coronary venous system ranges from 27% to 74%.[3–5,10] Unsuccessful ablation within the GCV is attributed to the inability to advance the catheter to the site of interest because of a small caliber vessel, inadequate power delivery secondary to high impedance in the vessel, close proximity to coronary arteries, or the left phrenic nerve, which precludes ablation.[1,3–5,7,11] In the authors' experience, the earliest site in the GCV is within 5 mm of a coronary artery in three-quarters of patients.[5] In general, catheter ablation is not recommended within 5 to 10 mm of a coronary artery because of the risk of vessel occlusion.[8,10,12,13] Hence, angiography is recommended to identify the origin and course of these coronaries before considering catheter ablation. The authors' experience is that low-power RF has not been successful in the elimination of GCV arrhythmias as at least some are likely intramural between the GCV and contiguous LV outflow tract structures. The authors, thus, avoid RF if the earliest site was within 5 mm of a coronary artery at any point in the cardiac cycle. Proximity to a coronary ostia or artery is also a concern for ablation in the aortic root. Some operators advocate intermittent hand coronary injection during catheter ablation of the VAs within the aortic sinuses to avoid and/or rapidly identify inadvertent catheter dislodgement and vessel injury.[14,15] Recently, ICE and electroanatomic mapping without the need for coronary angiography has been shown to be a reasonable substitute.[16] In both of the cases, the authors were able to satisfactorily locate the coronary ostia using ICE. During GCV ablation, the authors' preference is to perform coronary angiography with the catheter positioned at the site of origin in order to calculate the shortest distance between site of origin and the coronary arteries in multiple views. In the first case, however, ICE imaging reliably showed that the GCV site was intimately related to the left main coronary artery; hence, angiography was not performed. During ablation of the aortic

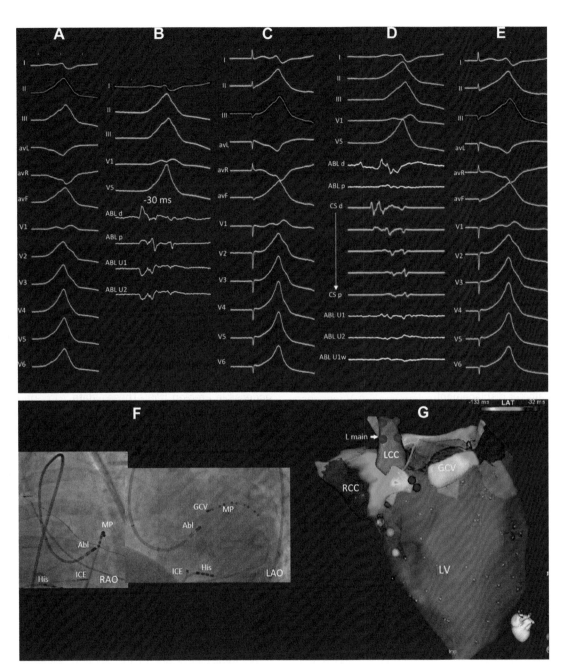

Fig. 6. (A) Spontaneous PVC of case 2; (B) activation was 30 milliseconds pre-QRS in the GCV with a near perfect pace match (C); however, this site was within 5 mm of the left anterior descending coronary artery. Activation mapping in the LCC-RCC junction (D) was even earlier, occurring 56 milliseconds pre-QRS with a perfect pace match (E). Note that the distal coronary sinus (CS) represents position of a multipolar catheter at the site of earliest activation in the distal GCV. (F) Fluoroscopic views of the ablation catheter (Abl) in the RAO and the LAO view. The catheter is at the LCC-RCC junction and the distal tip of the multipolar (MP) catheter is placed at the site of earliest activation in the distal GCV. (G) Site of ablation in the LCC-RCC junction and below the valve (*red dots*) where activation was earliest. This site was adjacent to the earliest activation in the GCV. ABL d, bipolar distal ablation signal; ABL p, bipolar proximal ablation signal; ABL U1, unipolar distal signal; ABL U1w, high pass unipolar filtered signal; ABL U2, unipolar proximal signal; LAO, left anterior oblique; RAO, right anterior oblique.

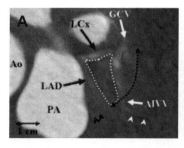
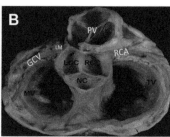

Fig. 7. (*A*) LV summit: defined based on fluoroscopy and coronary angiography as the region on the epicardial surface of the LV left main coronary artery (LM) bifurcation. The region is bounded by an arc (*black dotted line*) from the LAD superior to the first septal perforator (*black arrowheads*) to the region and anterior to the left circumflex (LCx) laterally. The GCV is said to bisect the LV summit into a superior inaccessible region and an inferolateral accessible region during epicardial ablation. White arrowheads indicate the first diagonal branch of the LAD. (*B*) Anatomy of the outflow regions and the atrioventricular valves, in a region often termed the LV ostium (defined as an elliptical opening at the base of the LV where the aortic and mitral valves (MVs) are direct apposition and attach). AIVV, anterior interventricular vein; Ao, aorta; NC, noncoronary cusp; PA, pulmonary artery; PV, pulmonary valve; RCA, right coronary artery; TV, tricuspid valve. (*Adapted from* [*A*] Yamada T, Litovsky SH, Kay GN. The left ventricular ostium: an anatomic concept relevant to idiopathic ventricular arrhythmias. Circ Arrhythm Electrophysiol 2008;1(5):398; with permission; and *From* [*B*] Tabatabaei N, Asirvatham SJ. Supravalvular arrhythmia: identifying and ablating the substrate. Circ Arrhythm Electrophysiol 2009;2(3):317; with permission.)

sinuses, the authors use ICE to identify coronary ostia and pay careful attention to catheter movement during ablation using fluoroscopy and the electroanatomic mapping to avoid inadvertent catheter displacement.

When one of the aforementioned factors prevents ablation in the coronary venous system, ablation can sometimes be successful from adjacent, directly opposed structures, including the LCC, LCC-RCC, LV endocardium in the AMC, and the most leftward aspect of the RVOT. Some of these sites may have a later local activation time or a poorer pace map than sites with the earliest activation. Caution must be exercised as can be in proximity to the left coronary artery, and there is also a risk of perforation if a steam pop occurs with ablation in this area.[5,8] When targeting the aortic sinuses, ablation is directed at the myocardial fibers that extend for a variable distance above the cusps.[10,17] The first case highlights this point whereby ablation at the AMC was performed to target the PVCs originating from the GCV. The second case shows that comprehensive mapping of surrounding structures is critical. Although a very early site was found in the GCV, activation mapping in the LCC-RCC junction revealed an even earlier site of activation where ablation was successful.

If attempts at ablation in the GCV or adjacent anatomic sites fail, ablation from the epicardium may abolish these arrhythmia with some important caveats. Yamada and colleagues considered the area lateral to the GCV accessible to epicardial catheter ablation; in contrast, the region superior to the GCV is deemed inaccessible because of its close proximity to the coronary arteries and the thick layer of epicardial fat that overlies the proximal portion of these vessels (see **Fig. 7**).[1] However, success rates of ablation from the epicardium are low (15%–44%) even from the accessible region.[1,5,7] These data, in part, tempered the authors' enthusiasm for epicardial mapping in the first case presented. In severely symptomatic cases that fail catheter ablation, a surgical cryoablation can be performed after dissection through the overlying fat and/or displacement of overlying coronary vessels.[5,18]

Electrocardiographic Considerations

Several signature EKG patterns, such as the qR characteristic of AMC origin,[19] the multiphasic M or W-type qrs pattern characteristic of LCC,[19,20] or a QS with notching on the downward deflection of V1 typical of origin from the LCC-RCC commissure,[21] were absent in the authors' case. VAs from the GCV generally have an RB branch block (RBBB) pattern; however, as the GCV-AIV junction is anatomically closer to the septum, either an RBBB or left bundle branch block pattern can be seen.[1] An important consideration for LV summit VAs is the MDI.[4] An MDI of 0.55 or greater may indicate that ablation from the epicardium was likely to be required.[4] In both of the authors' cases, MDI was 0.55 or greater; and one arrhythmia was transiently suppressed with ablation from the endocardium and the other successfully ablated from within an aortic sinus. Thus, the MDI is an initial guide; but mapping may identify nonepicardial ablation sites for ablation.[22] Finally, a useful observation by Bradfield and colleagues[23] was consistently observed in both of the authors' cases; these investigators found that the coupling interval variability of greater than 60 milliseconds differentiated PVCs from aortic sinuses of Valsalva and GCV from other ventricular foci. This finding was seen in both of the authors' cases.[23] This observation provides a putative mechanistic insight into PVCs from these regions whereby a lack of electronic interactions between poorly coupled myocytes may explain the random coupling intervals.

Predictors of Success

Several criteria have been associated with successful ablation. In the authors' experience, success rates depend highly on individual anatomy; each criterion has its limitations. Moreover, ablation can be successful despite demonstrating EKG findings known to be associated with failure in up to 41% of patients.[15] An appreciation of various criteria is, nevertheless, useful as it may facilitate planning of the procedure, especially the need for epicardial access, or the likelihood of success of ablation from endocardial sites:

1. An anatomic distance of less than 13.5 mm between the GCV/AIV and the left sinus of Valsalva or adjacent LV endocardium and a Q-wave ratio in avL/avR of less than 1.45 may identify GCV VAs that may be successfully ablated from the left sinus of Valsalva or adjacent LV endocardium.[8] Both criteria were observed in the authors' second case, with successful ablation from the LCC-RCC junction. In contrast, the first case also exhibited these criteria; however, ablation was unsuccessful.

2. An initial r wave in lead I and a difference in activation time between a non-GCV and a GCV site of 10 milliseconds or less[5,24] may identify successful ablation of GCV VA from an adjacent non-GCV site. In both of the authors' cases, an initial r wave was noted in lead I. The first case had a GCV–non-GCV interval of 6 milliseconds, but ablation was unsuccessful in follow-up.

3. Yamada and colleagues[10] found that an RBBB pattern, transition zone earlier than V1, avL/avR amplitude ratio greater than 1.1, and S waves in V5/V6 are likely to be successfully ablated from within the GCV, AIV, or the epicardial accessible area. A lead III/II amplitude ratio of greater than 1.25 and an aVL/aVR amplitude ratio of greater than 1.75 identified VA originates from the epicardial accessible area. When R-wave amplitude in the inferior leads is higher during spontaneous PVC compared with pacing in the GCV or AIV, the origin is likely in the inaccessible area and attempts at epicardial ablation are unlikely to be successful. In the authors' first case, the avL/avR and III/II amplitude ratio was lower than these cutoffs[10] and there was absence of S waves in V5/V6; furthermore, the paced R-wave amplitude was indeed lower than the spontaneous PVC R-wave amplitude. These findings suggest a PVC origin in the inaccessible area such that GCV or epicardial ablation was not likely to be successful.

4. Hachiya and colleagues[25] demonstrated that the latest peak in the inferior leads/total QRS duration (PDI) of greater than 0.6 identified ablation failure of outflow tract PVCs. Both of the authors' cases had a PDI greater than 0.6; however, one patient had successful ablation.

SUMMARY

These two cases illustrate important technical challenges posed by VA originating from structures surrounding the LV summit. The EKG with various electrocardiographic indices may give clues to the likely site of origin, but significant limitations exist. Systematic and comprehensive mapping of the septal RVOT, coronary venous system, and aortic sinuses is critical. Detailed understanding and imaging of the anatomy of this region, including the location of coronaries, is important. Activation mapping may reveal a site of origin within close proximity to the coronaries or the phrenic nerve. Ablation may target adjacently located aortic sinus or LV endocardial sites with variable success. EKG markers have limited ability to predict the site and outcome of ablation.

REFERENCES

1. Yamada T, McElderry HT, Doppalapudi H, et al. Idiopathic ventricular arrhythmias originating from the left ventricular summit: anatomic concepts relevant to ablation. Circ Arrhythm Electrophysiol 2010;3(6):616–23.

2. Tabatabaei N, Asirvatham SJ. Supravalvular arrhythmia: identifying and ablating the substrate. Circ Arrhythm Electrophysiol 2009;2(3):316–26.

3. Baman TS, Ilg KJ, Gupta SK, et al. Mapping and ablation of epicardial idiopathic ventricular arrhythmias from within the coronary venous system. Circ Arrhythm Electrophysiol 2010;3(3):274–9.

4. Daniels DV, Lu YY, Morton JB, et al. Idiopathic epicardial left ventricular tachycardia originating remote from the sinus of Valsalva: electrophysiological characteristics, catheter ablation, and identification from the 12-lead electrocardiogram. Circulation 2006;113(13):1659–66.

5. Nagashima K, Choi EK, Lin KY, et al. Ventricular arrhythmias near the distal great cardiac vein: challenging arrhythmia for ablation. Circ Arrhythm Electrophysiol 2014;7(5):906–12.

6. Obel OA, d'Avila A, Neuzil P, et al. Ablation of left ventricular epicardial outflow tract tachycardia from the distal great cardiac vein. J Am Coll Cardiol 2006;48(9):1813–7.

7. Santangeli P, Marchlinski FE, Zado ES, et al. Percutaneous epicardial ablation of ventricular arrhythmias arising from the left ventricular summit: outcomes and electrocardiogram correlates of success. Circ Arrhythm Electrophysiol 2015;8:337–43.

8. Jauregui Abularach ME, Campos B, Park KM, et al. Ablation of ventricular arrhythmias arising near the anterior epicardial veins from the left sinus of Valsalva region: ECG features, anatomic distance, and outcome. Heart Rhythm 2012;9(6):865–73.

9. Yamada T, Murakami Y, Yoshida N, et al. Preferential conduction across the ventricular outflow septum in ventricular arrhythmias originating from the aortic sinus cusp. J Am Coll Cardiol 2007;50(9):884–91.

10. Yamada T, Litovsky SH, Kay GN. The left ventricular ostium: an anatomic concept relevant to idiopathic ventricular arrhythmias. Circ Arrhythm Electrophysiol 2008;1(5):396–404.

11. Yamada T, Maddox WR, McElderry HT, et al. Radiofrequency catheter ablation of idiopathic ventricular arrhythmias originating from intramural foci in the left ventricular outflow tract; efficacy of sequential versus simultaneous unipolar catheter ablation. Circ Arrhythm Electrophysiol 2015;8(2):344–52.

12. Stavrakis S, Jackman WM, Nakagawa H, et al. Risk of coronary artery injury with radiofrequency ablation and cryoablation of epicardial posteroseptal accessory pathways within the coronary venous system. Circ Arrhythm Electrophysiol 2014;7(1):113–9.

13. Roberts-Thomson KC, Steven D, Seiler J, et al. Coronary artery injury due to catheter ablation in adults: presentations and outcomes. Circulation 2009; 120(15):1465–73.

14. Ouyang F, Fotuhi P, Ho SY, et al. Repetitive monomorphic ventricular tachycardia originating from the aortic sinus cusp: electrocardiographic characterization for guiding catheter ablation. J Am Coll Cardiol 2002;39(3):500–8.

15. Ouyang F, Mathew S, Wu S, et al. Ventricular arrhythmias arising from the left ventricular outflow tract below the aortic sinus cusps: mapping and catheter ablation via transseptal approach and electrocardiographic characteristics. Circ Arrhythm Electrophysiol 2014;7(3):445–55.

16. Hoffmayer KS, Dewland TA, Hsia HH, et al. Safety of radiofrequency catheter ablation without coronary angiography in aortic cusp ventricular arrhythmias. Heart Rhythm 2014;11(7):1117–21.

17. Gami AS, Noheria A, Lachman N, et al. Anatomical correlates relevant to ablation above the semilunar valves for the cardiac electrophysiologist: a study of 603 hearts. J Interv Card Electrophysiol 2011; 30(1):5–15.

18. Choi EK, Nagashima K, Lin KY, et al. Surgical cryoablation for ventricular tachyarrhythmia arising from the left ventricular outflow tract region. Heart Rhythm 2015;12(6):1128–36.

19. Lin D, Ilkhanoff L, Gerstenfeld E, et al. Twelve-lead electrocardiographic characteristics of the aortic cusp region guided by intracardiac echocardiography and electroanatomic mapping. Heart Rhythm 2008;5(5):663–9.

20. Yamada T, Yoshida N, Murakami Y, et al. Electrocardiographic characteristics of ventricular arrhythmias originating from the junction of the left and right coronary sinuses of Valsalva in the aorta: the activation pattern as a rationale for the electrocardiographic characteristics. Heart Rhythm 2008;5(2):184–92.

21. Bala R, Garcia FC, Hutchinson MD, et al. Electrocardiographic and electrophysiologic features of ventricular arrhythmias originating from the right/left coronary cusp commissure. Heart Rhythm 2010; 7(3):312–22.

22. Yokokawa M, Latchamsetty R, Good E, et al. Ablation of epicardial ventricular arrhythmias from nonepicardial sites. Heart Rhythm 2011;8(10):1525–9.

23. Bradfield JS, Homsi M, Shivkumar K, et al. Coupling interval variability differentiates ventricular ectopic complexes arising in the aortic sinus of Valsalva and great cardiac vein from other sources: mechanistic and arrhythmic risk implications. J Am Coll Cardiol 2014;63(20):2151–8.

24. Ito S, Tada H, Naito S, et al. Simultaneous mapping in the left sinus of Valsalva and coronary venous system predicts successful catheter ablation from the left sinus of Valsalva. Pacing Clin Electrophysiol 2005;28(Suppl 1):S150–4.

25. Hachiya H, Hirao K, Sasaki T, et al. Novel ECG predictor of difficult cases of outflow tract ventricular tachycardia: peak deflection index on an inferior lead. Circ J 2010;74(2):256–61.

Catheter Ablation of Ventricular Arrhythmias Arising from the Left Ventricular Summit

Pasquale Santangeli, MD*, David Lin, MD,
Francis E. Marchlinski, MD

KEYWORDS

• Catheter ablation • Ventricular arrhythmias • Left ventricular summit

KEY POINTS

• The left ventricular summit is a common site of origin of idiopathic ventricular arrhythmias.
• These arrhythmias are most commonly ablated within the coronary venous system or from other adjacent structures such as the right ventricular and left ventricular outflow tract or coronary cusp region.
• When ablation from adjacent structures fails, a percutaneous epicardial approach can be considered, but is rarely successful in eliminating the arrhythmias due to proximity to major coronary vessels and/or epicardial fat.

INTRODUCTION

The left ventricular summit (LVS) is the most superior aspect of the epicardial left ventricular outflow tract (LVOT) and represents a site of origin of idiopathic ventricular arrhythmias (VAs).[1] The LVS is a complex anatomic structure bounded by the bifurcation between the left anterior descending (LAD) and the left circumflex coronary (LCx) arteries, and transected laterally by the great cardiac vein (GCV) at its junction with the anterior interventricular vein (AIV).[2] Given the proximity to major epicardial coronary vessels and the presence of epicardial fat, catheter ablation of VAs originating from the LVS is particularly challenging. In most cases, effective ablation can be achieved from anatomically adjacent sites, such as the coronary venous system, the coronary cusp region, and/or the endocardial left ventricular (LV) or right ventricular (RV) outflow tracts.[3–5] When ablation from adjacent sites is unsuccessful, an epicardial approach may be considered, although typically with limited success.[6] In this article, a case of catheter ablation of a symptomatic frequent ventricular premature depolarizations (VPDs) arising from the LVS is reported, and the authors' approach to target these arrhythmias is discussed.

THE CASE

A 48-year-old woman with a 2-year history of frequent symptomatic monomorphic VPDs in the setting of a structurally normal heart was referred to the authors' institution for catheter ablation. Her most recent assessment of arrhythmia burden at a 48-hour electrocardiogram (ECG) Holter monitor showed a total VPD burden of 28%, despite treatment with metoprolol. The 12-lead ECG of the VPD (**Fig. 1**) demonstrates a right bundle branch block (RBBB) morphology, with an R/S wave ratio in lead V1 greater than 2.5, and a

Cardiovascular Division, Hospital of the University of Pennsylvania, 3400 Spruce Street, Philadelphia, PA 19104, USA
* Corresponding author. 9 Founders Pavilion – Cardiology, Hospital of the University of Pennsylvania, 3400 Spruce Street, Philadelphia, PA, 19104.
E-mail address: pasquale.santangeli@uphs.upenn.edu

Card Electrophysiol Clin 8 (2016) 99–107
http://dx.doi.org/10.1016/j.ccep.2015.10.011
1877-9182/16/$ – see front matter © 2016 Elsevier Inc. All rights reserved.

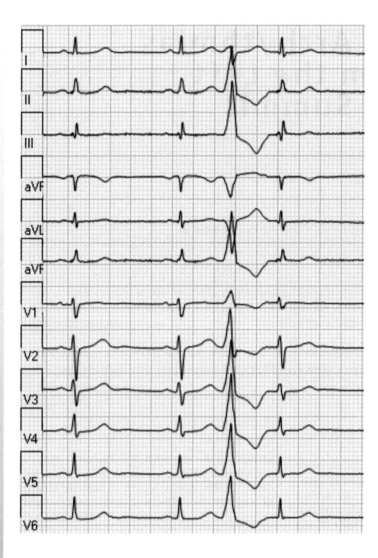

Fig. 1. Twelve-lead ECG of the frequent VPD.

very early precordial transition. Analysis of the augmented limb leads (aVL and aVR) and of the bipolar lead I indicates an origin leftward of the midline (Q wave in aVL significantly greater than Q wave in aVR, and predominantly negative deflection in lead I). In addition, the inferior leads show positive R waves, with a rightward axis (R wave in lead III greater than R wave in lead II). These features all point toward an origin from the LVS (see later discussion).[1,6] Using the CARTO Univu module (Biosense Webster, Diamond Bar, CA, USA), an open-irrigated ablation catheter was advanced to the ostium of the AIV with minimal use of fluoroscopy (**Fig. 2**A, B). Correct positioning at the AIV ostium was confirmed by injection of contrast from the ablation catheter (**Fig. 2**C, D). The local activation time in the AIV was 24 ms pre-QRS; pace mapping also revealed a near-perfect 12/12 ECG lead match (**Fig. 3**).

Coronary angiography was performed demonstrating a safe (>5 mm) distance from the major coronary vessels (**Fig. 4**). Radiofrequency energy could be delivered with a power up to 15 W for 20 seconds because of impedance increase and was initially successful in suppressing the VPD. During the waiting period and under infusion of 3 μg/min of isoproterenol, the VPD recurred. The ablation catheter was then maneuvered to the LV endocardium via a retrograde transaortic approach and positioned to a site just opposite to the earliest activation site recorded in the AIV region. The anatomic distance between the site of earliest activation in the AIV and the LV endocardium was 8 mm. Radiofrequency application (40 W) resulted in suppression of the VPD after 20 seconds (**Fig. 5**). The duration of radiofrequency application was extended to 2 minutes. No further VPD could be induced after a more

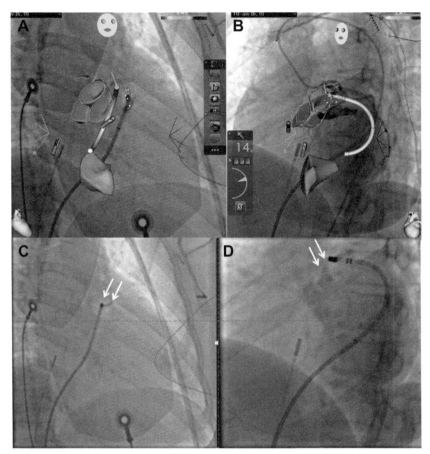

Fig. 2. (*A, B*) The mapping-ablation catheter is advanced to the ostium of the AIV with minimal use of fluoroscopy using the CARTO Univu module. Note the superimposed reconstruction of the coronary sinus ostium and of the coronary cusp region with the ICE and CARTOSOUND module. (*C, D*) Contrast injection from the ablation catheter shows correct positioning at the ostium of the AIV (*arrows*).

than 30-minute waiting period and under infusion of up to 6 μg/min of isoproterenol. The patient remained free from recurrent VPDs at 6-month follow-up.

DISCUSSION
Left Ventricular Summit Anatomy and Electrocardiography Correlates

A correct understanding of the LVS anatomy and ECG patterns associated with arrhythmias originating from this area is crucial both for preprocedural planning and to maximize the chances of success. The LVS is a triangular portion of the epicardial LVOT with the apex at the bifurcation between the LAD and the LCx coronary arteries, and the base formed by an arc connecting the first septal perforator branch of the LAD with the LCx. When viewed from an attitudinal orientation, the LVS lies posterior to the septal RVOT, and just inferior to left coronary cusp. On the 12-lead

ECG, this is reflected by an RBBB morphology and a rightward inferior axis, although there may be exception to the rule depending on the degree of heart rotation and the topographic relationship between the LVS and adjacent structures. In particular, in patients with significant clockwise rotation of the cardiac axis with a late precordial transition of the sinus rhythm ECG, arrhythmias originating from the LVS can still present with a left bundle branch block morphology in lead V1.[7] However, the precordial transition of the arrhythmia will invariably be earlier than that of the sinus rhythm QRS. In addition, LVS arrhythmias always manifest an inferior axis, with positive R waves in all of the 3 inferior leads (II, III, and aVF) and usually a more positive vector in lead III than II.

The LVS is bisected by the GCV in 2 main regions: the accessible area, which lies more laterally (base of the LVS triangle), and the inaccessible area, which lies septally to the GCV (apex of the

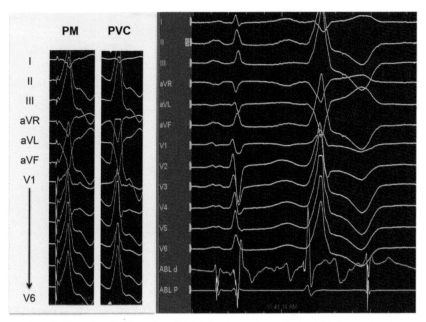

Fig. 3. Pace mapping (*left*) and activation time (*right*) in the ostium of the AIV. Pace mapping reveals a near-perfect 12/12 ECG lead match, and the local activation time is 24 ms pre-QRS. PM, pacemap; PVC, premature ventricular contraction.

LVS triangle) (**Fig. 6**). The definition of accessible versus inaccessible areas of the LVS is mainly based on the anatomic proximity to major coronary vessels (left main coronary artery and proximal bifurcation between LAD and LCx), and the terms indicate the likelihood of successful radiofrequency delivery due to either safe distance from major coronary vessels or lack of a thick layer of epicardial fat. In a recent study, the authors analyzed the ECG characteristics of LVS arrhythmia arising from the accessible versus inaccessible area. In this study, they included a series of 23 consecutive patients who underwent percutaneous epicardial mapping of LVS arrhythmias after a failed attempt at ablation from adjacent structures, including the LV and RV outflow tracts, the coronary cusp region, and coronary venous system. In this series, 5 patients were found to have arrhythmias originating from the accessible area, and the remaining 18 patients had arrhythmias mapped to the LVS inaccessible area mostly due to proximity to major coronary vessels or inability to deliver radiofrequency energy due to the presence of epicardial fat. The Q-wave ratio in leads aVL/aVR was significantly greater in patients with successful epicardial

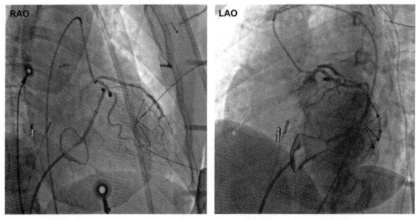

Fig. 4. Intraprocedural coronary angiography demonstrates safe distance between the major coronary vessels and the ostium of the AIV. RAO, right anterior oblique; LAO, left anterior oblique.

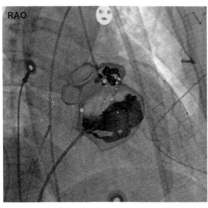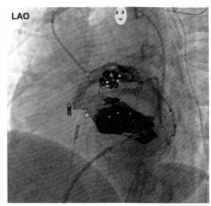

Fig. 5. Ablation set showing radiofrequency delivery in the AIV and from the adjacent LV endocardium. The anatomic distance between the 2 structures was 8 mm. RAO, right anterior oblique; LAO, left anterior oblique.

ablation compared with that in the unsuccessful group, with 4 of 5 (80%) successful ablation cases having a ratio greater than 1.85 (vs 2/18 [11%] unsuccessful cases, *P* = .008 for comparison). An R-wave to S-wave ratio in lead V1 greater than 2 was present in 4 of 5 (80%) patients in the successful group compared with 5 of 18 (28%) cases of unsuccessful ablation (*P* = .056 for comparison). None of the patients in the successful group had an initial q wave in lead V1 versus 6 of 18 (33%) in the unsuccessful group. These parameters reflect a more lateral site of origin of the VAs (distant from the midline and the apex of the LVS triangle). Of note, the presence of at least 2 of these 3 criteria predicted origin from the LVS

accessible area with 100% sensitivity and 72% specificity.[6] It is important to point out that the study included a select group of patients in whom epicardial access was performed after a failed attempt at ablation from adjacent structures such as the LV and RV outflow tracts, the coronary cusp region, and coronary venous system. This scenario is usually rare, as in most cases with VAs originating from the LVS inaccessible area successful ablation can still be achieved from adjacent structures. Successful ablation is particularly true when arrhythmias originate close to the true apex of the LVS triangle (see **Fig. 6**), which is anatomically adjacent to either the left coronary cusp or the most leftward aspect of the septal

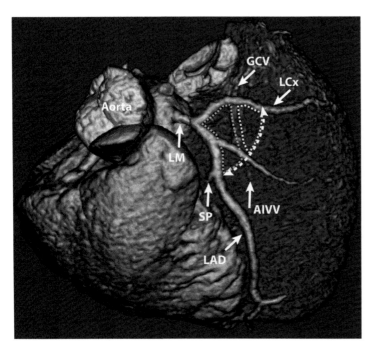

Fig. 6. Cardiac computed tomography reconstruction depicting the anatomic of the LVS. The LVS is a triangular region of the LV epicardium with the apex at the bifurcation between the LAD and LCx coronary arteries, and the base formed by an arc connecting the first septal perforator branch (SP) of the LAD with the LCx (*white dotted line* and *arrows*). The LVS is bisected by the GCV in 2 regions: (1) closer to the apex of the triangle (*blue dotted line*, inaccessible area), and (2) more lateral toward the base of the triangle (*yellow dotted line*, accessible area). LM, left main coronary artery.

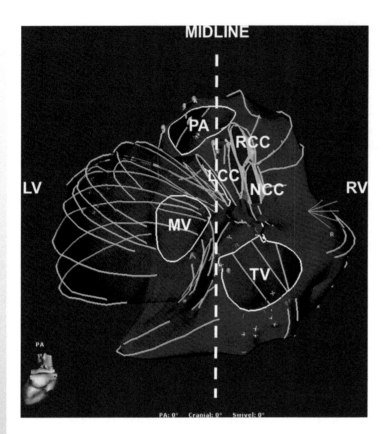

Fig. 7. CARTOSOUND reconstruction of the LV and RV shell and coronary cusp region in the posteroanterior view showing the attitudinal position of the cardiac structures with respect to the midline in the individual patient. LCC, left coronary cusp; MV, mitral valve; NCC, non-coronary cusp; PA, pulmonary artery; RCC, right coronary cusp; TV, tricuspid valve.

RVOT.[3,5] The authors' group has recently evaluated the ECG features of LVS arrhythmias that can be successfully targeted from the left coronary cusp in a group of 16 patients with LVS arrhythmias and early activation in the GCV/AIV in whom ablation was not attempted or aborted for ether proximity to a major coronary vessel, desire to avoid the potential risks of the transvenous and/or direct transcutaneous epicardial approach, and/or potential for higher power delivery from the coronary cusp region compared with the coronary venous system.[3] In this study, a Q-wave ratio in aVL/aVR less than 1.45 was associated with successful ablation from the adjacent left coronary cusp with 89% sensitivity and 75% specificity.[3] This parameter indicates the anatomic proximity between the GCV/AIV and the left coronary cusp (see also later discussion).

Approach to Catheter Ablation of Left Ventricular Summit Arrhythmias

As mentioned, pre-procedural ECG analysis is crucial to plan the most appropriate mapping approach of LVS arrhythmias. The authors' current approach for mapping LVS arrhythmias typically starts with a detailed anatomic reconstruction of the LV and RV outflow tract regions with intracardiac echocardiography (ICE) and the CARTOSOUND system (Biosense Webster) in order to define the anatomic relationships and distance between different adjacent sites, including LV endocardium, RVOT, and coronary cusp region (**Fig. 7**). A 7-Fr deflectable decapolar catheter (Bard, Lowell, MA, USA) is advanced to the GCV/AIV region under fluoroscopy guidance. In the case of difficulty in maneuvering the catheter to the GCV/AIV region, the coronary venous anatomy is defined with a retrograde angiogram using a standard pulmonary artery catheter in order to visualize the degree of vascular tortuosity and size of the coronary veins (**Fig. 8**). In the case of suitable anatomy, a long sheath (advanced to the proximal GCV) is typically used to increase the support and assist the advancement of the decapolar catheter to the GCV/AIV. If the size of the GCV/AIV is unsuitable to accommodate the 7-Fr decapolar mapping catheter, the coronary venous system can still be mapped with the aid of a 4-Fr decapolar catheter. The latter has a very soft body and may be difficult to maneuver within the coronary venous system unless the outer sheath is advanced distally to the GCV. In rare cases, the authors have used a

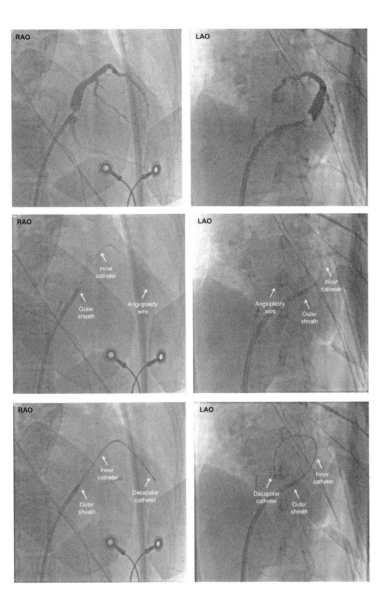

Fig. 8. (*top*) Example of coronary venous angiogram to define suitability of coronary venous system for mapping and ablation. (*middle*) In the case of vascular tortuosity and/or small caliber of the vessels, the AIV can be accessed with the aid of an angioplasty wire and an inner catheter advanced through a long outer sheath positioned at the GCV. (*bottom*) Once access to the AIV is obtained with the inner catheter, the wire is withdrawn, and a 4-Fr decapolar catheter is advanced through the inner to map the epicardial LVS from within the AIV. This approach is particularly helpful for mapping more distal portions of the AIV.

5-Fr inner catheter advanced to the ostium of the AIV over an angioplasty guidewire, which therefore facilitated the delivery of the 4-Fr decapolar catheter in the AIV region (see **Fig. 8**). This technique is particularly useful when it is necessary to map more distally in the AIV.

Once a catheter is deployed in the GCV/AIV region, it is important to assess the anatomic distance between the GCV/AIV and the other mappable adjacent structures, such as the LV and RV outflow tracts and the coronary cusp region. Pace mapping is performed from the GCV and AIV region to collect data on the paced 12-lead ECG morphologies and compared with the clinical VA. In the case of mismatch, a comparison of the paced QRS morphology at the GCV/AIV region

with the clinical VA is useful to anticipate the possible site of origin of the clinical VA. In this sense, a comparison of the R/S wave ratio in lead V1, of the Q-wave amplitude in lead I, and of the Q-wave ratio in aVL/aVR is useful to anticipate the site of origin septal or lateral to the GCV/AIV and guide further mapping.

Mapping is facilitated through the analysis the CARTOSOUND reconstruction of the anatomic shell of the RV and LV outflow tracts in the posteroanterior or anteroposterior views, which shows the attitudinal position of the heart (see **Fig. 7**) and helps identify the structures that are septal or lateral to the GCV/AIV in the individual patient. Further activation and pace mapping at anatomically adjacent sites, such as the septal

RVOT, coronary cusp region, and LV endocardium, are routinely performed to identify sites of earlier activation and collect the paced QRS morphologies at different sites. Catheter ablation is performed at the site of earliest activation and best pace map (12/12 ECG lead). In the case of discordant data between activation mapping and pace mapping, with different sites displaying early activation and best pace-map, ablation is always first delivered at the site of earliest activation and, if necessary, further ablation is performed at the site of best pace map. This phenomenon likely reflects preferential breakout sites due to either insulated strands of myocardial fibers or preferential conduction.[8] When the optimal site for ablation is defined to be at the GCV/AIV region, coronary angiogram should be performed in order to evaluate the distance between the GCV/AIV region and the major coronary vessels. Coronary angiography is also indicated when delivering energy at the most leftward aspect of the RVOT, especially when the selected site is 2 to 3 cm below the plane of the pulmonic valve in order to avoid injury to the LAD.[9] If the distance is greater than 5 mm (approximately 1.5 distal electrode tips of a standard open-irrigated ablation catheter with a 3.5-mm electrode tip size) in at least 2 different fluoroscopic projections, ablation energy can be safely delivered.[10] Coronary angiogram is not typically necessary for ablation in the endocardial LV or from the coronary cusp region (when performed under ICE guidance to define the ostium of the left main coronary artery).[11] However, there may be rare instances of an abnormal course of the LAD and LCx arteries, which can be missed with ICE and may account for collateral coronary artery injury with ablation in the coronary cusp region.

If ablation at the optimal site is not possible due to either proximity to major coronary vessels, inability to advance the ablation catheter to the site of origin (eg, GCV/AIV region), or inability to deliver sufficient power, ablation from anatomically adjacent sites should be considered. Criteria to define the optimal adjacent site to deliver additional radiofrequency energy are still a matter of active investigation at the authors' institution. Besides the ECG criteria discussed above, activation mapping is important to confirm that the selected site is the one with the earliest activation time compared with all of the anatomically adjacent sites. Another useful criterion is the anatomic distance between the site of origin and the selected adjacent site or sites. In the study by Jauregui Abularach and colleagues,[3] an anatomic distance less than 13.5 mm between the AIV and

the left coronary cusp identified patients with VAs with earliest activation from the AIV in whom successful ablation from the left coronary cusp was achieved. This anatomic distance is in line with experimental data showing that standard open irrigated catheters can deliver lesions up to 15 mm (high contact force, high power, and/or long duration).[12] When ablation from adjacent sites fails, a percutaneous epicardial approach may be considered, although rarely useful to achieve success (see later discussion). In the authors' experience, both the anterior and the posterior epicardial approaches are suitable to map the LVS region, and decision on the type of approach should be based on operator's preference and patient-specific risk assessment. An anterior approach provides direct access to the LVS region, whereas a posterior approach typically requires one to loop the catheter around the transverse sinus (unless steerable sheaths are used and/or the mapping/ablation catheter can be easily maneuvered laterally). In some instances, an enlarged left atrial appendage may prevent mapping of the LVS; caution should be exercised when mapping around the left atrial appendage in order to prevent catheter entrapment. Coronary angiography is always mandatory before ablation in the epicardial LVS; in the authors' experience, in about two-thirds of cases, radiofrequency delivery in the epicardial location was aborted due to proximity to major epicardial coronary vessels.[6]

Outcomes of Catheter Ablation of Left Ventricular Summit Arrhythmias

The outcome of catheter ablation of LVS arrhythmias largely depends on the likelihood of achieving success when ablating from adjacent structures, including the RV and LV outflow tracts, the coronary cusp region, and the coronary venous system.[1,3,5,6] Yamada and colleagues[1] studied 27 consecutive patients with VAs originating from the LVS. In this study, successful ablation was achieved from within the GCV/AIV in 14 of 27 (52%) cases.[1] When ablation from the GCV/AIV is not possible, success can still be achieved from anatomically adjacent structures. In the study by Jauregui Abularach and colleagues,[3] long-term success was achieved in 8 of 9 (89%) cases with early activation in the GCV/AIV from the adjacent left coronary cusp. As mentioned, when ablation from adjacent structures fails, a percutaneous pericardial approach can be considered but is of limited value. In particular, the authors recently reported a long-term success of only 17% in a consecutive series of cases of LVS arrhythmias undergoing an attempt at percutaneous epicardial mapping and ablation.[6]

SUMMARY

The LVS is a common site of origin of idiopathic VAs. These arrhythmias are most commonly ablated within the coronary venous system or from other adjacent structures such as the RV and LV outflow tract or coronary venous system. When ablation from adjacent structures fails, a percutaneous epicardial approach can be considered, but is rarely successful in eliminating the arrhythmias due to proximity to major coronary vessels and/or epicardial fat.

REFERENCES

1. Yamada T, McElderry HT, Doppalapudi H, et al. Idiopathic ventricular arrhythmias originating from the left ventricular summit: anatomic concepts relevant to ablation. Circ Arrhythmia Electrophysiol 2010;3:616–23.
2. McAlpine WA. Heart and coronary arteries. New York: Springer-Verlag; 1975.
3. Jauregui Abularach ME, Campos B, Park KM, et al. Ablation of ventricular arrhythmias arising near the anterior epicardial veins from the left sinus of Valsalva region: ECG features, anatomic distance, and outcome. Heart Rhythm 2012;9:865–73.
4. Obel OA, d'Avila A, Neuzil P, et al. Ablation of left ventricular epicardial outflow tract tachycardia from the distal great cardiac vein. J Am Coll Cardiol 2006;48:1813–7.
5. Frankel DS, Mountantonakis S, Dahu MI, et al. Elimination of ventricular arrhythmias originating from the anterior interventricular vein with ablation in the right ventricular outflow tract. Heart Rhythm 2014;11:S217.
6. Santangeli P, Marchlinski FE, Zado ES, et al. Percutaneous epicardial ablation of ventricular arrhythmias arising from the left ventricular summit: outcomes and ECG correlates of success. Circ Arrhythmia Electrophysiol 2015;8(2):337–43.
7. Betensky BP, Park RE, Marchlinski FE, et al. The V(2) transition ratio: a new electrocardiographic criterion for distinguishing left from right ventricular outflow tract tachycardia origin. J Am Coll Cardiol 2011;57:2255–62.
8. Yamada T, Murakami Y, Yoshida N, et al. Preferential conduction across the ventricular outflow septum in ventricular arrhythmias originating from the aortic sinus cusp. J Am Coll Cardiol 2007; 50:884–91.
9. Vaseghi M, Cesario DA, Mahajan A, et al. Catheter ablation of right ventricular outflow tract tachycardia: value of defining coronary anatomy. J Cardiovasc Electrophysiol 2006;17:632–7.
10. Stavrakis S, Jackman WM, Nakagawa H, et al. Risk of coronary artery injury with radiofrequency ablation and cryoablation of epicardial posteroseptal accessory pathways within the coronary venous system. Circ Arrhythmia Electrophysiol 2014;7: 113–9.
11. Hoffmayer KS, Dewland TA, Hsia HH, et al. Safety of radiofrequency catheter ablation without coronary angiography in aortic cusp ventricular arrhythmias. Heart Rhythm 2014;11:1117–21.
12. Ikeda A, Nakagawa H, Lambert H, et al. Relationship between catheter contact force and radiofrequency lesion size and incidence of steam pop in the beating canine heart: electrogram amplitude, impedance, and electrode temperature are poor predictors of electrode-tissue contact force and lesion size. Circ Arrhythmia Electrophysiol 2014;7: 1174–80.

Ventricular Tachycardia Arising from Cardiac Crux

Electrocardiogram Recognition and Site of Ablation

Leila Larroussi, MD, Nitish Badhwar, MD, FHRS*

KEYWORDS

- Ventricular tachycardia • Cardiac crux • Epicardial

KEY POINTS

- This case highlights idiopathic ventricular tachycardia (VT) can arise from crux of the heart.
- It is seen in patients without structural heart disease and can present as rapid hemodynamically unstable VT leading to cardiac arrest.
- 12 lead ECG showing RBBB with Q waves in inferior leads, precordial MDI >0.55 and R <S in V5 and V6 localize the VT to apical crux.
- The VT was successfully ablated in the epicardial cardiac crux through percutaneous pericardial access.

CLINICAL PRESENTATION

A 67-year-old man with a history of hypertension and hyperlipidemia presented to an outside hospital with a wide complex tachycardia (WCT) and altered mental status. One shock of 200 J converted him to normal sinus rhythm and he underwent a cardiac work-up. Transthoracic echocardiogram revealed a normal heart with no wall motion abnormalities or valvular dysfunction. A coronary angiogram showed nonobstructive coronary artery disease. Electrophysiologic study (EPS) confirmed inducible fast ventricular tachycardia (VT) and a single-chamber implantable cardioverter-defibrillator (ICD) was implanted for protection from sudden cardiac death. The patient was referred to our department for catheter ablation after receiving multiple shocks from his ICD despite being on β-blockers.

The patient has a single right ventricular lead ICD with 2 VT and 1 ventricular fibrillation (VF) therapy zones, respectively at cycle lengths (CLs) of 400 milliseconds, 320 milliseconds, and 260 milliseconds. On **Fig. 1**A, the first 3 beats are sinus, then the tachycardia starts with a CL of 387 milliseconds. The leadless electrocardiogram (ECG) and the recorded intracardiac electrogram (EGM) morphologies were similar to that of sinus rhythm, which is suggestive of a supraventricular arrhythmia origin. The tachycardia in **Fig. 1**B is faster (CL, 220 milliseconds) and has a different morphology on the leadless ECG and the recorded intracardiac EGM, suggesting that this is most likely VT.

During the EPS, 2 tachycardias were induced. The first was narrow QRS with a 1 to 1 AV conduction. It was proved to be atrial tachycardia based on VAAV response to ventricular overdrive pacing.

Disclosures: None.
Section of Cardiac Electrophysiology, Division of Cardiology, Department of Medicine, University of California, San Francisco, San Francisco, CA, USA
* Corresponding author. UCSF Medical Center, 500 Parnassus Avenue, MUE-431, San Francisco, CA 94143.
E-mail address: nitish.badhwar@ucsf.edu

cardiacEP.theclinics.com

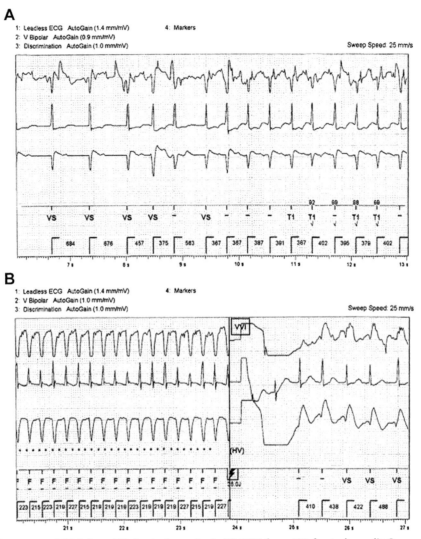

Fig. 1. (*A*) Electrogram (EGM) from ICD for tachycardia 1. (*B*) EGM from ICD for tachycardia 2.

As seen in **Fig. 2**, the P waves are narrow and the morphology (+/− in V1, with an early transition in V2; + in leads1 and aVL; − in leads II, III, and avF) is consistent with para-Hisian atrial tachycardia.[1] This tachycardia was mapped and successfully ablated in the para-Hisian region in the right atrium. With isoproterenol infusion, VT was induced (**Fig. 3**) that was consistent with the second tachycardia noted on the ICD interrogation.

Question: Based on the morphology of the VT in **Fig. 3**, what is the most likely site of origin?

This WCT is a VT with a CL of 220 milliseconds and QRS width of 130 milliseconds. The QRS morphology is right bundle branch block (RBBB) (R/s>1 in lead V1) with left superior axis. The poor precordial transition or reverse pattern is consistent with a midventricular or apical exit. The differential diagnosis includes a posterior fascicular VT, a posterior papillary muscle VT, or an apical crux VT.[2,3]

The presence of a QS in leads II and III, R greater than S in lead V5, and upright avR argue against fascicular VT and posterior papillary muscle VT.[2,3] The Maximum Deflection Index (MDI) is 86 milliseconds/130 milliseconds = 0.66 (>0.55) and there is a pseudodelta wave of 37 milliseconds. These QRS features are consistent with an epicardial origin, and suggest a diagnosis of crux VT. The RBBB morphology with R less than S in lead V6 favors an apical (as opposed to basal) crux VT.[2]

Intracardiac EGMs show that the earliest V signal recorded was at the coronary sinus distal (−18 milliseconds). During ventricular overdrive pacing (VOD) in tachycardia (**Fig. 4**A), the morphology is identical to ventricular pacing only (**Fig. 4**B), therefore no fusion is observed but the

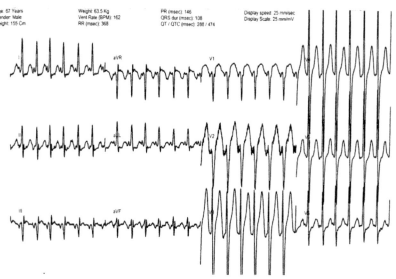

Fig. 2. Twelve-lead SVT.

tachycardia that continues after VOD is stopped. The lack of fusion is less compatible with reentry and suggests an automatic or a triggered mechanism. Moreover, this tachycardia seems to be catecholamine induced because the patient was stressed when he had it the first time and it required isoproterenol to be induced in the laboratory.

Question: What is the optimal ablation site for this VT?

The apical crux can be accessed by 2 different approaches: through the coronary sinus and middle cardiac vein (MCV) or through an epicardial access. In this case, the ablation catheter could not be advanced in the MCV and an epicardial access was performed.

The epicardial map showed no scar. Because of instability during VT, activation mapping could not be done in tachycardia. We used a pace-map technique to identify the best site for ablation. Two sites with 12/12 pace map were identified but could not be ablated because of close proximity to a posterolateral branch of the right coronary artery, as shown in **Fig. 5**. A very good pace map (11/12) was identified distally and radiofrequency ablation was applied there (**Fig. 6**). The VT was not inducible after the ablation. The patient has been free of VT at 6 months' follow-up.

Idiopathic epicardial VT arising from the crux of the heart has recently been described as a distinct entity with characteristic clinical and ECG findings.

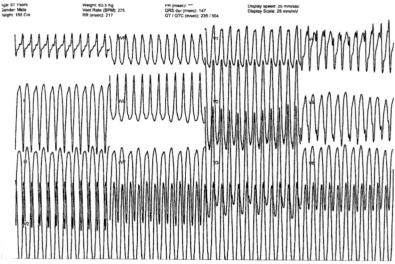

Fig. 3. Twelve-lead VT.

A   **B**

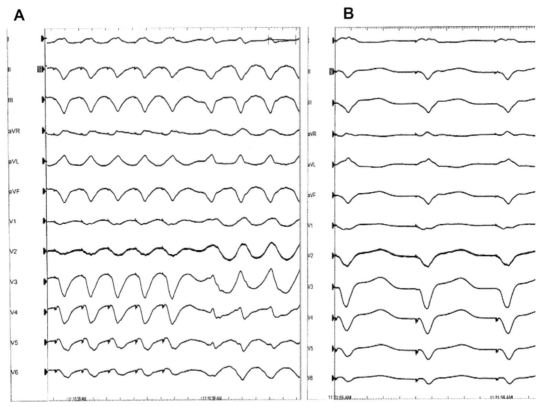

Fig. 4. (*A*) Right ventricular overdrive pacing during tachycardia. (*B*) Pure right ventricular pacing.

These patients present with very fast VT that can lead to syncope and cardiac arrest requiring resuscitation. Twelve-lead ECG shows morphology consistent with preexcited posteroseptal Wolff Parkinson White (WPW) pathway. They have left bundle branch block (LBBB) with early transition or RBBB morphology with QS pattern in leads II and III and precordial MDI greater than 0.55. It is further divided into basal crux VT that predominantly has LBBB pattern and has R greater than S in V6 and apical crux VT that can have LBBB or RBBB pattern with R less than S in V6. Basal crux VT can be successfully ablated in the proximal coronary sinus or the mouth of the MCV, whereas apical crux VT requires percutaneous pericardial access for successful ablation.[2]

SUMMARY

This case highlights the complex nature of some idiopathic VTs. First, this patient had 2 arrhythmias; 1 was supraventricular but because of its short CL it was treated as a VT by the ICD. The second was a VT in a structurally normal heart that was hemodynamically unstable. This VT had typical criteria for epicardial apical crux VT. The area could not be accessed from the coronary sinus and therefore needed an epicardial access. RF ablation was limited by epicardial structures such as coronary arteries and the close proximity of the phrenic nerve. However, with an almost

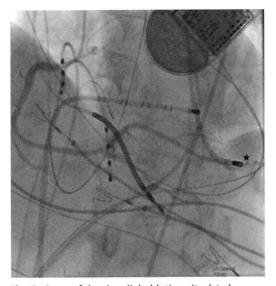

Fig. 5. Successful epicardial ablation site (*star*).

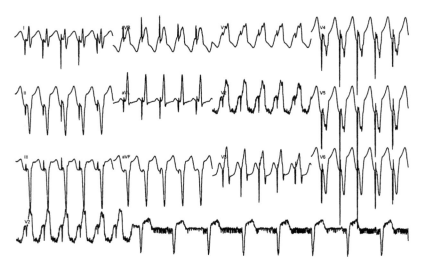

Fig. 6. Best pace map at the epicardial ablation site.

perfect pace-map site, the VT was rendered non-inducible after RF ablation.

REFERENCES

1. Iwai S, Badhwar N, Markowitz SM, et al. Electrophysiologic properties of para-Hisian atrial tachycardia. Heart Rhythm 2011;8(8):1245–53.
2. Kawamura M, Gerstenfeld EP, Vedantham V, et al. Idiopathic ventricular arrhythmia originating from the cardiac crux or inferior septum: an epicardial idiopathic ventricular arrhythmia. Circ Arrhythm Electrophysiol 2014;7(6):1152–8.
3. Kawamura M, Hsu JC, Vedantham V, et al. Clinical and electrocardiographic characteristics of idiopathic ventricular arrhythmias with right bundle branch block and superior axis-comparison of apical crux area and posterior-septal left ventricle. Heart Rhythm 2015; 12(6):1137–44.

Anatomical Ablation Strategy for Noninducible Fascicular Tachycardia

Ahmed Karim Talib, MD, PhD, Akihiko Nogami, MD, PhD*

KEYWORDS

- Fascicular tachycardia • Verapamil-sensitive ventricular tachycardia • Catheter ablation
- Anatomical approach

KEY POINTS

- The presence of structural heart disease does not exclude fascicular ventricular tachycardia (VT), especially if the VT is verapamil sensitive.
- An empirical anatomical approach is effective when fascicular VT is noninducible or if diastolic Purkinje potential (P1) cannot be recorded during VT mapping.
- Pace mapping at the successful ablation site is usually not effective because selective pacing of P1 is difficult and there is an antidromic activation of the proximal P1 potential.

CLINICAL PRESENTATION

A 22-year-old man presented to the emergency department with palpitation associated with wide QRS complex tachycardia (212 beats per minute), which was slowed and terminated by intravenous Verapamil (5 mg) injection (**Fig. 1**). The patient was kept on oral verapamil; however, he was still symptomatic and was referred to the authors' hospital for catheter ablation. The patient has a known history of Kawasaki disease and high-grade stenosis in the proximal segment of the left anterior descending artery associated with rich collaterals from both the left circumflex and right coronary arteries. During admission, coronary angiogram revealed no significant changes (ie, left anterior descending artery stenosis with rich collaterals) and the left ventriculography revealed normal ventricular wall motion.

Question 1: What Is the Most Likely Type of This Tachycardia?

Verapamil-sensitive fascicular tachycardia is characterized by right bundle branch block (RBBB)

configuration and left axis deviation.[1] It is typically idiopathic but can occur in patients with organic heart disease.[2] Although the patient had coronary lesion, left ventricular function and wall motion were normal. Moreover, 3-dimensional electroanatomical mapping revealed normal endocardial voltage.

VENTRICULAR TACHYCARDIA INDUCTION

Burst and programmed atrial and ventricular stimulation failed to induce clinical ventricular tachycardia (VT). Intravenous atropine administration followed by programmed atrial pacing resulted in wide QRS complexes (**Fig. 2**).

Question 2: What Are These Wide QRS Complexes and What Is the Role of Atropine?

During atrial pacing, His bundle was activated and His potential (H) was recorded in the distal His bipole. However, the wide QRS complexes were not preceded by His bundle activation; hence, aberrant conduction was ruled out. The wide QRS

Dr A. Nogami has received honoraria from St. Jude Medical and Boston Scientific and an endowment from Medtronic and Johnson & Johnson.
Cardiovascular Division, Faculty of Medicine, University of Tsukuba, Tsukuba, Japan
* Corresponding author. Cardiovascular Division, Faculty of Medicine, University of Tsukuba, 1-1-1 Tennodai, Tsukuba, Ibaraki 305-8575, Japan.
E-mail address: akihiko-ind@umin.ac.jp

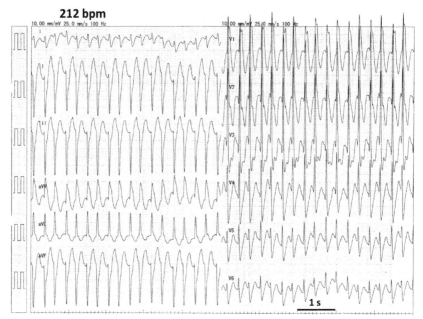

Fig. 1. Twelve-lead electrocardiogram (ECG) of clinically documented tachycardia. ECG exhibited right bundle branch block configuration and left axis deviation. QRS alternans was observed during ventricular tachycardia (VT). The VT was terminated by intravenous verapamil administration. bpm, beats per minute.

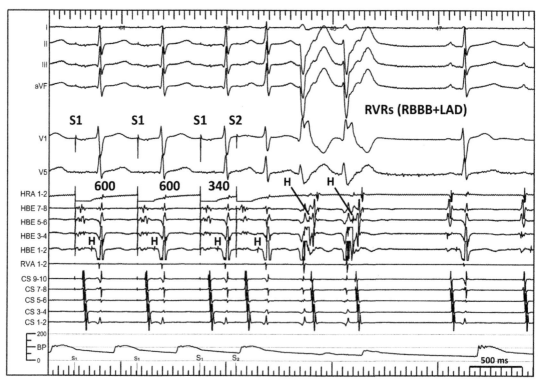

Fig. 2. Programmed atrial stimulation after intravenous atropine injection. Programmed atrial stimulation after intravenous atropine injection induced wide QRS complexes with RBBB configuration and left axis deviation, which is similar to the clinical VT. Negative His potential (H)-V interval was observed during these complexes. H-V interval during fascicular VT depends on the site of the upper turnaround. If the site of turnaround is high (or close to His bundle), H-V interval will be positive (but shorter than that during sinus rhythm) and vice versa (ie, if the lower turn-around site is more distal, the H-V interval will be negative). 1 to 2, distal bipole; 9 to 10, proximal bipole; CS, coronary sinus; HBE, His-bundle electrogram; HRA, high right atrium; LAD, left axis deviation; RBBB, right bundle branch block; RVA, right ventricular apex.

complexes exhibited RBBB configuration and left axis deviation, which is similar to the clinical VT; therefore, these beats are clinical repetitive ventricular responses. His were recorded after the QRS onset during the repetitive responses (see **Fig. 2**). The negative H-V interval during wide QRS complexes suggested the turnaround site is more distal, away from the His bundle.

Both isoproterenol and atropine are effective in inducing fascicular VT. However, the mechanism of VT induction is different. Although isoproterenol enhances the inducibility of the VT by affecting the VT circuit, atropine does not affect the circuit itself. One of the characteristics of verapamil-sensitive left fascicular VT is inducibility by atrial stimulation.[1] Atropine enhances the atrioventricular nodal conduction; therefore, it can increase the maximum stimulation rate to the Purkinje network during atrial stimulation. The authors usually use an intravenous injection of atropine 0.5 to 1.0 mg, if atrioventricular block occurs at a cycle length of longer than 300 milliseconds during atrial stimulation. Isoproterenol can also enhance the atrioventricular conduction; however, atropine has another benefit in the stability of mapping/ablation catheter. Unlike isoproterenol, atropine does not cause cardiac hyperkinetic contraction of the left ventricle.

Question 3: What Is the Ablation Strategy for This Case?

Because clinical VT could not be induced, an anatomical linear ablation[3] was decided. First, the exit site was defined by pace mapping. The ablation line is shown in **Fig. 3**A. Here, a linear lesion was designed to horizontally cross the distal one-fourth quarter point between the His-bundle recording site and the exit site. The line was supposed to create a block across the VT circuit.

After applying 5 radiofrequency (RF) energy applications to the exit site, which was determined by pace mapping and the anatomic linear lesion (see **Fig. 3**A), and before completing the ablation line, sustained VT initiated (**Fig. 4**) and became inducible by single atrial/ventricular extrastimulus.

Question 4: After it became inducible, where to ablate the Ventricular Tachycardia?

These RF energy applications might have created a slower conduction in the circuit and rendered VT more easily inducible. Left ventricular endocardium was mapped during VT (see **Fig. 3**B). However, the clear diastolic Purkinje potential (P1) could not be obtained during VT. Presystolic Purkinje potentials (P2) could be recorded during sinus rhythm and VT, and activation sequences of P2 were reversed (see **Fig. 4**). Although the low-voltage and low-frequency potentials were sometimes recorded in the diastolic phase (see **Fig. 4**, *arrows*), it was difficult to determine they were diastolic Purkinje potential (P1). The activation map revealed that the earliest activation was at the exit site in the infero-apical septum. In this

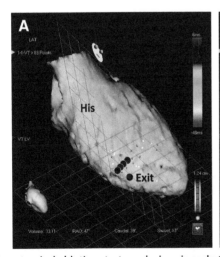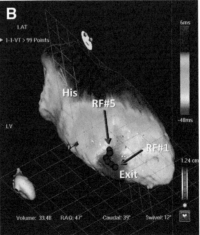

Fig. 3. First anatomical ablation strategy during sinus rhythm. A linear ablation strategy (*line represented by blue tags*) was initially planned at the distal one-fourth quarter point between the His-bundle recording site and the exit site to perpendicularly extend across the long axis of the left ventricle. The exit site (*red tag*) was defined as the best pace map site (*A*). After applying 5 radiofrequency (RF) ablation points including the exit site and the anatomic linear lesion (*B*), and before completing the ablation line, clinical VT initiated spontaneously. Ablation catheter placed at the left ventricular septum did not record any diastolic Purkinje potential, whereas activation mapping revealed that the early activation site was at the exit site.

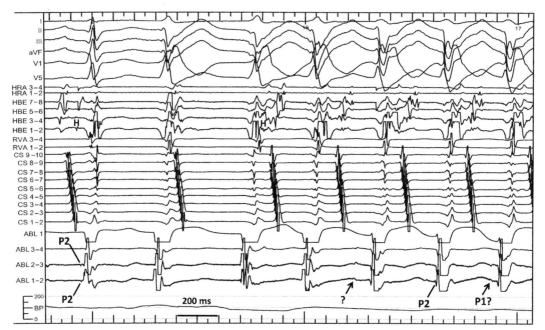

Fig. 4. Spontaneous initiation of VT after the initial anatomic linear RF lesion. After applying 5 RF ablation points including the exit site and the anatomic linear lesion, clinical VT (RBBB, left axis deviation) initiated spontaneously and became inducible by single atrial/ventricular extrastimulus. During sinus rhythm, the conduction propagated antegrade (proximal to distal) generating a presystolic potential (P2) immediately followed by the ventricular activation with short P2-QRS duration, which may indicate that the ablation catheter was positioned in the Purkinje-muscular junction. Presystolic Purkinje potentials (P2) could be recorded during sinus rhythm and VT, and activation sequences of P2 were reversed. Although the low-voltage and low-frequency potentials were sometimes recorded in the diastolic phase (*arrows*), it was difficult to determine they were diastolic Purkinje potential (P1). 1 to 2, distal bipole; 3 to 4, proximal bipole; ABL, ablation catheter; HBE, His bundle electrogram; HRA, high right atrium; RVA, right ventricular apex.

patient, the VT circuit seemed to be in a more basal site than the first linear lesion. Therefore, a second anatomical ablation line was created more proximally (**Fig. 5**), which resulted in VT termination and rendered the VT noninducible. Although a good pace map (94% match) was observed at the VT exit site, RF application was ineffective. On the other hand, the VT was terminated in a more basal site where there was less perfect pace map (88% match) with pacing latency, indicating a delay in capturing the Purkinje fiber at the lowest pacing threshold, which has a low possibility of capturing the surround myocardium (see **Fig. 5**). **Fig. 6** shows the entrainment pacing at the VT termination site. Fused presystolic P2 potential was recorded during VT, and P2 preceded the onset of the QRS by 10 milliseconds; however, P1 potential was not recognized. Entrained QRS waves exhibited minimal fusion with a 10-millisecond pacing delay. Postpacing interval (stimulus to returned P2) was 295 milliseconds, which was equal to the cycle length of VT.

DISCUSSION

In case of noninducible VT or if a good electrogram cannot be found during VT mapping, an anatomical approach is useful.[1,3] The distal third to a quarter point between His-bundle recording and the exit site, defined as the best QRS matched pace map, is usually selected for linear ablation (**Fig. 7**A). However, in this case, there might be a lower common pathway or a preferential pathway between the exit to the myocardium and the lower turnaround site of the VT circuit; therefore, the first linear ablation at the distal quarter was ineffective and a more proximal linear ablation was effective (see **Fig. 7**B). Local electrogram at the VT termination site exhibited fused P2 with myocardial electrogram, and entrainment pacing at this site showed minimal fusion with the short pacing delay; the postpacing interval was equal to the cycle length of VT (see **Fig. 6**). These findings suggest that this site is the outer loop near the lower turnaround (see **Fig. 7**B, *asterisk*).

The lower common pathway/preferential pathway is hypothetical. If the lower turnaround

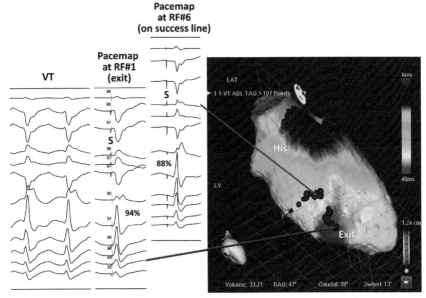

Fig. 5. Activation map during VT, pace mapping, and RF application sites. Electroanatomical map during VT exhibited a centrifugal pattern from the exit site, which was also determined by pace mapping. The second anatomic linear RF lesion (more proximal to the first RF line) was created and resulted in VT termination. Although a good pace map (94% match) was observed at the VT exit site, RF application was ineffective. On the other hand, the VT was terminated in a more basal site where less perfect pace map (88% matches) with a longer pacing latency, indicating a delay in capturing Purkinje fiber, was observed.

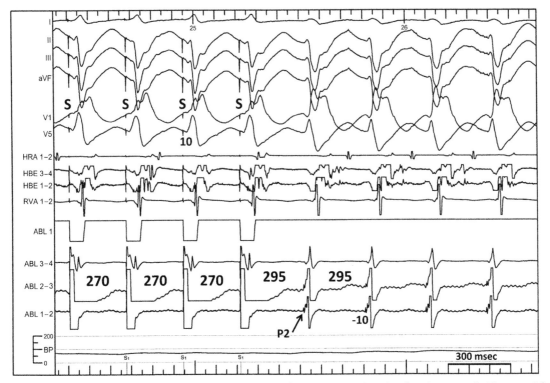

Fig. 6. Entrainment pacing at the VT termination site. At the VT termination site, fused presystolic P2 potential was recorded during VT and P2 preceded the onset of the QRS by 10 milliseconds; however, P1 potential was not recognized. Entrained QRS waves exhibited minimal fusion with 10-millisecond pacing delay. Postpacing interval (stimulus to returned P2) was 295 milliseconds, which was equal to the cycle length of VT. These findings suggest that this site is the outer loop near the lower turnaround (see **Fig. 7**B, *asterisk*).

A

Typical ILVT Circuit

B

ILVT Circuit with Lower Common Pathway

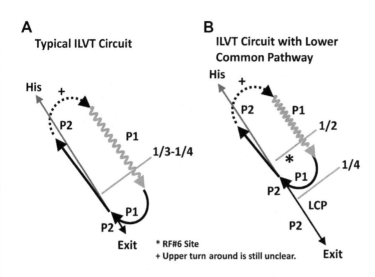

* RF#6 Site
+ Upper turn around is still unclear.

Fig. 7. Fascicular VT circuit and anatomic RF lines. (A) The distal third to a quarter point between His-bundle recording and the exit site, defined as the best QRS matched pace map, is usually selected for anatomic linear ablation. (B) In this case, the presence of a lower common pathway or a preferential pathway between the exit to the myocardium and the lower turnaround site of the VT circuit is hypothesized. First, a linear lesion was designed to horizontally cross the distal third to a quarter point between the His-bundle recording site and the exit site. The line was supposed to create a block across the VT circuit (left), however; in this case, there might be a lower common pathway or a preferential pathway between the exit and the lower turnaround site of the VT circuit (right); therefore, the first linear ablation, at the distal quarter, was ineffective but created slower conduction in the circuit and enhanced VT induction. A more proximal linear ablation successfully created a block across the VT circuit. Entrainment pacing at the site on this line (asterisk in B) exhibited minimal fusion with equal postpacing interval to the VT cycle length. ILVT, idiopathic left ventricular tachycardia.

point with the fusion of P1, P2, and ventricular myocardium could be found, there is no possibility of a lower common pathway. If the lower turnaround (pivot) was recorded but it was not fused with the ventricular activation, a lower common pathway/preferential pathway may be considered.

Pace mapping at the successful ablation site is usually not effective, because selective pacing of P1 is difficult and there is an antidromic activation of the proximal P1 potential.[1]

Far-field possible diastolic Purkinje potential (P1) can sometimes be recorded during VT and also during sinus rhythm, especially after the ablation. However, it is unclear whether those vague potentials are really related to the VT circuit. If the diastolic potentials with the same configuration were recorded during VT and sinus rhythm, and

the potential during sinus rhythm exhibits decrement properties and verapamil sensitivity, it can be proved that the potential is related to the circuit.[1]

REFERENCES

1. Nogami A. Purkinje-related arrhythmias part I: monomorphic ventricular tachycardias. Pacing Clin Electrophysiol 2011;34:624–50.
2. Hayashi M, Kobayashi Y, Iwasaki YK, et al. Novel mechanism of postinfarction ventricular tachycardia originating in surviving left posterior Purkinje fibers. Heart Rhythm 2006;3:908–18.
3. Lin D, Hsia HH, Gerstenfeld EP, et al. Idiopathic fascicular left ventricular tachycardia: linear ablation lesion strategy for noninducible or nonsustained tachycardia. Heart Rhythm 2005;2:934–9.

Ablation of Ventricular Tachycardia in Patients with Ischemic Cardiomyopathy

Paul Garabelli, MD, Stavros Stavrakis, MD, PhD,
Sunny S. Po, MD, PhD*

KEYWORDS

- Ablation • Ventricular tachycardia • Ischemic cardiomyopathy • Ventricular arrhythmia

KEY POINTS

- Ventricular tachycardias (VTs) occurring after prior myocardial infarction are usually caused by reentrant circuits formed by surviving myocardial bundles.
- Although part of the reentrant circuits may be located in the midmyocardium or epicardium, most of the VTs can be safely and successfully ablated by endocardial ablation targeting the late potentials/local abnormal ventricular activation, which are surrogates for the surviving myocardial bundles.
- A combination of activation, substrate, pace mapping, and entrainment mapping, as well as the use of contact force catheters, further improves ablation success and safety.

The management of ventricular arrhythmias following myocardial infarction is often limited by medication toxicities or treatment failure. Catheter ablation for ventricular tachycardia (VT) has emerged as a viable treatment of patients with recurrent arrhythmias, which often lead to shocks or antitachycardia pacing delivered by implantable cardiac defibrillators (ICDs). In the last 10 years, the use of VT ablation has increased from 2.8% in 2002 to 10.8% in 2011, reinforcing the importance of this option for managing such patients.[1]

CASE INTRODUCTION

A 70-year-old man with ischemic heart disease, previous 3-vessel coronary artery bypass graft, and ICD implantation for primary prevention developed recurrent monomorphic VT and multiple ICD shocks. He had a known basal-inferior scar. After maximizing antiarrhythmic therapy and ensuring no significant progression of his coronary artery disease, he was referred for ablation. His electrocardiogram (ECG) is shown in **Fig. 1**.

PREABLATION ASSESSMENT

Patients presenting for ischemic VT ablation are often ill and have several comorbidities, and optimization of medical management is often required. The presence of right heart failure also substantially increases procedure-related complications. At the authors' institution, reviewing the echocardiography and 12-lead ECGs of all clinical VTs constitutes the most important preablation assessment. Aneurysms, areas of wall motion abnormality, and wall thickness are carefully evaluated, and correlate with the scar identified by the voltage map acquired during the ablation procedure. The exit point of each clinical VT is predicted based on the criteria described later to guide pace mapping.

Department of Medicine, Heart Rhythm Institute, University of Oklahoma Health Sciences Center, 1200 Everett Drive, Oklahoma City, OK 73104, USA
* Corresponding author. Heart Rhythm Institute, 1200 Everett Drive (6E103), Oklahoma City, OK 73104.
E-mail address: sunny-po@ouhsc.edu

Card Electrophysiol Clin 8 (2016) 121–129
http://dx.doi.org/10.1016/j.ccep.2015.10.013
1877-9182/16/$ – see front matter © 2016 Elsevier Inc. All rights reserved.

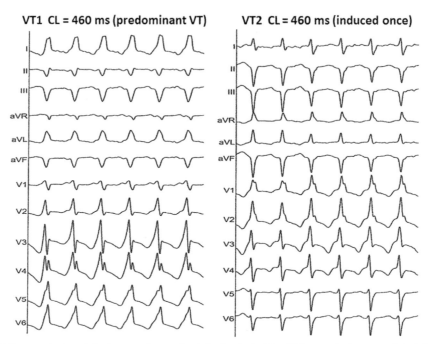

Fig. 1. Two VTs were induced during an electrophysiologic study. The QRS morphology predicted that the exit point of VT1 was septal, inferior, and basal left ventricle (LV). The exit point of VT2 was inferior and apical LV.

USING THE 12-LEAD AND QRS MORPHOLOGY TO DETERMINE EXIT OF VENTRICULAR TACHYCARDIA

Miller and colleagues[2] created an algorithm that gives a specific region of origin for ischemic VTs based on the 12-lead QRS characteristics. They divided the left ventricle (LV) into regions of origin, as seen in **Fig. 2**. Their data only included patients with a single site of infarction and was not perfect or universally applicable for VTs, such as those with multiple sites of infarction. Clinicians should also be suspicious for an epicardial exit because this can dramatically change the procedural plan. Berruezo and colleagues[3] reported on 3 specific characteristics that identify an epicardial exit of VT. These are a pseudodelta wave of greater than or equal to 34 milliseconds on the 12-lead ECG, an intrinsicoid deflection time of greater than or equal to 85 milliseconds, and an RS complex duration of greater than or equal to 121 milliseconds.

The QRS morphology of the recorded VT helps identify the exit of the ventricular tachycardia and can help plan the ablation approach and direct pace mapping maneuvers, if applicable. For example, as the exit site progresses closer to the left arm leads I and aVL, the lead polarity becomes more negative (progressive absence of an R wave). A VT with a left bundle branch block–like configuration usually originates in either the right ventricle (RV), LV septum, or is a form of bundle branch reentry. A VT with a right bundle branch block pattern (R > S in V1) originates from the LV, with few exceptions. A superiorly directly frontal plane axis (S > R in II, III, aVF) correlates with an exit at the inferior aspect of the ventricle. QRS progression is also used as a guide for exit. For example, dominant S waves in leads V3 and V4 suggest a more apical exit (away from the atrioventricular [AV] groove), whereas dominant R waves are associated with a more basal exit (near the AV groove).

CASE REVISITED

With this information, and by reviewing our 12-lead ECG, the exit point of VT1 and VT2 was predicted to be inferior-basal LV and inferior-apical LV, respectively.

MECHANISM OF ISCHEMIC VENTRICULAR TACHYCARDIA

Original research performed by de Bakker and colleagues[4,5] using Langendorff perfusion setup clarified the mechanisms and circuits for VT. Many VTs originate from circumscribed areas that can be as small as 1.4 cm². This finding is in contrast with the minority of cases in their electrophysiologic and histologic studies that showed only macroreentry around scar. Within the scar, multiple,

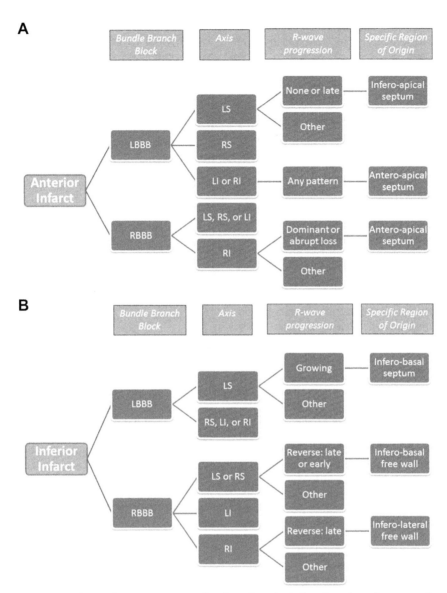

Fig. 2. (*A*, *B*) Algorithms for predicting exit point of VT based on the infarct location. The VT QRS bundle branch block pattern is the first branching point, followed by the axis. The third branching point is the precordial R-wave progression, which leads to the specific region of origin. I, inferior; L, left; LBBB, left bundle branch block; LI, left inferior; LS, left superior; R, right; RBBB, right bundle branch block; RI, right inferior; RS, right superior; S, superior. (*Modified from* Miller JM, Marchlinski FE, Buxton AE, et al. Relationship between the 12-lead ECG during ventricular tachycardia and endocardial site of origin in patients with coronary artery disease. Circulation 1988;77(4):764; with permission.)

discrete electrograms of low amplitude, termed presystolic potentials or late diastolic potentials, can be recorded. Histology of these endocardial resected preparations revealed separate zones of viable myocardium giving rise to these low-amplitude signals. These separate patchy zones of viable myocardial bundles can be intramural, subendocardial, or subepicardial. This finding suggested that reentry occurred between these myocardial bundles at the infarct border and between the remaining subendocardial muscle mass. The conduction velocity through these isolated tracts was slow (eg, 25 cm/s).

MAPPING TECHNIQUES

Four mapping techniques are used for VT ablation: activation mapping, substrate mapping, pace mapping, and entrainment mapping. These techniques are usually used in combination to improve ablation success.

Activation Mapping

As shown by the pioneering work of de Bakker and colleagues,[4,5] VT circuits usually have a vulnerable component, described as the slow conduction channel or isthmus. Assuming the patient tolerates VT well, without hemodynamic compromise, a three-dimensional (3D) electroanatomic activation map can help define the reentrant circuit for ablation. In contrast with mapping of reentrant atrial tachycardias, in which the complete reentrant circuit is usually obtained, a complete reentrant circuit of the VT often cannot be obtained. A portion of the reentrant circuit may be midmyocardial or epicardial. Importantly, most VTs are poorly tolerated and activation mapping is often not possible. For these patients, a substrate-based approach during sinus or paced rhythm is widely accepted as feasible.

Substrate Mapping

The substrate mapping approach defines the myocardial scar while in sinus or paced rhythm. Electrogram (EGM) voltage has proved to be the most useful index of scar. In approximately 95% of healthy left ventricular tissue sampling sites, a bipolar voltage of more than 1.5 mV is recorded.[6,7] However, some clinicians use a lower cutoff of 1.0 mV.[8] These areas are tagged on a corresponding 3D electroanatomic map and are used to further guide ablation. During this process, care must also be taken to ensure adequate electrode contact during mapping to avoid an underestimation of voltage.[8–10]

Different characteristics of local EGMs within scar can further refine appropriate targets for ablation. These abnormal EGMs, collectively described as local abnormal ventricular activation (LAVA), including multipotential EGMs, isolated diastolic potentials, and fractionated EGMs, are usually late potentials occurring after the end of the local ventricular signals or surface QRS complex.[11] These late potentials/LAVA within the scar are often viewed as the electrophysiologic signatures of viable myocardial bundles and potential circuits of VT. Late potentials are typically low-voltage signals (0.05–0.30 mV) that range from 100 to 400 milliseconds in duration. They can be separated from the local ventricular potential by an isoelectric interval.[12] They are more frequently seen in scar tissue of patients with documented VTs than in scar tissue in patients without VTs.[11–13] The presence of late potentials/LAVA

may vary based on anatomic locations and the wave front of activation; therefore, the distribution of late potentials/LAVA within a given scar may be different between ventricular-sensed rhythm and ventricular-paced rhythm.[14–16] Moreover, at the border of the scar, a local ventricular potential and late potentials may form a continuous potential. The former may represent the myocardial tissue outside the scar and the latter may represent the myocardial bundles at the edge of the scar.

Late potentials within the scar have been shown to be critical elements in the VT reentrant circuits.[12–16] However, they generally have poor specificity alone. For example, Brunckhorst and colleagues[12] showed that only 31% of late potentials identified within a scar were part of a critical isthmus. Two characteristics can improve this. A long, isolated late potential improves specificity.[11–16] Pace mapping from late potential sites that produce long stimulus-QRS (s-QRS) delays with good ECG match to VT also improves mapping accuracy.[14,15] Of note, a series of late potentials may not seem to participate in a given VT circuit but may form critical elements in the reentrant circuit of another VT. At the authors' institution, all late potentials are carefully tagged to serve as ablation targets. However, ablation does not start until the network of late potentials, presumably the network of potential VT circuits, has been mapped. Premature ablation, unless pressed by deterioration of the patient's condition, may produce conduction block to the downstream surviving myocardial bundles, leading to an underestimation of the potential VT circuits and a possibly less favorable ablation outcome.

Pace Mapping and Entrainment Mapping

Pacing during either sinus rhythm (pace mapping) or during VT (entrainment mapping) provides critical information about the proximity between the pacing site and the VT exit point. During pace mapping, 3 pieces of information are necessary: capture, paced QRS morphology, and s-QRS interval (indication of abnormal or slow conduction). Capture depends on electrically active tissue, and ideally the lowest current that captures tissue should be used. With that in mind, previous researchers have labeled unexcitable scar as areas with unipolar pacing thresholds greater than 10 mA at a 2-milliseond pulse width.[17] However, this definition needs to be interpreted with caution because some late potentials located in a dense scar cannot be captured at maximal current despite being a critical element in the reentrant circuit. Borders of a scar can be the exit points of multiple VTs and require detailed mapping as well. In pace mapping, a QRS morphology match to a clinical VT in all 12 leads usually approximates the exit point of the isthmus of a reentrant circuit.[18,19] However, a discrepancy between the paced QRS morphology and clinical VT does not exclude the possibility that the pace mapping site is in a critical area of the reentrant circuit, because the viable myocardial bundles within the scar form a complex network. Therefore, pacing at a given site can produce multiple morphologies, depending on the size of tissue captured, regions of conduction block, and multiple potential exits. It is common to observe that the paced QRS morphology from the successful ablation site failed to match the VT morphology but entrainment mapping during VT produced concealed fusion, indicating that this site is in the protected isthmus of the reentrant circuit.

In addition to the QRS morphology, entrainment during tachycardia requires comparison of the postpacing interval (PPI) with the VT cycle length

(TCL) as well as comparison of the s-QRS interval and the EGM-to-QRS (e-QRS) intervals. Overdrive pacing at an output as low as possible for consistent capture while avoiding far-field capture improves specificity. The PPI-TCL interval represents an estimate of the distance between the pacing site and the reentrant circuit. Manifest fusion usually indicates that the site of entrainment mapping is not located in a protected isthmus of the reentrant circuit and ablation there is unlikely to affect the VT. A short PPI-TCL interval (<30 milliseconds) suggests that the pacing catheter is in close proximity to the VT circuit. If the patient takes antiarrhythmic drugs that slow the conduction (eg, amiodarone), a longer PPI-TCL interval (eg, 50 milliseconds) does not exclude the pacing site's close proximity to the reentrant circuit. A longer s-QRS and e-QRS interval suggests a more proximal location, or entrance in the isthmus, which can be 51% to 70% of the s-QRS/TCL, depending on the location within the loop.[20] A shorter

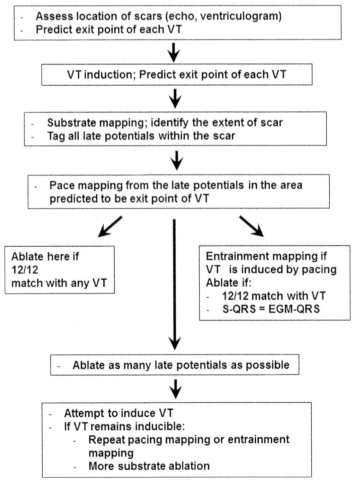

Fig. 3. The strategy of VT ablation in patients with ischemic cardiomyopathy in the electrophysiology laboratory of the University of Oklahoma.

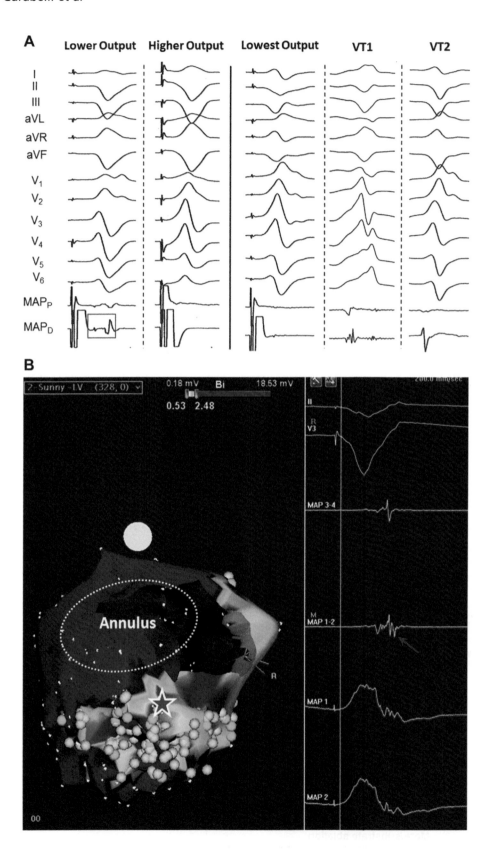

s-QRS interval and e-QRS interval suggest a more distal location, such as the exit, which is usually defined as less than 30% of the s-QRS/TCL. Common pitfalls of entrainment mapping include[1] pacing for too short a duration, or pacing at a cycle length (CL) that is too close to that of the VT to fully capture/entrain. Pacing with too low an output at a rate similar to the VT CL can also mislead physicians into thinking that capture occurred.

ENDOCARDIAL SUBSTRATE-BASED ABLATION

The strategy of ischemic VT ablation in the authors' laboratory is summarized in **Fig. 3**. Although substrate mapping has become the mainstay mapping strategy for VT ablation procedures, it is noteworthy that minimizing the noise level in the electrophysiology (EP) laboratory plays a determinant role in the success of such ablations. The amplitude of many of the late potentials is less than 0.1 mV. If the noise level in the EP laboratory is 0.1 mV, many of the viable myocardial bundles will be labeled as scars and will be missed, potentially leaving some VT circuits intact. In the authors' EP laboratory, ablation usually starts with targeting the late potentials in the predicted exit zone of the clinical VT. This zone is usually near the border of the scar and generally has a short QRS to late potential interval. After ablation begins, some of the late potentials previously recorded may disappear because ablation of a more proximal site in a channel may have an effect on the conduction of the downstream sites in the same channel.[21] If these sites are located in the predicted VT exit zone, we ablate these sites. These areas are potentially slow conduction zones if the activation wave front enters the scar from a different direction (eg, V-sensed rhythm vs V-paced rhythm).

CASE REVISITED

Two VTs were induced by RV burst pacing (see **Fig. 1**). Both had the same CL, and the predominant VT was VT1. An LV substrate map was created using the CARTO system (**Fig. 4**B). VT1 appeared to have a basal exit. High-output versus Low-output pacing at an inferior-basal LV site produced VT1-like and VT2-like morphology, respectively (**Fig. 4**A). In addition, pacing from this site with the lowest output that captured the myocardial tissue produced a QRS complex similar to VT2 (see **Fig. 4**A), which was predicted to have an apical exit. These findings suggest that part of the reentrant circuit of VT1 and VT2 may be in close proximity or overlap; higher pacing output may have captured the myocardial bundles that conduct through a long isthmus and exit at the basal aspect of the scar.

Entrainment was performed close to the annulus at the location shown in **Fig. 5**. The VT2 CL was 445 milliseconds, and the pacing CL was 415 milliseconds. Concealed entrainment with a PPI equal to the VT2 CL was produced. Note that pacing delivered at this site only captured part of the multicomponent late potential. The s-QRS and the e-QRS are equal at 365 milliseconds, accounting for 82% of the VT CL. Along with the findings of concealed entrainment, the entrainment site is either in an inner loop or at the entrance of a protected VT isthmus that may be long and convoluted. Because pace mapping (see **Fig. 4**A) suggests a long isthmus, radiofrequency current was delivered to this site and successfully eliminated this VT. Ablation targeting most of the late potentials were then performed. No VT was induced by RV pacing (burst pacing and programmed stimulation). The patient did not have VT recurrence for a 2-year follow-up period.

SUMMARY

VTs occurring after prior myocardial infarction are usually caused by reentrant circuits formed by surviving myocardial bundles. Although part of the reentrant circuits may be located in the midmyocardium or epicardium, most of the VTs can be safely and successfully ablated by endocardial ablation targeting the late potentials/LAVA, which are surrogates for the surviving myocardial bundles. A combination of activation, substrate, pace mapping, and entrainment mapping, as well

---

Fig. 4. (*A*) Pacing from a site showing a late potential located in the septal-basal aspect of the inferior wall scar produced 2 different morphologies. Lower bipolar pacing output likely captured only the local myocardium, producing an apical exit. Two potentials were not captured by pacing (*red box*). With high bipolar pacing output, more ventricular tissue was captured, leading to a more basal exit. Despite the inferior-basal location of the pacing site, the lowest pacing output capturing the local myocardium produced a QRS morphology that was predicted to be inferior-apical exit, nearly identical to VT2. (*B*) The red star indicates the site recording a late potential (*red arrow*) located in the inferior-basal aspect of the scar. Pink dots represent the sites showing late potentials. Blue dots represent pace mapping sites.

128

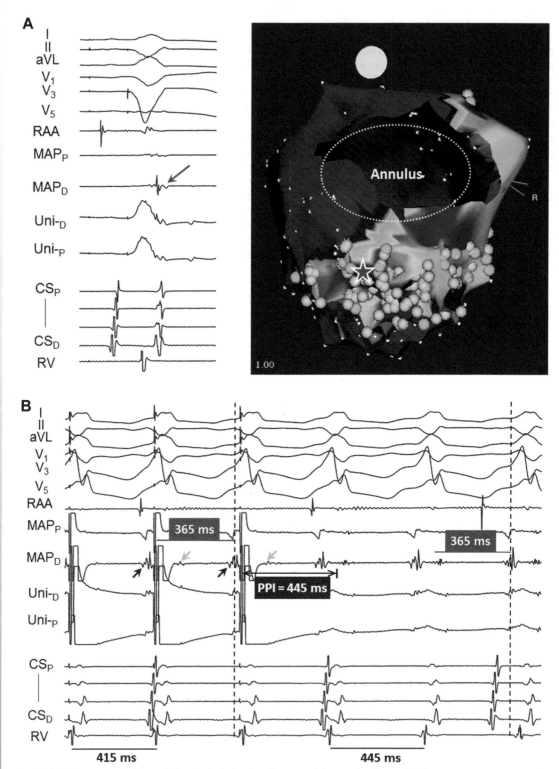

Fig. 5. (A) A late potential recorded at the inferior-basal aspect of the scar (*red arrow*). (B) Attempts at pace mapping induced VT2 (CL = 445 milliseconds). Entrainment (pacing CL = 415 milliseconds) delivered from this site produced concealed entrainment with a PPI equal to the VT2 CL. The stimulus-QRS was identical the EGM-QRS interval (365 milliseconds). Note that only part of the multicomponent late potential was captured by pacing. Electrograms, denoted by blue and green arrows, were not directly captured by the pacing electrode but were activated via slow-conducting myocardial bundles in the scar. Dotted vertical lines indicate the beginning of the QRS complex. Ablation at this site which is marked as a red star on the CARTO map, despite a very long stimulus-QRS or EGM-QRS interval, terminated VT in 2 seconds.

as use of contact force catheters, further improves ablation success and safety.

REFERENCES

1. Palaniswamy C, Kolte D, Harikrishnan P, et al. Catheter ablation of postinfarction ventricular tachycardia: ten-year trends in utilization, in-hospital complications, and in-hospital mortality in the United States. Heart Rhythm 2014;11(11):2056–63.
2. Miller JM, Marchlinski FE, Buxton AE, et al. Relationship between the 12-lead electrocardiogram during ventricular tachycardia and endocardial site of origin in patients with coronary artery disease. Circulation 1988;77(4):759–66.
3. Berruezo A, Mont L, Nava S, et al. Electrocardiographic recognition of the epicardial origin of ventricular tachycardias. Circulation 2004;109(15): 1842–7.
4. de Bakker JM, van Capelle FJ, Janse MJ, et al. Reentry as a cause of ventricular tachycardia in patients with chronic ischemic heart disease: electrophysiologic and anatomic correlation. Circulation 1988;77(3):589–606.
5. de Bakker JM, Coronel R, Tasseron S, et al. Ventricular tachycardia in the infarcted, Langendorff-perfused human heart: role of the arrangement of surviving cardiac fibers. J Am Coll Cardiol 1990; 15(7):1594–607.
6. Reddy VY, Neuzil P, Taborsky M, et al. Short-term results of substrate mapping and radiofrequency ablation of ischemic ventricular tachycardia using a saline-irrigated catheter. J Am Colle Cardiol 2003;41(12):2228–36.
7. Marchlinski FE, Callans DJ, Gottlieb CD, et al. Linear ablation lesions for control of unmappable ventricular tachycardia in patients with ischemic and nonischemic cardiomyopathy. Circulation 2000;101(11): 1288–96.
8. Zeppenfeld K, Kies P, Wijffels MC, et al. Identification of successful catheter ablation sites in patients with ventricular tachycardia based on electrogram characteristics during sinus rhythm. Heart Rhythm 2005;2(9):940–50.
9. Wrobleski D, Houghtaling C, Josephson ME, et al. Use of electrogram characteristics during sinus rhythm to delineate the endocardial scar in a porcine model of healed myocardial infarction. J Cardiovasc Electrophysiol 2003;14(5):524–9.
10. Callans DJ, Ren JF, Michele J, et al. Electroanatomic left ventricular mapping in the porcine model of healed anterior myocardial infarction. Correlation with intracardiac echocardiography and pathological analysis. Circulation 1999;100(16):1744–50.
11. Jaïs P, Maury P, Khairy P, et al. Elimination of local abnormal ventricular activities: a new end point for substrate modification in patients with scar-related ventricular tachycardia. Circulation 2012;125(18): 2184–96.
12. Brunckhorst CB, Stevenson WG, Jackman WM, et al. Ventricular mapping during atrial and ventricular pacing. Relationship of multipotential electrograms to ventricular tachycardia reentry circuits after myocardial infarction. Euro Heart J 2002; 23(14):1131–8.
13. Oza S, Wilber DJ. Substrate-based endocardial ablation of postinfarction ventricular tachycardia. Heart Rhythm 2006;3(5):607–9.
14. Arenal A, Glez-Torrecilla E, Ortiz M, et al. Ablation of electrograms with an isolated, delayed component as treatment of unmappable monomorphic ventricular tachycardias in patients with structural heart disease. J Am Coll Cardiol 2003;41(1):81–92.
15. Bogun F, Bahu M, Knight BP, et al. Response to pacing at sites of isolated diastolic potentials during ventricular tachycardia in patients with previous myocardial infarction. J Am Coll Cardiol 1997; 30(2):505–13.
16. Komatsu Y, Daly M, Sacher F, et al. Electrophysiologic characterization of local abnormal ventricular activities in postinfarction ventricular tachycardia with respect to their anatomic location. Heart Rhythm 2013;10(11):1630–7.
17. Soejima K, Stevenson WG, Maisel WH, et al. Electrically unexcitable scar mapping based on pacing threshold for identification of the reentry circuit isthmus: feasibility for guiding ventricular tachycardia ablation. Circulation 2002;106(13):1678–83.
18. Brunckhorst CB, Delacretaz E, Soejima K, et al. Identification of the ventricular tachycardia isthmus after infarction by pace mapping. Circulation 2004; 110(6):652–9.
19. Stevenson WG, Sager PT, Natterson PD, et al. Relation of pace mapping QRS configuration and conduction delay to ventricular tachycardia reentry circuits in human infarct scars. J Am Coll Cardiol 1995;26(2):481–8.
20. Stevenson WG, Friedman PL, Sager PT, et al. Exploring postinfarction reentrant ventricular tachycardia with entrainment mapping. J Am Coll Cardiol 1997;29(6):1180–9.
21. Tung R, Mathuria NS, Nagel R, et al. Impact of local ablation on interconnected channels within ventricular scar: mechanistic implications for substrate modification. Circ Arrhythm Electrophysiol 2013;6: 1131–8.

Pleomorphic Ventricular Tachycardias in Nonischemic Cardiomyopathy

CrossMark

Babak Nazer, MD, Henry H. Hsia, MD, FHRS*

KEYWORDS

- Ventricular tachycardia • Nonischemic cardiomyopathy • Myocardial substrate • Mapping
- Catheter ablation

KEY POINTS

- Two predominant regional scar distributions in nonischemic cardiomyopathy: basal inferolateral and anteroseptal locations.
- Myocardial depth of reentrant circuits contributes to the difficulties in VT ablation of in patients with nonischemic cardiomyopathy.
- Multiple morphologies of VT may be observed in patients with intramural septal substrate.
- Careful and systemic mapping is required to define the VT origin. Aggressive ablations are often required from both sides of the septum to achieve arrhythmia control.

CASE PRESENTATION

The patient is a 66-year-old man with a history of nonischemic cardiomyopathy (NICMP) and recurrent ventricular tachycardia (VT). His arrhythmia was refractory to multiple antiarrhythmic medications, including sotalol, procainamide, and mexiletine. The patient was also intolerant of quinidine and amiodarone because of side effects.

His past medical history was significant for hypertension, atrial fibrillation, and obstructive sleep apnea. He had previously presented with syncope and recurrent VT, and underwent implantation of a biventricular implantable cardioverter-defibrillator (ICD) for secondary prevention.

The patient had undergone 3 prior endocardial catheter ablations for recurrent VT over a 3-year period. Multiple morphologies of VTs were induced and mapped using pace mapping, activation mapping, and entrainment mapping. Voltage maps showed a dense left ventricular midanteroseptal scar. Extensive ablation with substrate modification was performed and resulted in complete heart block.

Echocardiogram showed left ventricular ejection fraction of 25% with global hypokinesis and regional variations. Moderate-to-severe mitral regurgitation was present with moderate left atrial enlargement. A computed tomography angiogram showed a globular left ventricle (LV) with prominent trabeculations, which was concerning for LV noncompaction. No myocardial delayed gadolinium enhancement was noted on MRI. Despite multiple ablations, the patient continued to experience incessant arrhythmias and ICD shocks. He is now referred for a repeat catheter ablation.

ELECTROPHYSIOLOGY STUDY AND CATHETER ABLATION

Electrophysiology study showed the presence of complete heart block. His bundle signal could not be recorded. Episodes of pleomorphic VT were reproducibly inducible with programmed

Cardiac Electrophysiology, University of California-San Francisco, San Francisco, CA, USA
* Corresponding author. Arrhythmia Service, VA San Francisco/MC, 111C-6, Building 203, Room 2A-52A, 4150 Clement Street, San Francisco, CA 94121.
E-mail address: henry.hsia@ucsf.edu

Card Electrophysiol Clin 8 (2016) 131–137
http://dx.doi.org/10.1016/j.ccep.2015.10.022
1877-9182/16/$ – see front matter Published by Elsevier Inc.

cardiacEP.theclinics.com

stimulation. The arrhythmia was hemodynamically tolerated, and therefore activation and entrainment mapping were performed.

The patient's initial electrocardiograms (ECGs) during VT showed variable QRS morphologies and cycle lengths (CLs), with a left bundle branch block (LBBB), inferior axis, and different precordial transition patterns (**Fig. 1**). Careful review of the ECG during sustained VT identified predominantly 2 distinct QRS morphologies with fusion beats (**Fig. 2**): VT 1 (LBBB, left inferior axis, late precordial transition at lead V5, CL 475 milliseconds) and VT 2 (LBBB, left inferior axis, early precordial transition at lead V3, CL 370–440 milliseconds).

Various electrocardiographic features may give clues to the likely site of origin.[1–4] The presence of LBBB pattern with inferior axis suggested arrhythmia originated from the outflow tract region. Based on specific ECG characteristics (QRS amplitude II > III, +aVL, late precordial transition), VT 1 was localized to the right ventricle (RV) septal region. Intracardiac echocardiography (CartoSound) was used for creation of the anatomic shells of the LV and RV. Mapping and radiofrequency (RF) ablation were performed using a 3.5-mm tip irrigated catheter (ThermoCool SF; Biosense Webster, Diamond Bar, CA) facilitated by an electroanatomic mapping system (CARTO 3; Biosense Webster). Bipolar electrogram (EGM) recordings were filtered at 30 to 500 Hz; unipolar EGM from the distal electrode was filtered at 0.05 to 150 Hz. Voltage map of the RV showed normal endocardial bipolar signal amplitudes. Activation mapping during VT showed an early (−40 milliseconds) bipolar EGM with QS pattern on unipolar recordings (**Fig. 3**) at the para-Hisian region. However, during episodes of

pleomorphism, the local EGM was not early for VT 2 (**Fig. 4**), which, along with the presence of fusion beats, suggested at least 2 exit sites from a septal/intramural focus or circuit. RF ablation from the RV targeting VT 1 at the para-Hisian location successfully terminated the arrhythmia after 6.0 seconds, and VT 1 was noninducible thereafter. However, monomorphic VT 2 remained inducible, although pleomorphism was no longer observed.

Mapping was subsequently focused on VT 2. Specific ECG characteristics (tall inferior lead amplitude, early precordial transition) suggested the site of origin to be the left ventricular outflow tract. LV bipolar voltage mapping showed a large area of septal scar (**Fig. 5**). During sustained VT 2, a low-amplitude, early (−149 milliseconds) mid-diastolic potential was noted at the basal septum at the left para-Hisian location (**Fig. 6**). Overdrive pacing at this site showed concealed fusion with a longer postpacing interval (PPI) of 560 milliseconds compared with the VT cycle length (488 milliseconds), and a longer stimulus-to-QRS (St-QRS) interval of 177 milliseconds compared with the EGM-QRS interval (142 milliseconds), that suggested an adjacent bystander site (**Fig. 7**). However, repeated pacing attempts at the same site revealed that the PPI was consistent with the longer of the spontaneous oscillating VT CLs (544 milliseconds) (**Fig. 8**). The longer St-QRS interval may be caused by additional conduction delay in the reentrant circuit during pacing, through an area of dense, previously ablated scar. Repeated entrainment attempts at the same site during stable VT CLs confirmed an isthmus site (see **Fig. 8**), and RF application at this point terminated VT 2 after 4.7 seconds. VT was noninducible at the end of the procedure.

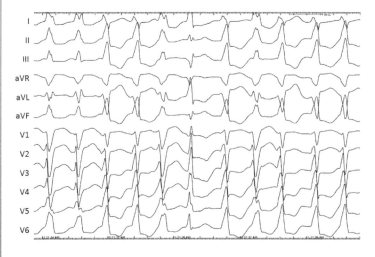

Fig. 1. Induced pleomorphic VT with variable QRS morphologies and cycle lengths. The predominant morphology has a left-bundle-branch block (LBBB), inferior axis with different precordial transition patterns.

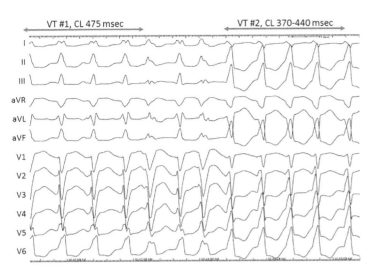

Fig. 2. During episodes of pleomorphism, predominantly two QRS morphologies were identified. VT #1 (LBBB-left-inferior axis, late precordial transition at lead V5, CL 475 ms) and VT #2 (LBBB-left-inferior axis, early precordial transition at lead V3, CL 370-440 ms).

DISCUSSION

Compared with patients with postinfarction VT undergoing ablation, patients with NICMP VT show higher recurrence rates of VT and ICD shocks, ranging 31% to 66% in long-term follow-up.[5–7] One possible explanation for higher VT recurrence rates among patients with NICMP is disease progression with formation of new scar and potential reentry circuits (as opposed to static scar in patients with postinfarct VT). Another difference that may explain this difference in outcomes is the distribution of scar. Because of coronary perfusion gradients, the infarct distribution of patients with ischemic cardiomyopathy is predominantly subendocardial, corresponding with large areas of scar on endocardial electroanatomic bipolar voltage mapping.[8] By contrast, scar in patients with NICMP is more often located in the midmyocardium or epicardium, and is associated with smaller areas of endocardial bipolar voltage map scar[8,9] and larger areas of epicardial bipolar voltage map scar than scar in patients with postinfarct VT.[8,10] Endocardial unipolar voltage mapping may also be used to predict areas of epicardial scar.[11] Accordingly, NICMP VT isthmuses are more commonly associated with epicardial than endocardial scar,[12] and epicardial mapping is commonly used in patients with NICMP VT requiring catheter ablation.

Among patients with NICMP VT, detailed multimodality imaging, such as MRI[13] and

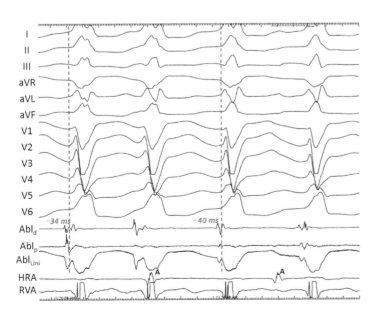

Fig. 3. Activation mapping at the para-Hisian region. Recordings during VT #1 QRS demonstrated early (−34 to −40 msec) pre-QRS bipolar electrograms with a QS pattern on the unipolar signals, suggesting an exit site.

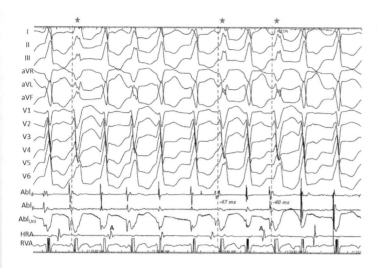

Fig. 4. Pleomorphic QRS with alternating VT #1 and VT #2 morphologies and fusion. Notice that the local bipolar and unipolar electrograms were early for VT #1 QRS (*stars*) but late for VT #2 QRS.

electroanatomic mapping studies,[14] has shown 2 predominant regional scar distributions: basal inferolateral (47%–49% of patients) and basal anteroseptal (42%–51%). Among the latter group, the subset with predominantly septal scar poses particular challenges. Patients with NICMP VT with septal scar have high long-term VT recurrence rates of 32% to 60%,[14,15] and often require multiple ablations targeting the septal substrate. One contributing factor may be that septal scar can be located intramurally, effectively shielded from RF energy delivered from either the RV or LV. Midseptal substrate, as suggested by normal bipolar but low unipolar voltage maps of the septum, was detected in 29% of septal VT cases.[15] In contrast with patients with NICMP with the predominant inferolateral scar distribution pattern, epicardial mapping and ablation is of low yield in this population.

The case described earlier shows many of the unique challenges facing patients with NICMP VT. This patient's voltage maps were most consistent with the basal anteroseptal pattern, and prior ablations had targeted this area. His presenting pleomorphic VT was consistent with variable fusion from multiple exit sites involving a septal reentrant circuit, and a local EGM that was early with 1 QRS, but not the other. Despite a normal RV endocardial bipolar voltage (>1.5 mV), 1 of the exits was located at the RV septum, because a single ablation lesion at this site eliminated QRS fusion and rendered the VT monomorphic. This finding is consistent with the observation that subendocardial, intramural scar may not be detectable using bipolar EGM recording.[16] LV mapping revealed a large, dense, basal septal scar across from the RV para-Hisian exit (see **Fig. 5**).

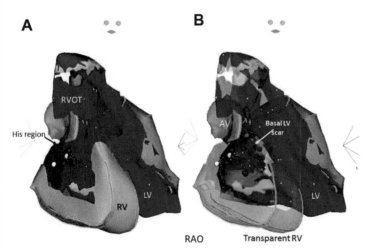

Fig. 5. Electroanatomical mapping coupled with the endocardial shells constructed using ICE. (*A*) showed voltage maps of the RV and RVOT superimposed on the LV. The color scheme depicts "Normal" tissue with signal amplitude >1.5 mV (*purple*), "Dense scar" with signal amplitude <0.5 mV (*red*), and the "Border" as transition zone between dense scar and normal tissue (0.5 to 1.5 mV). The RV endocardial voltage map showed no endocardial low voltage area/scar. Early pre-QRS recording was marked by the yellow dot at the para-Hisian site. Red dots represent ablation lesions. (*B*)showed a transparent RV/RVOT map. LV bipolar voltage map demonstrated a large basal septal scar. ICE, intracardiac echocardiogram; RVOT, right ventricular outflow tract; AV, aortic valve; RV, right ventricle; LV, left ventricle.

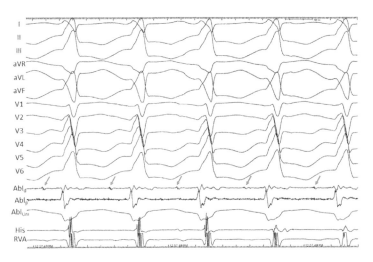

Fig. 6. During persistently inducible slower LBB-LI VT #2, CL 490 msec, a low amplitude early (−149 ms) bipolar potential (*arrow*) was recorded at the basal septum. The unipolar recording was at the QRS onset (∼0 msec).

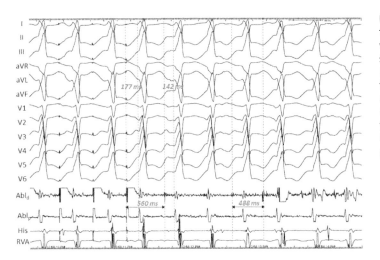

Fig. 7. Overdrive pacing during sustained LBB-LI VT #2. Entrainment with concealed fusion was demonstrated with a longer post-pacing interval (PPI=560 msec) compared to the VT cycle length (488 msec), and a longer stimulus-to-QRS (St-QRS=177 msec) interval compared to the electrogram-to-QRS (EGM-QRS=142 msec) interval that suggested an adjacent bystander site.

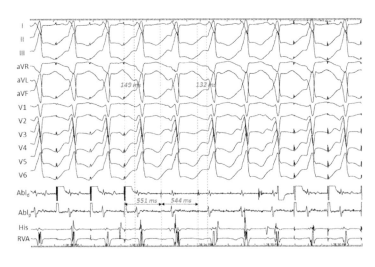

Fig. 8. Repeated pacing attempts at the same site during LBB-LI VT #2 demonstrated concealed fusion. The post-pacing interval (PPI) of 551 msec nearly equaled the VT cycle length of 544 msec during rate oscillations. The stimulus-to-QRS interval (st-QRS) was 149 msec, similar to the electrogram-to-QRS interval (egm-QRS) of 132 msec that suggested an isthmus site.

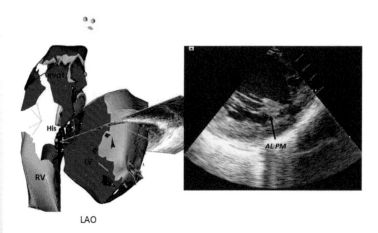

LAO

Fig. 9. Electroanatomical maps of both RV and LV, demonstrating ablation lesions (*red dots*) on both sides of the septum. The intracardiac echocardiographic (ICE) view revealed a short-axis image of LV, depicting the anterolateral papillary muscle (AL PM) and prominent trabeculations (*red arrows*) suggestive of non-compaction.

Entrainment mapping of VT 2 was also misleading, and the initial interpretation suggested the presence of an adjacent bystander site (with PPI > TCL and St-QRS > EGM-QRS). However, significant baseline cycle length oscillation was noted, most likely caused by the presence of dense septal scar with multiple prior ablations. Overdrive pacing can cause further conduction delay that contributed to a longer PPI. With careful analysis and patience, an LV isthmus site for VT 2 was eventually identified and successfully ablated.

Myocardial depth of reentrant circuits contributes to the difficulties in ablating NICMP VT, particularly the subset with isolated septal substrate. Aggressive ablations are often required from both sides of the septum to achieve arrhythmia control (**Fig. 9**). This clinical shortcoming has stimulated research and development of novel ablation technologies for ablating deep, three-dimensional VT substrates, such as RF needle catheter,[17] bipolar RF ablation from RV to LV,[18] and high-intensity focused ultrasonography.[19] Until these tools are readily available, these deep, three-dimensional substrates must be systematically mapped and ablated from both the RV and LV sides, with careful attention to multiple exit sites.

REFERENCES

1. Yamauchi Y, Aonuma K, Takahashi A, et al. Electrocardiographic characteristics of repetitive monomorphic right ventricular tachycardia originating near the His-bundle. J Cardiovasc Electrophysiol 2005; 16:1041–8.

2. Hutchinson MD, Garcia FC. An organized approach to the localization, mapping, and ablation of outflow tract ventricular arrhythmias. J Cardiovasc Electrophysiol 2013;24(10):1189–97.

3. Jadonath RL, Schwartzman DS, Preminger MW, et al. Utility of the 12-lead electrocardiogram in localizing the origin of right ventricular outflow tract tachycardia. Am Heart J 1995;130:1107–13.

4. Yoshida N, Inden Y, Uchikawa T, et al. Novel transitional zone index allows more accurate differentiation between idiopathic right ventricular outflow tract and aortic sinus cusp ventricular arrhythmias. Heart Rhythm 2011;8:349–56.

5. Tung R, Michowitz Y, Yu R, et al. Epicardial ablation of ventricular tachycardia: an institutional experience of safety and efficacy. Heart Rhythm 2013;10: 490–8.

6. Schmidt B, Chun KRJ, Baensch D, et al. Catheter ablation for ventricular tachycardia after failed endocardial ablation: epicardial substrate or inappropriate endocardial ablation? Heart Rhythm 2010;7: 1746–52.

7. Tokuda M, Tedrow UB, Kojodjojo P, et al. Catheter ablation of ventricular tachycardia in nonischemic heart disease. Circ Arrhythm Electrophysiol 2012;5: 992–1000.

8. Nakahara S, Tung R, Ramirez RJ, et al. Characterization of the arrhythmogenic substrate in ischemic and nonischemic cardiomyopathy. Implications for catheter ablation of hemodynamically unstable ventricular tachycardia. J Am Coll Cardiol 2010;55:2355–65.

9. Hsia HH, Callans DJ, Marchlinski FE. Characterization of endocardial electrophysiological substrate in patients with nonischemic cardiomyopathy and monomorphic ventricular tachycardia. Circulation 2003;108:704–10.

10. Cano O, Hutchinson M, Lin D, et al. Electroanatomic substrate and ablation outcome for suspected epicardial ventricular tachycardia in left ventricular nonischemic cardiomyopathy. J Am Coll Cardiol 2009;54:799–808.

11. Hutchinson MD, Gerstenfeld EP, Desjardins B, et al. Endocardial unipolar voltage mapping to detect

epicardial ventricular tachycardia substrate in patients with nonischemic left ventricular cardiomyopathy. Circ Arrhythm Electrophysiol 2011;4:49–55.

12. Soejima K, Stevenson WG, Sapp JL, et al. Endocardial and epicardial radiofrequency ablation of ventricular tachycardia associated with dilated cardiomyopathy: the importance of low-voltage scars. J Am Coll Cardiol 2004;43:1834–42.

13. Piers SRD, Tao Q, van Huls van Taxis CFB, et al. Contrast-enhanced MRI-derived scar patterns and associated ventricular tachycardias in nonischemic cardiomyopathy: implications for the ablation strategy. Circ Arrhythm Electrophysiol 2013;6:875–83.

14. Oloriz T, Silberbauer J, MacCabelli G, et al. Catheter ablation of ventricular arrhythmia in nonischemic cardiomyopathy: anteroseptal versus inferolateral scar sub-types. Circ Arrhythm Electrophysiol 2014; 7:414–23.

15. Haqqani HM, Tschabrunn CM, Tzou WS, et al. Isolated septal substrate for ventricular tachycardia in nonischemic dilated cardiomyopathy: incidence, characterization, and implications. Heart Rhythm 2011;8:1169–76.

16. Dickfeld T, Tian J, Ahmad G, et al. MRI-guided ventricular tachycardia ablation integration of late gadolinium-enhanced 3D scar in patients with implantable cardioverter-defibrillators. Circ Arrhythm Electrophysiol 2011;4:172–84.

17. Sapp JL, Beeckler C, Pike R, et al. Initial human feasibility of infusion needle catheter ablation for refractory ventricular tachycardia. Circulation 2013; 128(21):2289–95.

18. Koruth JS, Dukkipati S, Miller MA, et al. Bipolar irrigated radiofrequency ablation: a therapeutic option for refractory intramural atrial and ventricular tachycardia circuits. Heart Rhythm 2012;9:1932–41.

19. Koruth JS, Dukkipati S, Carrillo RG, et al. Safety and efficacy of high-intensity focused ultrasound atop coronary arteries during epicardial catheter ablation. J Cardiovasc Electrophysiol 2011;22:1274–80.

Ventricular Tachycardia in a Patient with Biventricular Noncompaction

Jaime E. Gonzalez, MD, Wendy Tzou, MD,
William H. Sauer, MD, Duy Thai Nguyen, MD*

KEYWORDS

• Catheter ablation • Ventricular tachycardia • Noncompaction • Epicardial ablation

KEY POINTS

- Patients with ventricular noncompaction are susceptible to developing ventricular tachycardia.
- Commonly, the origin of ventricular tachycardia is endocardial; however, epicardial origins and scar cannot be excluded and should be considered when poor endocardial mapping is present.
- Other cardiomyopathies, such as arrhythmogenic right ventricular cardiomyopathy, can coexist with ventricular noncompaction and should be excluded in these patients.

INTRODUCTION

A 19-year-old woman with a history of biventricular noncompaction and ventricular tachycardia (VT) presented with recurrent VT despite antiarrhythmic therapy. She had 2 prior endocardial VT ablations targeting the low septal right ventricular outflow tract (RVOT) with acute success. Several months later, she had recurrence with VT storm and multiple implantable cardioverter-defibrillator shocks after failed antitachycardia pacing. She presented in sinus rhythm (**Fig. 1**) and was referred for a repeat VT ablation.

ELECTROPHYSIOLOGY STUDY AND ABLATION

Venous access was obtained in the standard fashion and a quadripolar catheter and an irrigated-tip, contact force–sensing ablation catheter were advanced into the right ventricle. An endocardial voltage map was performed in sinus rhythm, and areas of scar were noted around the tricuspid valve and in the low anterior RVOT,

where her prior ablations were performed (**Fig. 2**). Next, programmed ventricular extrastimulation induced VT1 with a left bundle branch block (LBBB) morphology, inferior axis (II > III), and precordial transition by V4 (**Fig. 3**). Activation mapping during VT localized the earliest activation at the lateral superior tricuspid annulus, within the previously delineated area of low voltage. A near exit site was identified using entrainment mapping (**Fig. 4**), and ablation performed near this site resulted in termination of the VT. Further consolidation of the ablation lesions was performed.

VT2, which also had an LBBB-type QRS morphology with an inferior axis, was then induced. Earliest activation was mapped to areas of scar within the low lateral RVOT, near previous ablation sites. Ablation resulted in termination of this VT and additional consolidation lesions were also applied. Ventricular extrastimulation was again performed that induced a faster VT3, with a left bundle branch morphology, left inferior axis, and a precordial transition by V5 (see **Fig. 3**). This VT was not hemodynamically tolerated despite vasopressors, and attempts at pace

Cardiac Electrophysiology, Cardiology Division, University of Colorado, Denver, Anschutz Medical Campus, 12401 East 17th Avenue, B-132, Aurora, CO 80045, USA
* Corresponding author.
E-mail address: duy.t.nguyen@ucdenver.edu

Card Electrophysiol Clin 8 (2016) 139–144
http://dx.doi.org/10.1016/j.ccep.2015.10.014

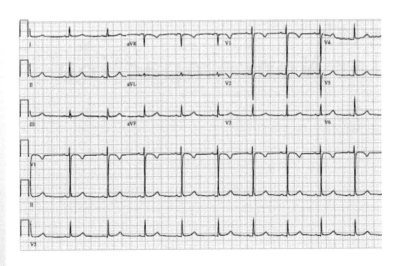

Fig. 1. Sinus rhythm electrocardiogram showing T-wave inversions in V1 and V2.

termination changed the VT to other untolerated VTs (VT4–VT8; see **Fig. 3**) that eventually required cardioversion. Brief endocardial activation mapping had no areas of early activation of VT3. Pace mapping was performed throughout the right ventricular endocardium and coronary sinus without good pace maps for any of the VTs.

QUESTION

What is the next step in mapping unstable VTs with a left bundle branch morphology in patients with ventricular noncompaction?

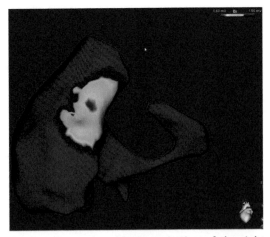

Fig. 2. Left anterior oblique projection of the right ventricular voltage map showing the low septal RVOT scar, consistent with the areas targeted for ablation during the patient's prior VT ablations. Areas of dense scare in red are defined as a voltage of less than 0.5 mV. Areas of normal myocardium are purple and defined as a voltage of greater than 1.5 mV.

The morphologies of VT3 to VT8, LBBB with a late precordial transition, suggested a right ventricular origin of the VT. These hemodynamically untolerated VTs had wider QRS durations than VT1 and VT2 targeted in the endocardium (QRS >174 ± 37 milliseconds) and had longer maximum deflection indices (>0.55) and pseudo-R waves (>34 milliseconds) (**Table 1**).[1] These electrocardiogram (ECG) morphologic features, along with poor endocardial activation and pace maps, suggest a right ventricular epicardial origin of the VTs.[2] Given that multiple VTs were still inducible, and given her history of VT storm and prior unsuccessful endocardial ablations, epicardial access was obtained via the subxyphoid anterior approach.

Epicardial voltage mapping in sinus rhythm was performed that showed a large area of right ventricular epicardial scar notable for sparing of the left ventricle. Within the scar, there were multiple channels, where electrograms in sinus rhythm showed late potentials (**Figs. 5** and **6**). These channels were defined using color thresholds of greater than 1.0 mV for normal tissue and less than 0.5 mV for dense scar. Programmed stimulation was once again performed inducing VT4. Mid-diastolic potentials (MDPs) were noted within these channels (see **Fig. 5**). Attempts to entrain the MDPs were unsuccessful, and the patient was defibrillated because of hemodynamic instability.

DISCUSSION

Ventricular noncompaction results from alterations in myocardial morphogenesis that leads to prominent endocardial trabeculations, most commonly in the left ventricle. The thickened noncompacted

Ventricular Tachycardias

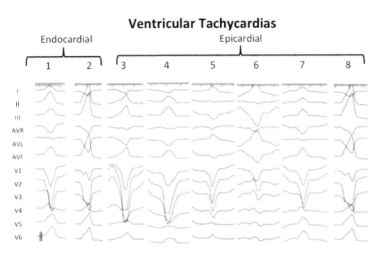

Fig. 3. QRS morphologies of the 8 different VTs that were induced throughout the study. VT1 and VT2 were endocardial VTs. VTs 3 to 8 were epicardial VTs.

endocardium is thought to predispose patients to endocardial ventricular arrhythmias. The pathophysiology of VT in noncompaction is not completely understood. There is pathologic evidence of scar in the subendocardium of patients with noncompaction that could act as substrate for ventricular arrhythmias.[3] However, there have been a few case reports of epicardial left VTs in patients with noncompaction.[4–6] There are also rare reports of combined arrhythmogenic right ventricular cardiomyopathy (ARVC) and noncompaction.[3,4] Desmoplakin gene mutations, present

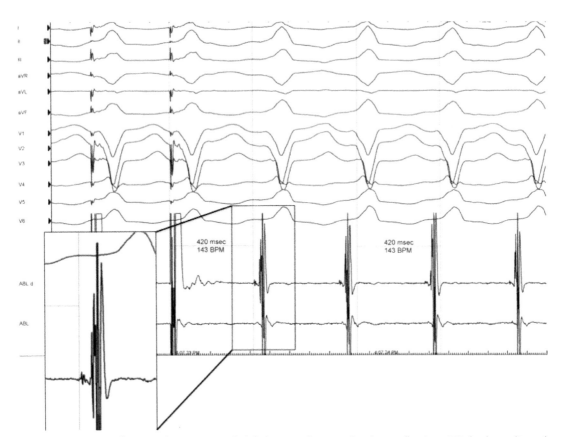

Fig. 4. Entrainment of VT1 with near-concealed fusion, PPI (post pacing interval) minus TCL (tachycardia cycle length) of 0 milliseconds, and S-QRS/TCL less than 30% indicated a site near the VT exit.

Table 1
VT characteristics

VT	QRS Duration	Pseudodelta	Maximum Deflection Index
1	144	30	0.65
2	157	28	0.33
3	178	88	0.74
4	191	82	0.76
5	191	81	0.62
6	163	43	0.72
7	147	46	0.44
8	174	58	0.69

in patients with ARVC, have also been noted to occur in particularly aggressive forms of arrhythmogenic left ventricular cardiomyopathy and noncompaction.[5] This finding suggests that there could be epicardial substrate for ventricular arrhythmias in patients with noncompaction.

The patient's cardiac MRI was clearly consistent with noncompaction with a noncompacted to compacted myocardium ration of 3.7, much greater than the diagnostic MRI threshold of 2.3[7] (see **Fig. 6**B, C). Even though our voltage map is

suspicious for ARVC, her sinus rhythm ECG showed no major criteria for ARVC (see **Fig. 1**) and she currently only meets 1 major criterion for ARVC (induced left bundle superiorly directed VT). Genetic testing has been pursued but financial issues and patient reluctance have delayed this evaluation.

Hemodynamically unstable VTs are challenging to target because entrainment and localization of the critical isthmus during tachycardia is difficult. Other strategies for targeting unmappable VTs include substrate modification, electrical scar isolation, and ablation of local abnormal ventricular activity (LAVA).[7–10] Substrate modification involves pace mapping near the border zones of the scar in order to identify potential exit or isthmus sites of the VT and perform linear ablation at these sites.[7] Electrical isolation entails performing circumferential ablation around the areas of scar in order to achieve electrical isolation of the scar, which is proved by pacing inside the scar without global ventricular capture.[8] To perform LAVA ablation, ablation is performed targeting low-amplitude signals recorded in areas of delayed conduction that may represent the site of the VT's critical isthmus.[9,10] Other options, not pursued in this case, include the use of ventricular assist devices, such as an Impella or

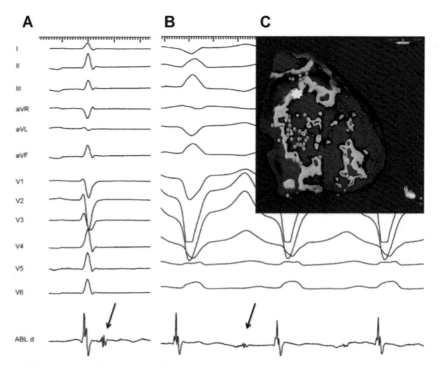

Fig. 5. Epicardial late potentials and local abnormal ventricular activity (*arrow*) in sinus rhythm are shown (*A*), with corresponding mid-diastolic potential (*arrow*) in VT (*B*). Location of late potentials (*yellow star*) on the epicardial map is shown (*C*).

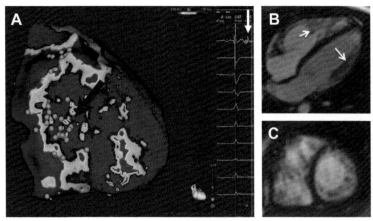

Fig. 6. (*A*) Right anterior oblique (RAO) projection of epicardial voltage map. Red areas indicate dense scar with a voltage of less than 0.5 mV. Purple areas indicate normal myocardium with a voltage of greater than 1.0 mV. Blue lesion tags represent areas with late potentials (*white arrow*). The black arrow points to a lesion tag representing the late potential shown in the side panel. (*B* and *C*) Short-axis and long-axis views of MRI with white arrows showing areas of noncompacted myocardium. Left ventricle noncompacted to compacted ratio of 3.7 (values >2.3 are diagnostic of noncompaction).

extracorporeal mechanical oxygenation, to provide hemodynamic support during VT.[11]

In our case, epicardial pace mapping was performed near the scar channels and there was an excellent pace match to 1 of the unstable VTs (**Fig. 7**). Extensive epicardial ablation was performed around the areas of scar eliminating all channels, late potentials, and LAVAs, which was confirmed by remapping over these areas. Pacing was performed around the areas of ablation and additional radiofrequency lesions were delivered at sites of pace capture. Noninvasive programmed stimulation down to 400 triple extrastimulation performed several days after ablation was unable to induce any VT. The patient has not had recurrence of VT during follow-up.

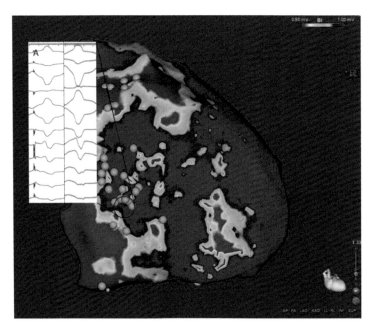

Fig. 7. RAO projection of epicardial voltage map. Red areas indicate dense scar with a voltage of less than 0.5 mV. Purple areas indicate normal myocardium with a voltage of greater than 1.0 mV. Blue lesion tags represent areas with late potentials. The inset panel A shows a near 12/12 pace map of VT6 on the left with VT6 on the right, highlighting the possible location of this VT.

SUMMARY

Patients with ventricular noncompaction are susceptible to developing VT. Commonly, the origin of VT is endocardial; however, epicardial origins and scar cannot be excluded and should be considered when poor endocardial mapping is present. Other cardiomyopathies, such as ARVC, can coexist with ventricular noncompaction and should be excluded in these patients.

REFERENCES

1. Berruezo A, Mont L, Nava S, et al. Electrocardiographic recognition of the epicardial origin of ventricular tachycardias. Circulation 2004;109:1842–7.
2. Martinek M, Stevenson WG, Inada K, et al. QRS characteristics fail to reliably identify ventricular tachycardias that require epicardial ablation in ischemic heart disease. J Cardiovasc Electrophysiol 2012;23:188–93.
3. Chinushi M, Iijima K, Furushima H, et al. Suppression of storms of ventricular tachycardia by epicardial ablation of isolated delayed potential in noncompaction cardiomyopathy. Pacing Clin Electrophysiol 2013;36:e115–9.
4. Lim HE, Pak HN, Shim WJ, et al. Epicardial ablation of ventricular tachycardia associated with isolated ventricular noncompaction. Pacing Clin Electrophysiol 2006;29:797–9.
5. López-Ayala JM, Gómez-Milanés I, Sánchez Muñoz JJ, et al. Desmoplakin truncations and arrhythmogenic left ventricular cardiomyopathy: characterizing a phenotype. Europace 2014;16: 1838–46.
6. Petersen SE, Selvanayagam JB, Wiesmann F, et al. Left ventricular non-compaction: insights from cardiovascular magnetic resonance imaging. J Am Coll Cardiol 2005;46:101–5.
7. Soejima K, Suzuki M, Maisel WH, et al. Catheter ablation in patients with multiple and unstable ventricular tachycardias after myocardial infarction: short ablation lines guided by reentry circuit isthmuses and sinus rhythm mapping. Circulation 2001;104:664–9.
8. Tilz RR, Makimoto H, Lin T, et al. Electrical isolation of a substrate after myocardial infarction: a novel ablation strategy for unmappable ventricular tachycardias–feasibility and clinical outcome. Europace 2014;16:1040–52.
9. Jaïs P, Maury P, Khairy P, et al. Elimination of local abnormal ventricular activities: a new end point for substrate modification in patients with scar-related ventricular tachycardia. Circulation 2012;125:2184–96.
10. Sacher F, Lim HS, Derval N, et al. Substrate mapping and ablation for ventricular tachycardia: the LAVA approach. J Cardiovasc Electrophysiol 2014; 26(4):464–71.
11. Reddy YM, Chinitz L, Mansour M, et al. Percutaneous left ventricular assist devices in ventricular tachycardia ablation: multicenter experience. Circ Arrhythm Electrophysiol 2014;7:244–50.

Section 3: Atrial Fibrillation and Flutter

Editor: Edward P. Gerstenfeld

Concomitant Isolation of the Pulmonary Veins and Posterior Wall Using a Box Lesion Set in a Patient with Persistent Atrial Fibrillation and Variant Pulmonary Venous Anatomy

CrossMark

Jason D. Roberts, MD, Edward P. Gerstenfeld, MD*

KEYWORDS

- Pulmonary vein • Isolation • Atrial fibrillation • Variant pulmonary venous anatomy • Adenosine

KEY POINTS

- Variant pulmonary venous anatomy is common and its pre-procedural recognition through cardiac imaging facilitates a personalized approach to ablation tailored to the individual patient.
- Close juxtaposition of the right and left pulmonary veins is an anatomic variation that serves as an ideal substrate for creation of a single box lesion set that concomitantly isolates the pulmonary veins and posterior wall.
- Isolation of the posterior wall may be an effective adjunctive ablative therapy among patients with persistent atrial fibrillation.
- Routine assessment for dormant conduction with adenosine serves as a valuable tool to assess for durability of ablation lesions and may improve clinical outcomes.

CLINICAL HISTORY

A 61-year-old man with a mildly reduced left ventricular ejection fraction was evaluated for symptomatic persistent atrial fibrillation. Because of the additional presence of marked sinus bradycardia and a prolonged QT interval, he was thought to be a poor candidate for medical therapy and was referred for catheter ablation. Preprocedure computed tomography and intraprocedural electroanatomic mapping revealed that the right and left pulmonary veins were closely juxtaposed on the posterior wall (**Fig. 1**).

CLINICAL QUESTION

How should ablation for atrial fibrillation be approached in this patient with variant pulmonary vein anatomy?

CLINICAL COURSE

Our standard approach to pulmonary vein isolation consists of wide-area circumferential ablation, encircling each pair of pulmonary veins together as a unit. Given the close proximity of the right-sided and left-sided veins in the current patient, this

Section of Cardiac Electrophysiology, Division of Cardiology, Department of Medicine, University of California San Francisco, San Francisco, CA, USA
* Corresponding author. 500 Parnassus Avenue, San Francisco, CA 94143.
E-mail address: egerstenfeld@medicine.ucsf.edu

Card Electrophysiol Clin 8 (2016) 145–149
http://dx.doi.org/10.1016/j.ccep.2015.10.015
1877-9182/16/$ – see front matter © 2016 Elsevier Inc. All rights reserved.

Fig. 1. Cranial (*left*) and posteroanterior (PA; *right*) computed tomography images of the left atrium showing the close proximity of the left-sided and right-sided pulmonary veins.

approach is likely to result in an intersection of our ablation lines along the posterior wall. As an alternative, we elected to isolate the pulmonary veins and posterior wall as a unit by a drawing a box lesion set (**Fig. 2**). In addition to facilitating electrical isolation of the pulmonary veins, isolation of the posterior wall may also be advantageous given its suggested importance in maintaining persistent atrial fibrillation.

Following creation of the box lesion set, there was apparent entrance block involving the posterior wall and all 4 pulmonary veins (**Fig. 3**). Electrical cardioversion to sinus rhythm was then performed and pacing along the 20 poles of the circular mapping catheter within the posterior wall was consistent with exit block (**Fig. 4**). Exit block was also evident in the left-sided and right inferior pulmonary veins, but a residual connection was observed in the right superior pulmonary vein. Further ablation along the left atrial roof just medial to the right superior pulmonary vein

resulted in entrance and exit block. However, following administration of 6 mg of intravenous adenosine, transient reconnection was noted (**Fig. 5**). On performing subsequent ablation along the roof line near the right superior pulmonary vein, no further evidence of reconnection was observed in response to further infusions of adenosine.

DISCUSSION

Variant pulmonary venous anatomy is common, with prior reports suggesting its presence in approximately 30% to 40% of patients undergoing ablation for atrial fibrillation.[1,2] The most common anatomic variations are a common left trunk and right-sided accessory veins, whereas less common variants include aberrant pulmonary vein ostia arising from the roof and posterior wall. The presence of variant anatomy may require an alternative approach to ablation in order to

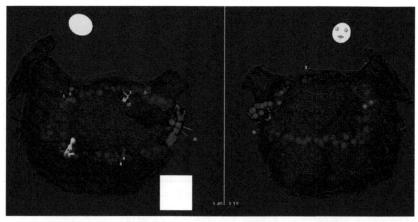

Fig. 2. PA (*left*) and anteroposterior (*right*) electroanatomic images of the box lesion set encompassing the left-sided and right-sided pulmonary veins, along with the posterior wall. The points 1,2,3,4 are landmark points used from registration of the computed tomographic scan to the electroanatomic map.

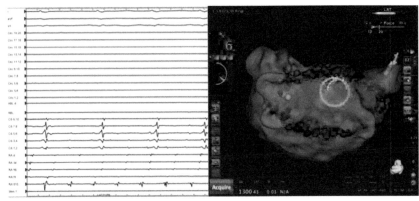

Fig. 3. Electrically silent circular mapping catheter (Circ) on the posterior wall consistent with entrance block. CS, coronary sinus; RA, right atrium.

isolate each vein; however, there is discord in the literature regarding its impact on procedural outcomes.[3,4]

The box lesion set that concomitantly isolated the pulmonary veins and posterior wall took advantage of the rare variant anatomy observed in our patient involving the close proximity of the right-sided and left-sided veins along the posterior wall. The posterior wall has been suggested to be capable of harboring organized high-frequency activity that may play a critical role in the maintenance of persistent forms of the arrhythmia.[5,6] This notion highlights the potential value of isolating the posterior wall among these patients, an approach that has been successfully used in the context of surgical ablation for atrial fibrillation.[7,8] Our box lesion set may not be suitable for most patients, but it could serve as an ideal approach to ablation among individuals with this form of variant anatomy that may facilitate the procedure and could conceivably be associated with improved outcomes. This approach also limited lesions along the posterior wall, which increase the risk of esophageal injury.

Our case also serves to show the value of using adenosine to examine for the presence of dormant conduction across ablation lesions, which is associated with an increased risk of pulmonary vein reconnection and recurrent atrial fibrillation following apparent successful ablation. Pulmonary vein reconnection is thought to be an important contributor to poor outcomes among patients

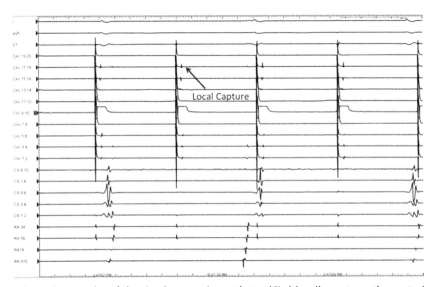

Fig. 4. Pacing along the 20 poles of the circular mapping catheter (Circ) locally captures the posterior wall; however, the electrical impulse fails to reach the surrounding atria, which is consistent with exit block. Ventricular beats 1 and 3 are junctional in origin.

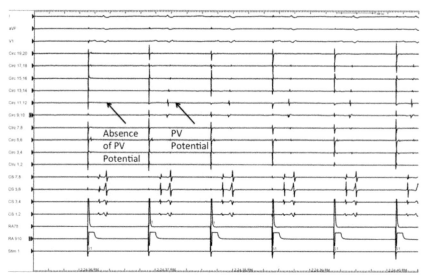

Fig. 5. Transient reconnection of potentials inside the right superior pulmonary vein (PV) following administration of 6 mg of intravenous adenosine.

undergoing atrial fibrillation ablation.[9,10] Radiofrequency catheter ablation induces cellular necrosis through delivery of thermal energy that results in extreme membrane depolarization and ensuing cellular inexcitably.[11] When insufficient thermal energy is delivered to achieve cellular necrosis, membrane depolarization may occur and cells may become dormant. Adenosine has been shown to hyperpolarize dormant cells, rendering them reexcitable and capable of conducting, which may manifest clinically as transient pulmonary vein reconnection.[11] Insight into this phenomenon has led to the use of intraprocedural adenosine to identify pulmonary veins at increased risk of reconnection, alerting the operator to the need to perform additional ablation in order to ensure a durable long-term result.[12,13] Given the known high prevalence of pulmonary vein reconnection after catheter ablation, we think that routine use of adenosine after ablation is important. Preablation imaging remains important to identify variant anatomy, as described in this case.

REFERENCES

1. Kato R, Lickfett L, Meininger G, et al. Pulmonary vein anatomy in patients undergoing catheter ablation of atrial fibrillation: lessons learned by use of magnetic resonance imaging. Circulation 2003; 107:2004–10.

2. Mansour M, Holmvang G, Sosnovik D, et al. Assessment of pulmonary vein anatomic variability by magnetic resonance imaging: implications for catheter ablation techniques for atrial fibrillation. J Cardiovasc Electrophysiol 2004;15:387–93.

3. Hof I, Chilukuri K, Arbab-Zadeh A, et al. Does left atrial volume and pulmonary venous anatomy predict the outcome of catheter ablation of atrial fibrillation? J Cardiovasc Electrophysiol 2009;20:1005–10.

4. Hunter RJ, Ginks M, Ang R, et al. Impact of variant pulmonary vein anatomy and image integration on long-term outcome after catheter ablation for atrial fibrillation. Europace 2010;12:1691–7.

5. Mandapati R, Skanes A, Chen J, et al. Stable microreentrant sources as a mechanism of atrial fibrillation in the isolated sheep heart. Circulation 2000;101: 194–9.

6. Kalifa J, Tanaka K, Zaitsev AV, et al. Mechanisms of wave fractionation at boundaries of high-frequency excitation in the posterior left atrium of the isolated sheep heart during atrial fibrillation. Circulation 2006;113:626–33.

7. Cox JL, Schuessler RB, Boineau JP. The development of the Maze procedure for the treatment of atrial fibrillation. Semin Thorac Cardiovasc Surg 2000;12:2–14.

8. Todd DM, Skanes AC, Guiraudon G, et al. Role of the posterior left atrium and pulmonary veins in human lone atrial fibrillation: electrophysiological and pathological data from patients undergoing atrial fibrillation surgery. Circulation 2003;108:3108–14.

9. Ouyang F, Antz M, Ernst S, et al. Recovered pulmonary vein conduction as a dominant factor for recurrent atrial tachyarrhythmias after complete circular isolation of the pulmonary veins lessons from double lasso technique. Circulation 2005;111:127–35.

10. Callans DJ, Gerstenfeld EP, Dixit S, et al. Efficacy of repeat pulmonary vein isolation procedures in patients with recurrent atrial fibrillation. J Cardiovasc Electrophysiol 2004;15:1050–5.

11. Datino T, Macle L, Qi X-Y, et al. Mechanisms by which adenosine restores conduction in dormant canine pulmonary veins. Circulation 2010;121:963–72.

12. Macle L, Khairy P, Verma A, et al, ADVICE Study Investigators. Adenosine following pulmonary vein isolation to target dormant conduction elimination (ADVICE): methods and rationale. Can J Cardiol 2012;28:184–90.

13. Andrade JG, Pollak SJ, Monir G, et al. Pulmonary vein isolation using a pace-capture-guided versus an adenosine-guided approach: effect on dormant conduction and long-term freedom from recurrent atrial fibrillation–a prospective study. Circ Arrhythm Electrophysiol 2013;6:1103–8.

Acquired Pulmonary Vein Isolation in a Patient with Friedreich Ataxia

Matthew M. Zipse, MD*, Ryan G. Aleong, MD*

KEYWORDS

• Atrial fibrillation • Friedreich ataxia • Arrhythmia • Cardiomyopathy

KEY POINTS

• The electrophysiologic nature of atrial fibrillation (AF) and related atrial arrhythmias in Friedreich ataxia has not previously been characterized.
• In the presented case, dense atrial scar had progressed to the point of acquired pulmonary vein (PV) isolation before the delivery of a single radiofrequency lesion.
• AF was still induced, and ultimately organized spontaneously into a microreentrant atrial tachycardia.
• Other atrial tachycardias were also identified near scar border zones; these potentially served as triggers for AF in this patient, independent of the PVs.
• This extreme example of atrial fibrosis emphasizes the need to address non-PV substrate, even if AF has only been paroxysmal, in some patients undergoing catheter ablation of AF.

CLINICAL PRESENTATION

A 38-year-old man with Friedreich ataxia and associated cardiomyopathy with moderate left ventricular dysfunction was referred for evaluation and management of atrial fibrillation (AF). The patient first experienced AF at age 21 years, and since has continued to have paroxysmal AF that has been highly symptomatic and refractory to multiple antiarrhythmic drugs. The patient is limited by weakness and is wheelchair bound as a result of his neuromuscular disease, but lives independently. Pulmonary function testing had been performed and was normal. With AF, associated symptoms of palpitations, fatigue, and malaise have become more frequent. After discussion, the patient opted to proceed with catheter ablation of AF.

The patient was brought to the electrophysiology laboratory in normal sinus rhythm, where general anesthesia was administered and femoral access obtained. After performing double transseptal puncture, placement of a circular mapping catheter in each of the pulmonary veins (PVs) revealed 4-vein electrical isolation with entrance and exit block at baseline. Left atrial voltage mapping revealed extensive posterior wall dense scar, involving the PV ostia (**Fig. 1**).

CLINICAL QUESTION

What is the approach to patients referred for catheter ablation of AF who are found to have 4-vein isolation at the start of the procedure?

CLINICAL COURSE

With PV isolation (PVI) at baseline, high-dose isoproterenol was administered to assess for spontaneous non-PV triggers for AF, but none

Disclosures: None of the authors have any conflicts to disclose relevant to this article.
Cardiac Electrophysiology, Cardiology Division, University of Colorado, Denver, Anschutz Medical Campus, 12401 East 17th Avenue, B-132, Aurora, CO 80045, USA
* Corresponding authors.
E-mail addresses: matthew.zipse@ucdenver.edu; ryan.aleong@ucdenver.edu

Card Electrophysiol Clin 8 (2016) 151–153
http://dx.doi.org/10.1016/j.ccep.2015.10.016
1877-9182/16/$ – see front matter © 2016 Elsevier Inc. All rights reserved.

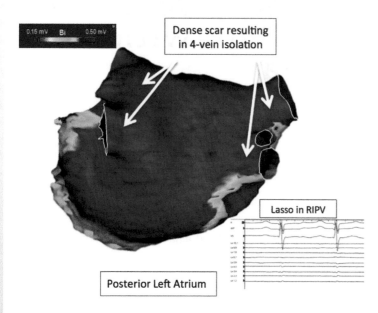

Fig. 1. A left atrial voltage map performed at the outset of the procedure shows dense posterior wall scar (*red*), resulting in acquired PVI × 4 at baseline. The circular mapping catheter (Lasso, Biosense-Webster, Inc, Diamond Bar, CA) was placed in each vein (right inferior PV [RIPV], pictured inset), with confirmation of entrance and exit block.

were identified. Atrial burst pacing was subsequently performed, and AF was induced. After only a brief period, this rhythm spontaneously organized. Activation mapping suggested a focal origin of an atrial tachycardia (AT), and entrainment mapping revealed a region adjacent to scar on the septal aspect of the anterior wall to be in the tachycardia circuit. Ablation lesions

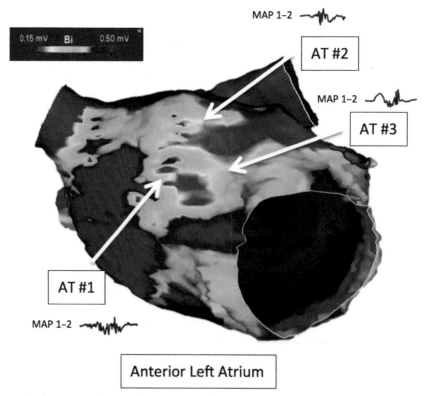

Fig. 2. A left atrial voltage map showing the anterior left atrium and sites near scar border zones where ATs were targeted with catheter ablation. Local electrograms during ATs observed on the mapping catheter at the sites of successful ablation are shown as well.

delivered to this area terminated the AT and sinus rhythm was restored. Additional ATs were induced and targeted in this fashion (**Fig. 2**). Activation and entrainment mapping were performed as tachycardia stability allowed, and these ATs also seemed to be focal in origin and microreentrant in mechanism. After targeted ablation of inducible ATs, further atrial burst pacing on and off isoproterenol could sustain neither AT nor AF. The procedure was concluded without complication, and the patient has done well without arrhythmia recurrence after more than 1 year of follow-up.

DISCUSSION

Friedreich ataxia is an autosomal recessive neurodegenerative disorder caused by a trinucleotide expansion on chromosome 9q13 involving the gene that encodes frataxin,[1] a protein responsible for mitochondrial iron handling. The disorder results in free radical–mediated cell damage to susceptible myocardial and central nervous system tissue, manifesting clinically as weakness, ataxia, and areflexia. Myocardial involvement in Friedreich ataxia, when present, can lead to either a hypertrophic or dilated cardiomyopathy phenotype.[2] In some patients, ventricular arrhythmias predominate, although early onset AF and AT have been described in this population as well, all resulting from early and progressive fibrosis.[3–6]

Despite this, the electrophysiologic nature of AF and related atrial arrhythmias in Friedreich ataxia has not previously been characterized. In the presented case, dense atrial scar had progressed to the point of acquired PVI before the delivery of a single radiofrequency lesion. AF was still induced, and ultimately organized spontaneously into a microreentrant AT. Other ATs were also identified near scar border zones; these potentially served as triggers for AF in this patient, independent of the PVs. This extreme example of atrial fibrosis emphasizes the need to address non-PV substrate, even if AF has only been paroxysmal, in some patients undergoing catheter ablation of AF.

REFERENCES

1. Child JS, Perloff JK, Bach PM, et al. Cardiac involvement in Friedreich's ataxia: a clinical study of 75 patients. J Am Coll Cardiol 1986;7:1370–8.
2. Kipps A, Alexander M, Colan SD, et al. The longitudinal course of cardiomyopathy in Friedreich's ataxia during childhood. Pediatr Cardiol 2009;30:306–10.
3. Raman SV, Phatak K, Hoyle JC, et al. Impaired myocardial perfusion reserve and fibrosis in Friedreich ataxia: a mitochondrial cardiomyopathy with metabolic syndrome. Eur Heart J 2011;32:561–7.
4. Panas M, Gialafos E, Spengos K, et al. Prevalence of interatrial block in patients with Friedreich's ataxia. Int J Cardiol 2010;145:386–7.
5. Asaad N, El-Menyar A, Al Suwaidi J. Recurrent ventricular tachycardia in patient with Friedreich's ataxia in the absence of clinical myocardial disease. Pacing Clin Electrophysiol 2010;33:109–12.
6. Lee JMS, Turner I, Agarwal A, et al. An unusual atrial tachycardia in a patient with Friedreich ataxia. Europace 2011;13:1660–1.

Ablation of Atrial Fibrillation in a Patient with a Mechanical Mitral Valve

Matthew M. Zipse, MD, Duy Thai Nguyen, MD*

KEYWORDS

- Atrial fibrillation • Catheter ablation • Mechanical mitral valve

KEY POINTS

- Clinicians must be mindful of the left ventricular lead when cannulating the coronary sinus with a decapolar catheter or an ablation catheter.
- Left atrial catheter ablation for the treatment of atrial fibrillation in patients with a mechanical mitral valve, when approached carefully, can be performed safely and effectively.
- Block across linear lines should be confirmed using differential activation and/or differential pacing to decrease risks of proarrhythmias.

CLINICAL PRESENTATION

A 69-year-old man was referred for evaluation of recurrent atrial fibrillation (AF). He had a history of surgical mechanical prostheses in the aortic and mitral positions for valvular stenosis related to rheumatic heart disease. He also had a history of a nonischemic dilated cardiomyopathy with severe left ventricular systolic dysfunction and left bundle branch block, and a biventricular implantable cardioverter-defibrillator was implanted. With cardiac resynchronization, his left ventricular ejection fraction normalized.

In the intervening time, he developed AF and underwent catheter ablation at an outside institution. Review of the patient's prior procedure report revealed that, in addition to pulmonary vein isolation (PVI), he also had linear radiofrequency ablations (RFAs) across the cavotricuspid isthmus, the left atrial roof, and a mitral annular line from the left inferior pulmonary vein (PV) to the mitral annulus.

He is now referred, several years later, for repeat ablation after AF and atrial flutter recurrence. His persistent AF has been highly symptomatic and refractory to multiple antiarrhythmic drugs and electrical cardioversions. Furthermore, in AF, appropriate biventricular pacing has decreased to 50%.

CLINICAL QUESTION

What is the approach to AF ablation in a patient with a mechanical mitral prosthesis and prior linear ablations?

CLINICAL COURSE

The patient presented to the electrophysiology laboratory for repeat PVI, assessment of prior ablation lines, and ablation of any inducible atrial flutters. Venous access was obtained, and a double transseptal puncture was performed under intracardiac ultrasonography and fluoroscopy. An open-irrigated, force-sensing ablation catheter was placed through a deflectable sheath (Agilis, St Jude Medical) into the left atrium (LA), and a circular mapping catheter (CMC) was placed through an SL1 long sheath to the LA. At baseline, the right

Disclosures: The authors have no disclosures relevant to this article.
Cardiac Electrophysiology, Cardiology Division, University of Colorado, Anschutz Medical Campus, Denver, 12401 East 17th Avenue, B-132, Aurora, CO 80045, USA
* Corresponding author.
E-mail address: duy.t.nguyen@ucdenver.edu

Card Electrophysiol Clin 8 (2016) 155–159
http://dx.doi.org/10.1016/j.ccep.2015.10.017
1877-9182/16/$ – see front matter © 2016 Elsevier Inc. All rights reserved.

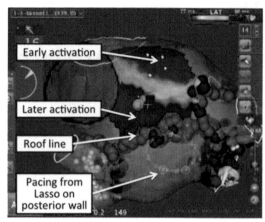

Fig. 1. Assessment of block across the left atrial roof line. This pattern of activation, when pacing the posterior wall, is consistent with block in the posterior to anterior direction. Pacing from the anterior side, and confirming an inferior to superior activation along the posterior LA, confirmed block in the anterior to posterior direction (data not shown).

superior and left inferior PVs were isolated, but the right inferior and left superior PVs had reconnected, as assessed by the CMC. Care was taken with manipulation of the CMC to avoid entrapment within the mechanical mitral prosthesis. When not being used, the CMC was retracted into the long sheath, with a small tail remaining out of the sheath, to minimize the risk of it inadvertently being displaced toward the valve because of interaction with the ablation catheter.

A left atrial voltage map was created to help identify the locations of the prior circumferential antral lines of ablation, LA roof line, and posterolateral mitral annular line. Additional ablation around PV antra was guided both by early signals on

the CMC and by areas of pace capture when pacing the line.[1] Four-vein entrance and exit block was achieved in this manner, and pharmacologic challenge with adenosine after a waiting period showed no evidence of dormant conduction.[2]

Bidirectional block was not present across the left atrial roof line at baseline. Additional RFA was delivered in areas of pace capture on the left atrial roof. After ablation of gaps in the roof line, the CMC was positioned on the posterior wall, and the ablation catheter was positioned anterior to the roof line. With pacing from the CMC, activation mapping was performed with the ablation catheter. The latest activation was observed anteriorly just adjacent to the roof line (Fig. 1). The process was repeated with the catheters reversed, again showing latest activation just opposite to the roof line from the site paced, confirming bidirectional block across the left atrial roof. Differential pacing was also used to further confirm bidirectional block.

Next, bidirectional block was found to also not be present across the posterolateral mitral annular line. Using intracardiac echocardiography, fluoroscopy, and electroanatomic mapping, the ablation catheter was carefully advanced to the mitral annulus (Fig. 2), where additional lesions were delivered in areas of pace capture. Ultimately, block across the mitral annular line could only be achieved after the ablation catheter was advanced into the coronary sinus (CS) (Fig. 3) and RFA was delivered opposite the endocardial lesion set. Bidirectional block was confirmed with assessment of differential activation, akin to the technique used to assess the roof line. In this case, the distal pole of the CS catheter was paced and activation was latest just adjacent to the pacing poles on the opposite side of the line

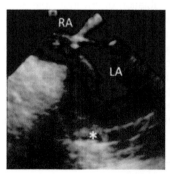
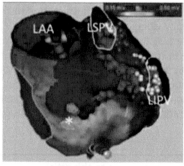
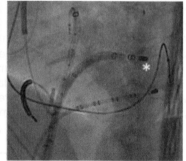

Fig. 2. Multiple imaging modalities were used to avoid catheter entrapment in the mechanical mitral valve with ablation near the mitral annulus. (Left) ICE showing the ablation catheter tip projected (asterisk) at the mitral annulus. (Middle) Electroanatomic map with contact force sensing. Gray lesion tags represent scar, or areas of noncapture with pacing. Additional RFA (red lesion tags) was guided by areas of pace capture along the posterolateral mitral annular line. (Right) Fluoroscopy in left anterior oblique (LAO) projection. ICE, intracardiac echocardiography; LAA, left atrial appendage; LIPV, left inferior PV; LSPV, left superior PV; RA, right atrium.

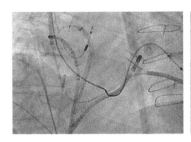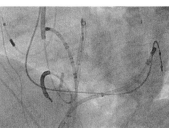

Fig. 3. Fluoroscopic views showing the relationship between the ablation catheter and the mechanical mitral prosthesis in right anterior oblique (*left*) and LAO (*right*) projections.

(**Fig. 4**). Pacing from the ablation catheter, placed next to the mitral annular line opposite the distal CS, showed a proximal-to-distal activation pattern on the CS decapolar catheter (**Fig. 5**), confirming bidirectional block across the mitral annular line. Again, differential pacing was also used to further confirm bidirectional block as shown by differential activation.

Having performed left atrial ablation to achieve PVI and bidirectional block across the roof and mitral annular lines, AF was induced but could not be sustained after multiple attempts at atrial burst pacing down to atrial refractoriness, on and off isoproterenol. No other atrial flutters were induced. Catheters were withdrawn to the right atrium; after confirming block across the

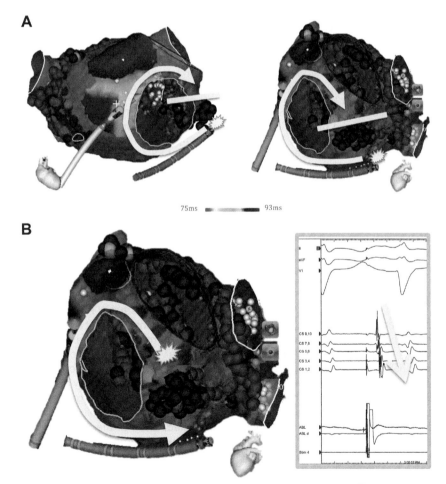

Fig. 4. Assessment of block across the posterolateral mitral annular line using differential activation. (*A*) The distal CS is paced, and activation points are taken along the mitral annulus. The latest activation is immediately opposite the line, consistent with block. (*B*) The ablation catheter is paced just anterior to the mitral annular line, and CS activation is proximal to distal, consistent with block. The yellow markings indicate the direction of electrical propagation.

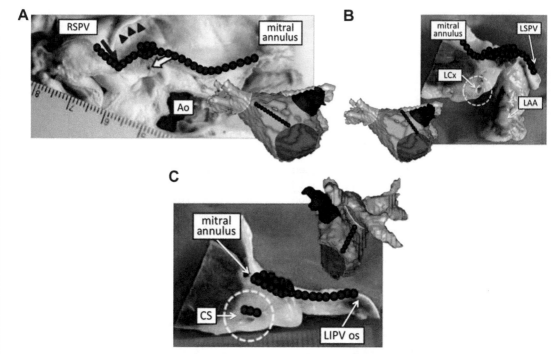

Fig. 5. Representative electroanatomic maps with lesion sets for 3 possible mitral annular lines and corresponding cross-sectional gross pathologic specimens. (*A*) Anteroseptal line. Ridges (*arrowheads*), diverticula (*dark arrow*), and the sinoatrial artery (*white arrow*) are sometimes present along this line, which can limit RFA effectiveness. This line commonly is the longest of the 3. (*B*) Anterolateral line. This line general requires RFA to be delivered over the thickest tissue of the 3 lines. Also, the left circumflex artery can limit lesion effectiveness. (*C*) Posterolateral line. The shortest of the 3 lines, but frequently requires RFA within the CS to achieve block. Ao, aorta; LCx, left circumflex coronary artery; RSPV, right superior PV. (*Adapted from* Cho Y, Lee W, Park EA, et al. The anatomical characteristics of three different endocardial lines in the left atrium: evaluation by computed tomography prior to mitral isthmus block attempt. Europace 2012;14:1104–11; with permission.)

previously ablated cavotricuspid isthmus, the procedure was concluded. The patient tolerated the procedure well and has been arrhythmia free for more than 8 months of follow-up.

DISCUSSION

There are several factors to consider when performing left atrial ablation in patients with AF and mechanical mitral valves. First, because of the higher perceived risk of performing catheter ablation for AF in patients with mechanical valves, these patients are often referred late in their clinical course. Frequently, this means multiple failed antiarrhythmic drugs and cardioversions and longstanding persistent AF. These factors immediately stratify these patients into a group known to have lower arrhythmia-free survival after undergoing catheter ablation[3] with a high incidence of left atrial tachycardias and atrial flutters when they do recur.[4] However, multiple studies have shown safety and efficacy of catheter ablation for AF in patients with a mechanical mitral valve,[5–7]

suggesting that these higher perceived risks may be unwarranted when the procedure is performed by high-volume operators at an experienced center. The use of a deflectable sheath can minimize extension of the ablation catheter shaft into the LA and decrease the risk of its entrapment in the mitral prosthesis. Furthermore, careful use of the CMC to ensure that it is oriented posteriorly or use of a Pentarray (not available for this case) can minimize risks of a mapping catheter being entangled in the mitral valve.

Mitral annular flutter may also occur in patients with prior mitral valve surgery.[8,9] If so, in addition to performing PVI, a mitral annular line may be indicated. Each of the 3 standard mitral annular lines (the anteroseptal line, the anterolateral line, and the posterolateral line; see **Fig. 5**) have their advantages and disadvantages. The anteroseptal line tends to be the longest and may have ridges, diverticula, and an underlying sinoatrial nodal artery, which can limit RFA effectiveness. The anterolateral line most commonly has the thickest underlying myocardium, whereas the posterolateral line often requires ablation within the CS to achieve block, as was required in this case.[10] However, the posterolateral line is a reasonable choice in patients with a mechanical mitral valve, because the CS provides an anatomic approach to the mitral annulus without risk of catheter entrapment or valve damage, provided the CS is patent after surgery. Ultimately, regardless of the mitral annular line performed, bidirectional block is paramount and should be confirmed by differential activation and differential pacing. Without block across the line, mitral annular lines have considerable proarrhythmic potential.[11,12]

Our patient's endovascular leads also presented additional obstacles for catheter ablation. Although the risk of dislodgment of a CS lead in patients with a biventricular device has not been reported with AF ablation, one series has reported a 2.4% risk of atrial lead dislodgment in patients with dual-chamber devices.[13] Clinicians must be mindful of the left ventricular lead when cannulating the CS with a decapolar catheter or an ablation catheter. In this case, the decapolar catheter was placed in the superior vena cava for most of the procedure, and only carefully advanced into the CS when needed.

In summary, left atrial catheter ablation for the treatment of AF in patients with a mechanical mitral valve, when approached carefully, can be performed safely and effectively. Block across linear lines should be confirmed using differential activation and/or differential pacing to decrease risks of proarrhythmias.

REFERENCES

1. Steven D, Sultan A, Reddy V, et al. Benefit of pulmonary vein isolation guided by loss of pace capture on the ablation line: results from a prospective 2-center randomized trial. J Am Coll Cardiol 2013; 62:44–50.
2. Arentz T, Macle L, Kalusche D, et al. "Dormant" pulmonary vein conduction revealed by adenosine after ostial radiofrequency catheter ablation. J Cardiovasc Electrophysiol 2004;15:1041–7.
3. Ganesan AN, Shipp NJ, Brooks AG, et al. Long-term outcomes of catheter ablation of atrial fibrillation: a systematic review and meta-analysis. J Am Heart Assoc 2013;2:e004549.
4. Haïssaguerre M, Hocini M, Sanders P, et al. Catheter ablation of long-lasting persistent atrial fibrillation: clinical outcome and mechanisms of subsequent arrhythmias. J Cardiovasc Electrophysiol 2005;16: 1138–47.
5. Hussein AA, Wazni OM, Harb S, et al. Radiofrequency ablation of atrial fibrillation in patients with mechanical mitral valve prostheses safety, feasibility, electrophysiologic findings, and outcomes. J Am Coll Cardiol 2011;58:596–602.
6. Lakkireddy D, Nagarajan D, di Biase L, et al. Radiofrequency ablation of atrial fibrillation in patients with mitral or aortic mechanical prosthetic valves: a feasibility, safety, and efficacy study. Heart Rhythm 2011; 8:975–80.
7. Bai R, di Biase L, Mohanty P, et al. Catheter ablation of atrial fibrillation in patients with mechanical mitral valve: long-term outcome of single procedure of pulmonary vein antrum isolation with or without nonpulmonary vein trigger ablation. J Cardiovasc Electrophysiol 2014;25:824–33.
8. Viles-Gonzalez JF, Enriquez AD, Castillo JG, et al. Incidence, predictors, and evolution of conduction disorders and atrial arrhythmias after contemporary mitral valve repair. Cardiol J 2014;21:569–75.
9. Chen H, Yang B, Ju W, et al. Long-term outcome following ablation of atrial tachycardias occurring after mitral valve replacement in patients with rheumatic heart disease. Pacing Clin Electrophysiol 2013;36:795–802.
10. Cho Y, Lee W, Park E-A, et al. The anatomical characteristics of three different endocardial lines in the left atrium: evaluation by computed tomography prior to mitral isthmus block attempt. Europace 2012;14:1104–11.
11. Essebag V, Baldessin F, Reynolds MR, et al. Noninducibility post-pulmonary vein isolation achieving exit block predicts freedom from atrial fibrillation. Eur Heart J 2005;26:2550–5.
12. Chugh A, Oral H, Lemola K, et al. Prevalence, mechanisms, and clinical significance of macroreentrant atrial tachycardia during and following left atrial ablation for atrial fibrillation. Heart Rhythm 2005;2: 464–71.
13. Lakkireddy D, Patel D, Ryschon K, et al. Safety and efficacy of radiofrequency energy catheter ablation of atrial fibrillation in patients with pacemakers and implantable cardiac defibrillators. Heart Rhythm 2005;2:1309–16.

Atrial Fibrillation Ablation Without Pulmonary Vein Isolation in a Patient with Fontan Palliation

Emily Sue Ruckdeschel, MD, Joseph Kay, MD,
William H. Sauer, MD, Duy Thai Nguyen, MD*

KEYWORDS

• Atrial fibrillation • Pulmonary vein isolation • Fontan palliation • Superior vena cava

KEY POINTS

• Two triggers were identified that initiated atrial fibrillation (AF) from the superior vena cava (SVC) and the right atrium.
• SVC triggers are more common in patients with a normal-sized left atrium.
• Eliminating these triggers prevented AF from being sustained in this patient and thus pulmonary vein isolation was not pursued.
• The patient has remained AF free for 3 years without medications or repeat ablation.
• Targeting of potential right-sided triggers for AF ablation, before pulmonary vein isolation, should be considered; such an approach may reduce risks in these complex patients.

CLINICAL HISTORY

A 32-year-old woman with a history of tricuspid atresia and ventricular septal defect who had a Bjork-type modification of the Fontan procedure (right atrial appendage to right ventricle anastomosis) developed persistent atrial fibrillation (AF) and symptoms of heart failure. She was initially treated with medical therapy but had recurrence of AF and symptoms and was therefore referred for an ablation. Preprocedure imaging showed a normal-sized left atrium and a very enlarged right atrium.

CLINICAL QUESTION

How should ablation for AF be approached in patients with a Fontan correction?

CLINICAL COURSE

AF ablation in patients with a Fontan palliation is rare. In the few reported cases, patients with AF had intra-atrial reentrant tachycardias (IARTs) and triggers from the right atrium (RA) caused by the abnormal RA substrate; when these triggers were targeted, the patients' AF improved. Hence, given our patient's complex anatomy, the decision was made to search for RA triggers and then to assess for AF recurrence thereafter. If she had AF recurrence, we would then proceed to pulmonary vein isolation (PVI) and left-sided ablations. Her presentation predated the advent/availability of focal impulse and rotor mapping.

The patient presented to the electrophysiology laboratory in AF. A decapolar catheter was placed

Cardiac Electrophysiology, Cardiology Division, University of Colorado, Aurora, CO, USA
* Corresponding author. University of Colorado, 12401 East 17th Avenue, Leprino Building, 5th Floor, Mailstop B-132, Aurora, CO 80045-2548.
E-mail address: duy.t.nguyen@ucdenver.edu

Card Electrophysiol Clin 8 (2016) 161–164
http://dx.doi.org/10.1016/j.ccep.2015.10.018
1877-9182/16/$ – see front matter © 2016 Elsevier Inc. All rights reserved.

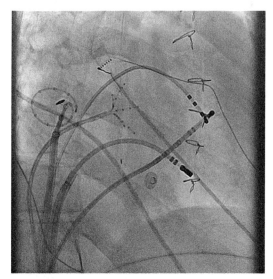

Fig. 1. Fluoroscopic image in left anterior oblique projection showing a rotated and enlarged right atrium with the decapolar catheter in the coronary sinus, Pentarray catheter on the RA posterior-lateral wall, a Lasso catheter in the SVC, and an irrigated-tip catheter in the atrial portion of the Fontan.

in the coronary sinus, a Pentarray catheter (Biosense Webster) on the RA posterolateral wall, and a circular mapping catheter in the superior vena cava (SVC). An irrigated-tip ablation catheter was placed in the atrial portion of the Fontan (**Fig. 1**). To map potential AF triggers, cardioversion was performed twice. Premature atrial beats

from the RA posterior wall (**Fig. 2**, arrows) and SVC (**Fig. 3**, arrows) reinitiated AF.

Hence, it was decided to target these triggers before PVI. Ablation around the SVC resulted in exit and entrance block. Complex fractionated atrial electrograms were ablated along the RA posterior wall, terminating AF. An intercaval line, from the SVC to the inferior vena cava (IVC), was completed through the posterior RA to prevent development of atrial flutter as a result of our posterior RA ablations (**Fig. 4**). AF was initiated multiple times with isoproterenol and programmed stimulation (atrial burst pacing down to atrial refractoriness), but AF could not be sustained and self-terminated. Given these results, no PVI was performed. After 3 years of follow-up, the patient has remained free of AF and is on no medications.

DISCUSSION

Adults with congenital heart disease now outnumber children with congenital heart disease.[1] Complex repairs in childhood improve survival but are associated with long-term morbidities. Surgical palliation of single-ventricle physiology has been the mainstay of treatment for the last 3 decades. Staged single-ventricle palliation (Fontan) is a series of procedures by which systemic venous return is routed either directly to the pulmonary arteries or through the hypoplastic subpulmonary ventricle.[2]

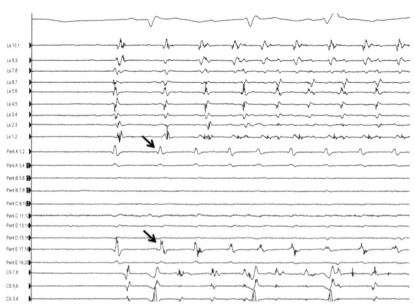

Fig. 2. Premature atrial beats from the RA posterior wall (*black arrows*), as seen from electrograms from the Pentarray catheter, reinitiated AF after a short period of postcardioversion sinus rhythm.

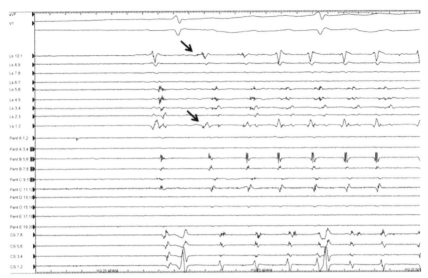

Fig. 3. Premature atrial beats from the SVC (*black arrows*), as seen from electrograms from the circular mapping catheter, reinitiated AF after a short period of postcardioversion sinus rhythm.

Arrhythmias are frequent in patients with adult congenital heart disease and are a common cause of sudden cardiac death.[3] Furthermore, in patients with Fontan circulation, atrial arrhythmias can lead to systemic ventricular dysfunction.[4] Atrial arrhythmias may be the result of hemodynamic changes from obstruction, worsening atrial dilatation, or

scar. Treatment of atrial arrhythmias in Fontan patients can be challenging because of their complex anatomy. AF may be related to right atrial substrates, rather than typical AF triggers, such as the pulmonary veins.[5] Although less common than IART, AF does occur regularly in patients with palliated congenital heart disease.[6]

Ablation in this patient population is challenging for a variety of reasons. Surgical manipulation of the atria leaves significant scar as well as setting up anatomic and electrical barriers. Different types of Fontan palliation allow different levels of access to native atrial tissue. Transbaffle puncture or retrograde approaches may be required when addressing the origins of atrial arrhythmias.[7]

In this case, we identified 2 triggers that initiated AF from the SVC and the RA. SVC triggers are more common in patients with a normal-sized left atrium, which was the case for our patient, as well as in patients with concurrent right atrial flutter, which our patient was not known to have but was at risk of having.[8] Eliminating these triggers prevented AF from being sustained in our patient and thus PVI was not pursued. She has remained AF free for 3 years without medications or repeat ablation. Hence, given the underlying RA disorder in Fontan patients, targeting of potential right-sided triggers for AF ablation, before PVI, should be considered; such an approach may reduce risks in these complex patients. With the introduction of focal impulse and rotor mapping, these may be additional tools to identify electrophysiologic RA triggers of AF in Fontan patients.

Fig. 4. Electroanatomic map (CARTO, Biosense Webster) of the posterior RA. A Fontan anastomosis connects the RA appendage to the right ventricle (not shown). Ablation (*red lesion tags*) around the SVC resulted in entrance and exit block. Ablation of the posterior RA targeted complex fractionated atrial electrograms, which terminated AF. An intercaval line was completed to prevent development of atrial flutter.

REFERENCES

1. Marelli AJ, Mackie AS, Ionescu-Ittu R, et al. Congenital heart disease in the general population: changing prevalence and age distribution. Circulation 2007; 115(2):163–72.
2. Khairy P, Poirier N, Mercier LA. Univentricular heart. Circulation 2007;115(6):800–12.
3. Nieminen HP, Jokinen EV, Sairanen HI. Causes of late deaths after pediatric cardiac surgery: a population-based study. J Am Coll Cardiol 2007;50(13):1263–71.
4. Deal BJ, Mavroudis C, Backer CL. Arrhythmia management in the Fontan patient. Pediatr Cardiol 2007; 28(6):448–56.
5. Takahashi K, Shoda M, Manaka T, et al. Successful radiofrequency catheter ablation of atrial fibrillation late after modified Fontan operation. Europace 2008; 10(8):1012–4.
6. Kirsh JA, Walsh EP, Triedman JK. Prevalence of and risk factors for atrial fibrillation and intra-atrial reentrant tachycardia among patients with congenital heart disease. Am J Cardiol 2002; 90(3):338–40.
7. Correa R, Walsh EP, Alexander ME, et al. Transbaffle mapping and ablation for atrial tachycardias after Mustard, Senning, or Fontan operations. J Am Heart Assoc 2013;2(5):e000325.
8. Miyazaki S, Taniguchi H, Kusa S, et al. Factors predicting an arrhythmogenic superior vena cava in atrial fibrillation ablation - insight into the mechanism. Heart Rhythm 2014;11(9):1560–6.

Section 4: Troubleshooting Device Function

Editor: Byron Lee

A Case of Cough-induced Ventricular Tachycardia in a Patient with a Left Ventricular Assist Device

Emily Sue Ruckdeschel, MD, Eugene Wolfel, MD,
Duy Thai Nguyen, MD*

KEYWORDS

• Left ventricular assist device (LVAD) • Ventricular tachycardia • Cough

KEY POINTS

- In this case, the patient's ventricular tachycardia (VT) was specifically induced by coughing, which has not previously been described.
- Decreasing the rotational speed of the left ventricular assist device (LVAD) and increasing preload by stopping the patient's nitrates and reducing diuretic dose allowed improved filling of the left ventricle (LV) and increased LV volumes.
- When coughing recurred, the effects on the LV cavity were less pronounced and thus VT was reduced.
- Although ventricular arrhythmias are common after LVAD placement, this is a unique case in which VT was caused by coughing, which is ordinarily not considered arrhythmogenic.

CLINICAL PRESENTATION

A 69-year-old man with history of severe ischemic cardiomyopathy, who underwent left ventricular assist device (LVAD) placement (Heart Mate II) 1 year previously, presented with increasing shortness of breath, fatigue, and several defibrillation shocks from his internal cardioverter-defibrillator (ICD). In addition, he reported frequent episodes of cough and upper respiratory symptoms for the prior 10 days. At a clinic visit several weeks prior he had been started on low-dose nitrates and his dose of diuretic had been increased. His LVAD interrogation revealed stable parameters for him at 9400 rotations per minute (rpm) with a flow of 5.4 L/min, pulsatility index of 4.5, and power consumption of 6.6 W. He did not have any abnormal alarms, changes in flow or power, or evidence of a suction event. His dual-chamber ICD (Boston Scientific) was interrogated and revealed 11 episodes of monomorphic ventricular tachycardia (VT), with rates in the ventricular fibrillation (VF) zone (>240 beats per minute [bpm]), for which he received 1 defibrillation shock and 1 successful episode of antitachycardia pacing (ATP); 9 episodes spontaneously terminated and therapies were diverted. Furthermore, he had 9 episodes of monomorphic VT in the VT zone (rates >200 bpm) for which he received 2 successful defibrillation shocks and 3 successful ATP therapies; 4 episodes were self-terminated and therapies were diverted. There were also 30 episodes in the VT-1 zone (rates >160 bpm), all of which were successfully treated with ATP.

Disclosures: There are no disclosures.
Section of Electrophysiology, Cardiology Division, University of Colorado, Aurora, CO, USA
* Corresponding author. University of Colorado, Denver, Anschutz Medical Campus, 12401 East 17th Avenue, B-132, Aurora, CO 80045.
E-mail address: duy.t.nguyen@ucdenver.edu

CLINICAL QUESTION

How does coughing cause VT in a patient with an LVAD?

CLINICAL COURSE

While the patient was being examined, he was noted to have episodes of VT on telemetry coinciding with his fits of coughing. When the patient was asked to cough spontaneously, he had recurrent VT. A 12-lead electrocardiogram was obtained during 1 coughing episode (**Fig. 1**). The VT morphology was a right bundle branch pattern with a left superior axis, consistent with an origin from the inferolateral left ventricle (LV). This finding raised concerns that the inflow cannula of the LVAD may be causing myocardial irritation and arrhythmia that was exacerbated by the coughing episodes.

The patient was placed on cough suppressants, which reduced his coughing and subsequently his VT burden. He also underwent a transesophageal echocardiogram (TEE) to further assess the location of the LVAD inflow cannula. The TEE revealed a small left ventricular cavity (LV end-diastolic dimension of 2.5 cm) with the LVAD inflow cannula tip abutting the LV inferolateral wall during systole, consistent with the origin of the monomorphic VT. When the LVAD speed was decreased from 9200 rpm (**Fig. 2**A) to 8600 rpm (see **Fig. 2**B), the LV cavity appeared larger (LV end-diastolic dimension of 3.4 cm) and there was less interaction of the LVAD inflow cannula with the LV inferolateral wall. In order to further increase the size of the LV cavity, the patient's nitrates were discontinued and his diuretic dose was decreased. This combination of interventions minimized the interaction of the inflow cannula with the LV inferolateral wall during coughing, VT events significantly decreased, and the patient received no further ICD therapies.

DISCUSSION

LVADs have been in use since the 1980s and have undergone significant changes in design since their inception.[1] Blood flow through the LVAD starts in the inflow cannula, which is located in the left ventricular apex, and returns to the body through the outflow cannula in the ascending aorta. Initial ventricular assist devices were pulsatile but were large, significantly audible, and required a moderate body surface area to implant. More importantly, they did not have significant longevity and most required replacement before 2 years of use. Current LVADs are continuous flow devices, which have been found to have superior outcomes compared with pulsatile devices.[1,2]

The incidence of ventricular arrhythmias in ambulatory patients with LVADs is high.[3] Small studies have shown that 52% of patients with continuous flow LVADs have sustained VT or VF, most commonly in the first 4 weeks after implantation.[4,5] Although they cause symptoms, ventricular arrhythmias are generally better tolerated in patients with LVADs because of the hemodynamic support of the LVAD.[6] Cardioversion or defibrillation is often required to terminate the ventricular arrhythmias, if the arrhythmias do not spontaneously terminate or if ATP is unsuccessful.

Ventricular arrhythmias may be related to a variety of underlying issues, including scar-based arrhythmia, ischemia, and suction events.[5,7,8] Development of new, sustained, monomorphic VT after LVAD placement is more likely than resolution of previous VT before LVAD placement.[4] The underlying disease process may contribute to ongoing ventricular arrhythmias, and a history of previous ventricular arrhythmias predicts risk of appropriate ICD shock after LVAD placement.[9] Suction events have also been a well-documented cause of ventricular arrhythmias.[7]

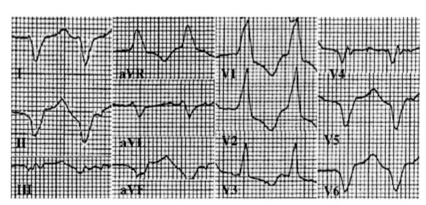

Fig. 1. Electrocardiogram tracing of monomorphic VT associated with coughing. The right bundle branch pattern with a left superior axis was consistent with an origin from the inferolateral wall.

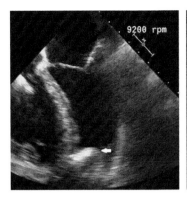
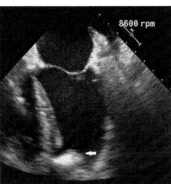

Fig. 2. Transesophageal echocardiogram images of LV showing the relationship between LVAD inflow cannula (*white arrow*) and the ventricular walls at 9200 rpm (*left*) and 8600 rpm (*right*).

Continuous flow LVADs generally have a constant speed mode that is not readily able to adjust to changes in venous return.[7] A suction event occurs when the speed remains constant but venous flow is decreased. The left ventricular volume is therefore significantly decreased, causing movement of the intraventricular septum toward the inflow cannula and inducing ventricular arrhythmias.

In this case, the patient's VT was specifically induced by coughing, which has not previously been described. The exact mechanism for this case of cough-induced VT is not fully known but is likely mechanical. It is probable that, during episodes of coughing, the intrathoracic pressure is significantly increased and venous return impaired.[10] Poor venous return would result in a smaller LV cavity, which could lead to possible suction events but also to direct mechanical contact of the LV cannula with the LV wall. This process may have been exacerbated by the rapid upward movement of the diaphragm with coughing and subsequent upward mechanical movement of the LVAD inflow cannula at the apex of the heart. Given that no suction events were documented in this case, it is most likely that the LV cavity was already small from the flow of the LVAD; decreased venous return from prolonged coughing caused the LV cavity to decrease further, allowing contact between the cannula and LV wall, and thus causing mechanical irritation of the LV wall and subsequent VT. Decreasing the rotational speed of the LVAD and increasing preload by stopping the patient's nitrates and reducing diuretic dose allowed improved filling of the LV and increased LV volumes. When coughing recurred, the effects on the LV cavity were less pronounced and thus VT was reduced.

In summary, although ventricular arrhythmias are common after LVAD placement, this is a unique case in which VT was caused by coughing, which would ordinarily not be considered arrhythmogenic.

REFERENCES

1. Caccamo M, Eckman P, John R. Current state of ventricular assist devices. Curr Heart Fail Rep 2011;8(2):91–8.
2. Slaughter MS, Rogers JG, Milano CA, et al. Advanced heart failure treated with continuous-flow left ventricular assist device. N Engl J Med 2009; 361(23):2241–51.
3. Ambardekar AV, Allen LA, Lindenfeld J, et al. Implantable cardioverter-defibrillator shocks in patients with a left ventricular assist device. J Heart Lung Transplant 2010;29(7):771–6.
4. Ziv O, Dizon J, Thosani A, et al. Effects of left ventricular assist device therapy on ventricular arrhythmias. J Am Coll Cardiol 2005;45(9):1428–34.
5. Andersen M, Videbaek R, Boesgaard S, et al. Incidence of ventricular arrhythmias in patients on long-term support with a continuous-flow assist device (HeartMate II). J Heart Lung Transplant 2009; 28(7):733–5.
6. Oz MC, Rose EA, Slater J, et al. Malignant ventricular arrhythmias are well tolerated in patients receiving long-term left ventricular assist devices. J Am Coll Cardiol 1994;24(7):1688–91.
7. Vollkron M, Voitl P, Ta J, et al. Suction events during left ventricular support and ventricular arrhythmias. J Heart Lung Transplant 2007;26(8):819–25.
8. Refaat M, Chemaly E, Lebeche D, et al. Ventricular arrhythmias after left ventricular assist device implantation. Pacing Clin Electrophysiol 2008;31(10):1246–52.
9. Brenyo A, Rao M, Koneru S, et al. Risk of mortality for ventricular arrhythmia in ambulatory LVAD patients. J Cardiovasc Electrophysiol 2012;23(5):515–20.
10. Benditt DG, Samniah N, Pham S, et al. Effect of cough on heart rate and blood pressure in patients with "cough syncope". Heart Rhythm 2005;2(8):807–13.

An Approach to Endovascular Ventricular Pacing in a Patient with Ebstein Anomaly and a Mechanical Tricuspid Valve

Matthew M. Zipse, MD*, Daniel W. Groves, MD,
Amber D. Khanna, MD, Duy Thai Nguyen, MD*

KEYWORDS

- Ebstein anomaly • Cardiac pacing • Mechanical tricuspid valve

KEY POINTS

- In the presence of a mechanical tricuspid valve, endocardial right ventricular pacing is contraindicated, and permanent pacing is usually achieved via a surgically implanted epicardial lead.
- In this case of a patient with Ebstein anomaly, a mechanical tricuspid valve, and complete heart block, transvenous pacing was achieved by implantation of a pace-sense lead in a coronary sinus ventricular branch, obviating cardiac surgery.
- Noninvasive cardiac imaging can provide invaluable information regarding anatomic variation in patients with congenital heart disease or when there are anticipated challenges to lead placement.
- With this preprocedural planning and careful execution, endovascular pacing in patients with a mechanical tricuspid valve is feasible and can safely be performed.

CLINICAL PRESENTATION

A 72-year-old man with a history of Ebstein anomaly had previously undergone surgical implantation of a mechanical tricuspid valve. He also had prophylactic placement of 2 epicardial left ventricular (LV) pacing leads (1 serving as a backup), which were tunneled to a left prepectoral pocket, where a dual-chamber pacemaker and an endovascular atrial lead were later implanted (**Fig. 1**). He subsequently developed complete atrioventricular block and failure of both epicardial leads with increasing pacing thresholds. The patient reported presyncope corresponding with intermittent ventricular noncapture despite increased pacing output. Furthermore, increased pacing output was complicated by diaphragmatic capture. Lead revision to allow reliable ventricular capture with pacing was indicated.

CLINICAL QUESTIONS

Is there a nonsurgical, endovascular option for lead revision?

Is there a role for preprocedural cardiac imaging to improve the safety and efficacy of lead revision?

CLINICAL COURSE

In order to avoid repeat cardiac surgery, the decision was made to attempt placement of an endovascular ventricular pace-sense lead via a

Disclosures: None of the authors have any conflicts to disclose relevant to this article.
Cardiac Electrophysiology, Cardiology Division, University of Colorado, Denver, Anschutz Medical Campus, 12401 East 17th Avenue, B-132, Aurora, CO 80045, USA
* Corresponding authors.
E-mail addresses: matthew.zipse@ucdenver.edu; duy.t.nguyen@ucdenver.edu

Card Electrophysiol Clin 8 (2016) 169–171
http://dx.doi.org/10.1016/j.ccep.2015.10.020
1877-9182/16/$ – see front matter © 2016 Elsevier Inc. All rights reserved.

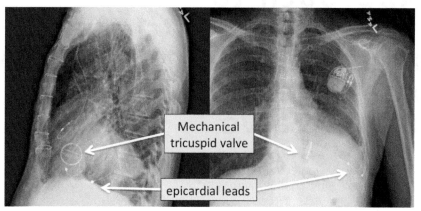

Fig. 1. The patient's chest radiograph following implantation of a dual-chamber pacemaker, showing 2 epicardial LV leads (1 redundant serving as backup), a prepectoral generator, and an endovascular atrial lead. A mechanical prosthesis is present in the tricuspid position.

coronary sinus (CS) branch. To assess CS anatomy and feasibility of lead placement, preprocedural cardiac computed tomography (CT) was obtained with postprocessing three-dimensional reconstruction (**Fig. 2**). Imaging revealed not only the mechanical tricuspid valve in an ebsteinoid position with ventricular displacement but also a significantly rotated heart, such that the ventricular apex projected posterolaterally and the right atrium anteriorly. Intravenous contrast injection phased for CS opacification was able to confirm CS patency, but, because of the rotation, the CS takeoff was more posteriorly directed than its usual position. Multiple possible targets for CS lead placement were identified, including a large middle cardiac vein fed by several smaller lateral branches, as well as an anterolateral branch off of the great cardiac vein beyond the valve of Vieussens.

Having reviewed the cardiac CT images, the patient was brought to the electrophysiology laboratory for CS lead placement. Because of the anticipated challenges presented by anatomic variation and the mechanical tricuspid prosthesis,

femoral venous access was obtained before opening the pocket. Using a deflectable sheath, the CS was cannulated from below with care to avoid the mechanical valve, and a wire advanced into the CS body to serve as a fluoroscopic landmark (**Fig. 3**, left panel). Venography was performed through the sheath and an anterolateral branch was identified as suitable for lead placement.

Attention was then turned to the pocket, which was opened and access was obtained with standard technique. Through a multipurpose outer sheath, a deflectable inner sheath was used to cannulate the CS os, again with care to avoid the mechanical valve, and was then advanced into the CS body over a 0.89-mm (0.035-inch) wire. With the inner sheath and wire advanced well into the CS to provide adequate support, the multipurpose outer sheath was advanced into the mid-CS. The deflectable inner sheath was removed and replaced with a splitable 90° inner sheath, which was able to subselectively engage an anterolateral CS branch over a wire. A quadripolar LV lead was successfully advanced through the outer and inner sheaths into the CS branch of interest.

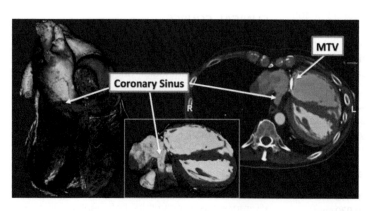

Fig. 2. Preprocedural imaging by cardiac CT, with three-dimensional full-volume reconstruction (*left* and *middle*) and two-dimensional axial (*right*) images. MTV, mechanical tricuspid valve.

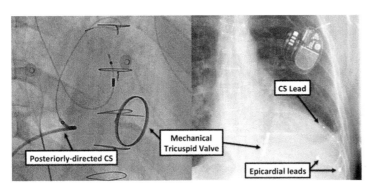

Fig. 3. (*Left*) Intraprocedural fluoroscopy in right anterior oblique projection, highlighting the posterior takeoff of the CS when cannulated from below with a deflectable sheath. (*Right*) Postprocedure chest radiograph, showing final CS lead placement.

The lead was advanced to an apical position to afford maximal stability (and because the patient had no clear indication for resynchronization, for which a more basal position would be desirable, although the proximal poles on his quadripolar lead were more basal). The patient has done well in follow-up, with consistent ventricular capture and no further diaphragm capture.

DISCUSSION

In the presence of a mechanical tricuspid valve, endocardial right ventricular pacing is contraindicated, and permanent pacing is usually achieved via a surgically implanted epicardial lead. In this case of a patient with Ebstein anomaly, a mechanical tricuspid valve, and complete heart block, transvenous pacing was achieved by implantation of a pace-sense lead in a CS ventricular branch, obviating cardiac surgery. Noninvasive cardiac imaging can provide invaluable information regarding anatomic variation in patients with congenital heart disease or when there are anticipated challenges to lead placement, such as a mechanical tricuspid valve.[1,2] With this preprocedural planning and careful execution, endovascular pacing in patients with a mechanical tricuspid valve can be feasibly and safely performed.

REFERENCES

1. Van de Veire NR, Marsan NA, Schuijf JD, et al. Noninvasive imaging of cardiac venous anatomy with 64-slice multi-slice computed tomography and noninvasive assessment of left ventricular dyssynchrony by 3-dimensional tissue synchronization imaging in patients with heart failure scheduled for cardiac resynchronization therapy. Am J Cardiol 2008;101: 1023–9.

2. Alikhani Z, Li J, Merchan JA, et al. Coronary sinus anatomy by computerized tomography, overlaid on live fluoroscopy can be successfully used to guide left ventricular lead implantation: a feasibility study. J Interv Card Electrophysiol 2013;36:217–22.

Implantable Cardioverter-Defibrillator Discharge in a Patient with Dilated Cardiomyopathy
What Is the Mechanism?

Jermey Docekal, MD, David K. Singh, MD*

KEYWORDS

- SVT • AVNRT • Implantable cardioverter-defibrillator

KEY POINTS

- Careful interrogation of implantable cardioverter defibrillator tracings can provide clues about the underlying arrhythmia.
- Antitachycardic pacing may result in entrainment of the underlying arrhythmia.
- The response to entrainment can be used to establish a diagnosis, particularly in the case of supraventricular tachycardia.

INTRODUCTION

A 51-year-old man with a history of dilated cardiomyopathy caused by prior methamphetamine abuse presented for routine follow-up to our device clinic. In 2005 he underwent implantation of an implantable cardioverter-defibrillator (ICD) for primary prevention. In 2011, the device was upgraded to a Boston Scientific biventricular ICD following the development of left bundle branch block. On questioning, he stated that approximately 5 months before his visit, he felt his ICD discharge. He did not seek medical attention for this event. Further questioning revealed that he experienced frequent palpitations, occurring up to 4 times a day. The patient's device was interrogated, and the rhythm strip from the ICD discharge is presented in **Fig. 1**.

WHAT IS THE RHYTHM THAT LED TO THE PATIENT'S IMPLANTABLE CARDIOVERTER-DEFIBRILLATOR SHOCK?
Commentary

Interrogation of ICDs has become a routine matter in clinics around the world, and is usually straightforward even in the setting of an ICD discharge. Typically, examination of the atrio-ventricular (A-V) relationship yields a speedy diagnosis. A rhythm with ventriculo-atrial (VA) dissociation is almost always consistent with ventricular tachycardia. When confronted with a tachycardia with a 1:1 A-V relationship, as in this tracing, the differential diagnosis includes a supraventricular rhythm or ventricular tachycardia with 1:1 V-A conduction. In this tracing, the first premature beat arises in the atrium, strongly suggesting the presence of a supraventricular rhythm. Initially, the SVT appears to be a long R-P tachycardia (**Fig. 2**). Examination of the initial complexes of the tachycardia reveals a lengthening A-V relationship. In addition, during the first 10 beats of the tachycardia, it appears that slight changes in the atrial cycle length generally precede changes in the ventricular cycle length. This finding strongly suggests atrial tachycardia (AT).

On the 11th complex, the A-V pattern changes and the A and V complexes appear to occur simultaneously. This pattern is commonly referred to as an A-on-V tachycardia. The differential diagnosis for an A–on-V tachycardia includes AT with a

Section of Electrophysiology, Cardiology Division, Queens Medical Center, Honolulu, HI, USA
* Corresponding author. Electrophysiology Division, Queens Heart Physician Practice, 550 South Beretania Street, Suite 601, Honolulu, HI 96813.
E-mail address: dsingh@queens.org

Card Electrophysiol Clin 8 (2016) 173–176
http://dx.doi.org/10.1016/j.ccep.2015.10.023
1877-9182/16/$ – see front matter © 2016 Elsevier Inc. All rights reserved.

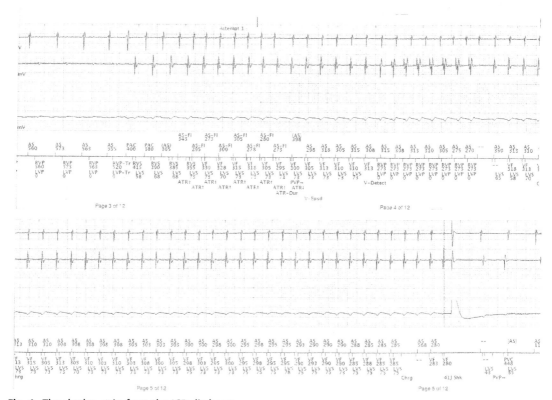

Fig. 1. The rhythm strip from the ICD discharge.

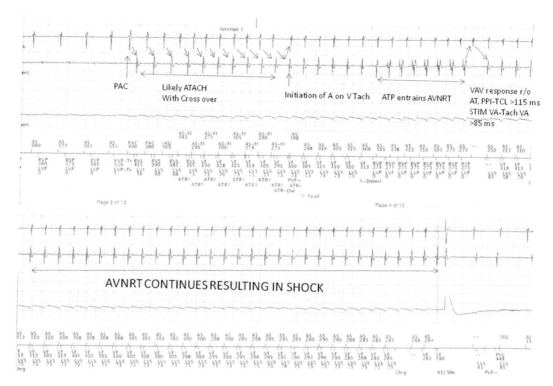

Fig. 2. The first premature beat arises in the atrium, strongly suggesting the presence of a supraventricular rhythm. Initially, the SVT appears to be a long R-P tachycardia.

long AV conduction time, junctional tachycardia (JT), and typical slow-fast atrioventricular nodal reciprocating tachycardia (AVNRT). Although JT is a possibility, it is rare and typically maneuvers are used in the electrophysiology laboratory to distinguish AT from AVNRT. A-on-V tachycardias are not likely to be the result of orthodromic atrioventricular reciprocating tachycardia (AVRT) given that the atria and ventricle are depolarized in series, usually resulting in a short RP tachycardia rather than an A–on-V tachycardia.

The tachycardia rate is in the ventricular fibrillation (VF) zone of the device. Usually ICDs do not use SVT discriminators in a VF zone and therapies are activated according to prespecified settings. After several beats, antitachycardia pacing (ATP) starts. Careful examination of the atrial electrogram reveals that the atrial rate is accelerated to the ATP cycle length. In the event of a focal AT, this overdrive suppresses the focus. In the setting of AVNRT, ATP can result in entrainment of the arrhythmia. The response to ventricular pacing can therefore be used to differentiate AVNRT from AT. With cessation of ATP, a single atrial electrogram is seen between the final pacing stimulus and the subsequent native ventricular complex. This VAV response proves the participation of the AV node as part of the circuit and establishes typical AVNRT as the diagnosis.[1] A VAAV response is typically seen in patients with AT.

In addition, the parameters established by Michaud and colleagues[2] can be used as further evidence to support the diagnosis of AVNRT. Although this maneuver is more commonly used to distinguish septal AVRT from AVNRT, it nonetheless provides further evidence supporting AVNRT as the diagnosis. Because the circuit is remote from the pacing stimulus in AVNRT, the postpacing interval is usually long (>115 milliseconds). In addition, it is important to recognize that the atria and ventricles are activated in parallel in AVNRT and in series with ventricular overdrive pacing (VOD). As a result, the stimulation-atrial electrogram (SA) interval during VOD should be longer than the ventricular-atrial electrogram (VA) interval during tachycardia. The SA-VA should therefore generally exceed 85 milliseconds[2]. Examination of the ICD tracing shows both of the features to be present. The tachycardia continues until the device delivers a 41-J shock that terminates the arrhythmia.

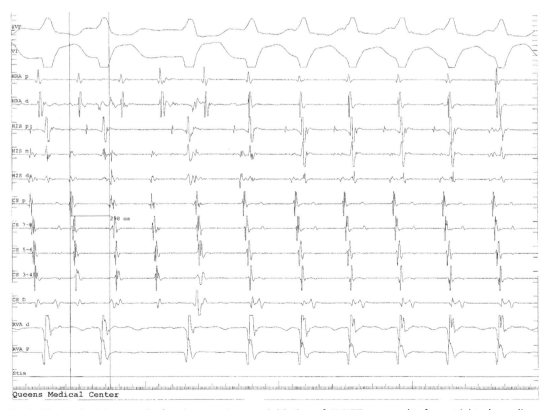

Fig. 3. Electrophysiology study showing spontaneous initiation of AVNRT as a result of an atrial tachycardia.

Several weeks later, the patient was brought to the electrophysiology laboratory. A similar phenomenon was observed whereby the patient was noted to spontaneously develop AT that subsequently initiated an A-on-V tachycardia (**Fig. 3**). Response to VOD (not shown) yielded a VAV response confirming the diagnosis. Modification of the AV nodal slow pathway resulted in elimination of the AVNRT.

SUMMARY

The response to ATP can sometimes reveal clues about tachycardia mechanisms. In this case, the diagnosis of typical AVNRT could be firmly established from the ICD interrogation alone.

REFERENCES

1. Knight BP, Ebinger M, Oral H, et al. Diagnostic value of tachycardia features and pacing maneuvers during paroxysmal supraventricular tachycardia. J Am Coll Cardiol 2000;36:574–82.
2. Michaud GF, Tada H, Chough S, et al. Differentiation of atypical atrioventricular node re-entrant tachycardia from orthodromic reciprocating tachycardia using a septal accessory pathway by the response to ventricular pacing. J Am Coll Cardiol 2001;38:1163–7.

Inappropriate Implantable Cardioverter-Defibrillator Shock from QRS Double Counting in the Setting of Hyperkalemia

Akash Dadlani, Jonathan W. Dukes, MD,
Nitish Badhwar, MD, FHRS*

KEYWORDS

• ICD • Inappropriate shock • Hyperkalemia

KEY POINTS

- This case shows the complexity of arrhythmia management in patients with implantable cardioverter-defibrillators (ICDs) who present with hyperkalemia.
- In order to prevent inappropriate ICD shock, consideration should be given to the suspension of ICD therapies while intensive care treatment of extreme electrolyte derangements is being pursued.
- Patients in these setting should be closely monitored until their electrocardiograms have normalized, after which the device can safely be reactivated.

CLINICAL PRESENTATION

A 57-year-old man with a history of coronary artery disease, ischemic cardiomyopathy following biventricular implantable cardioverter-defibrillator (ICD) implantation, and end-stage renal disease presented to the emergency department with generalized pain, chills, shortness of breath, and fatigue. His medications included carvedilol 3.125 mg twice daily, amiodarone 400 mg daily, aspirin 81 mg daily, furosemide 40 mg daily, and a renal multivitamin. On arrival, he was noted to have an increased potassium level of 6.8 mmol/L. His electrocardiogram (ECG) showed an atrioventricularly paced rhythm at a rate of 70 beats per minute (bpm) with QRS duration of 208 milliseconds and peaked T waves (**Fig. 1**). Shortly after admission, he was noted on telemetry to develop a wide complex tachycardia at 120 bpm. This tachycardia was followed by a single ATP (antitachycardia pacing) burst and a 36-J ICD shock.

CLINICAL QUESTION

Can an inappropriate ICD shock occur in the setting of hyperkalemic ECG changes?

CLINICAL COURSE

An ICD interrogation performed shortly after the event revealed that the ventricular tachycardia (VT) and ventricular fibrillation zones were programmed to deliver therapies at cycle lengths of less than 375 milliseconds and 330 milliseconds respectively. An event was recorded in the ventricular fibrillation therapy zone that corresponded with the ICD shock. The intracardiac electrogram from that event showed VT with A-V dissociation at 500 milliseconds as measured on the leadless ECG telemetry (**Fig. 2**). The device-measured marker channel showed clear double counting of the ventricular signal during the QRS complex on most tachycardic beats. This

Division of Electrophysiology, Department of Medicine, University of California, San Francisco, 500 Parnassus Avenue, San Francisco, CA 94143, USA
* Corresponding author. University of California, San Francisco, 500 Parnassus Avenue, MU East 431, Box 1354, San Francisco, CA 94143.
E-mail address: badhwar@medicine.ucsf.edu

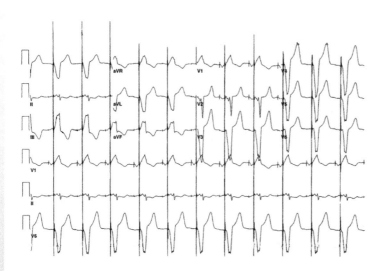

Fig. 1. ECG showing an atrioventricularly paced rhythm at 70 bpm. QRS duration of 208 milliseconds, QTc interval of 596 milliseconds, with potassium levels of 6.8 mmol/L.

double counting resulted in the device registering the tachycardia cycle length to be between 130 and 367 milliseconds, resulting in an ICD discharge.

A chest radiograph following the event showed normal lead positions and no mechanical lead disruptions. The patient was treated for the hyperkalemia with calcium chloride, sodium bicarbonate, and glucose followed by hemodialysis. Following hemodialysis there were no further episodes of ICD discharge. His postdialysis ECG revealed both a narrowing of the QRS duration to 184 milliseconds and T-wave normalization (**Fig. 3**).

DISCUSSION

Prior studies in patients with ICDs have shown an inappropriate shock rate of 12% to 16% following device implantation.[1,2] Patients who receive such shocks have increased rates of mortality, anxiety, and posttraumatic stress disorder compared with other patients with ICDs.[3] Inappropriate ICD shocks can occur for numerous reasons, including supraventricular tachycardia, atrial fibrillation, inadequate lead positions, and electrolyte derangements.

This article presents a case in which hyperkalemia caused an inappropriate shock because of QRS double counting from ventricular oversensing as a result of hyperkalemia and amiodarone use. In this case, double counting of the wide QRS complex of the slow VT resulted in an inappropriate shock. Correction of the hyperkalemia through hemodialysis resulted in normalization of the device sensing and cessation of the inappropriate device therapies.

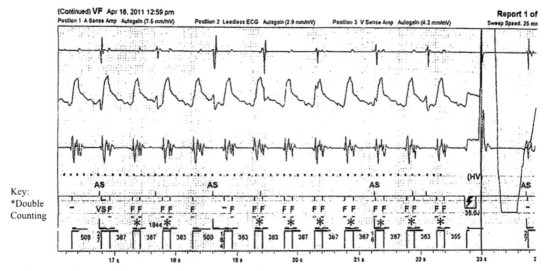

Fig. 2. Device interrogation report from the time of ICD discharge showing a slow VT with a cycle length of 500 milliseconds. As shown on the sensing channel, most QRS complexes are counted twice, resulting in a device-measured tachycardia cycle length of up to 130 milliseconds.

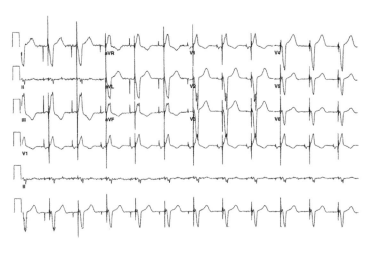

Fig. 3. Postdialysis ECG showing sinus rate of 69 bpm, with reduction in the QRS width to 184 milliseconds and the QTc to 567 milliseconds.

Hyperkalemia (potassium level >5.0 mmol/L) is associated with multiple ECG abnormalities, including peaked T waves, decreased QRS complex amplitude, widened QRS complex, prolonged PR interval and shortened QT interval.[4,5] These changes are the result of potassium effects on the cardiac action potential. Hyperkalemia decreases the resting membrane potential and the upstroke velocity of phase 0 (depolarization), causing slow intraventricular conduction leading to widening of the QRS. At the same time, hyperkalemia decreases the gradient between intracellular and extracellular fluid, which increases the velocity and slope of the phase 3 (repolarization), thereby shortening ventricular repolarization. This process causes the tall, narrow, peaked T waves and shortens the QT interval.

Prior studies have shown inappropriate shocks in the setting of hyperkalemia.[6–8] In 2 of these cases, increased T waves in the presence of hyperkalemia were the cause of inappropriate ICD shocks caused by T wave oversensing. In contrast, our case shows ventricular oversensing caused by double counting of the QRS complex. One study found QRS double and triple counting in a patient with a wide complex rhythm during a cardiac arrest.[7] Our case showed inappropriate shocks in a fairly stable patient with hyperkalemia on amiodarone, with resolution of the inappropriate therapies after hemodialysis.

This case shows the complexity of arrhythmia management in patients with ICDs who present with hyperkalemia. In order to prevent inappropriate ICD shock, consideration should be given to the suspension of ICD therapies while intensive care treatment of extreme electrolyte derangements is being pursued. Patients in these settings should be closely monitored until their ECGs have normalized, after which the device can safely be reactivated.

REFERENCES

1. Daubert JP, Zareba W, Cannom DS, et al. Inappropriate implantable cardioverter-defibrillator shocks in MADIT II: frequency, mechanisms, predictors, and survival impact. J Am Coll Cardiol 2008;51:1357–65.
2. van Rees JB, Borleffs CJ, de Bie MK, et al. Inappropriate implantable cardioverter-defibrillator shocks: incidence, predictors, and impact on mortality. J Am Coll Cardiol 2011;57:556–62.
3. Prudente LA, Reigle J, Bourguignon C, et al. Psychological indices and phantom shocks in patients with ICD. J Interv Card Electrophysiol 2006;15:185–90.
4. Ettinger PO, Regan TJ, Oldewurtel HA. Hyperkalemia, cardiac conduction, and the electrocardiogram: a review. Am Heart J 1974;88:360–71.
5. Surawicz B. Relationship between electrocardiogram and electrolytes. Am Heart J 1967;73:814–34.
6. Oudit GY, Cameron D, Harris L. A case of appropriate inappropriate device therapy: hyperkalemia-induced ventricular oversensing. Can J Cardiol 2008;24:e16–8.
7. Guenther M, Rauwolf TP, Bock M, et al. A rare type of ventricular oversensing in ICD therapy–inappropriate ICD shock delivery due to triple counting. Pacing Clin Electrophysiol 2010;33:e17–9.
8. Koul AK, Keller S, Clancy JF, et al. Hyperkalemia induced T wave oversensing leading to loss of biventricular pacing and inappropriate ICD shocks. Pacing Clin Electrophysiol 2004;27:681–3.

A Confused Pacemaker

Bernard Abi-Saleh, MD, FHRS, Mohammad ElBaba, MD,
Maurice Khoury, MD, Marwan M. Refaat, MD, FHRS, FESC*

KEYWORDS

- Pacemaker • Heart • Cardiac • Electrocardiogram

KEY POINTS

- The electrocardiogram (ECG) raises the question of inappropriate device behavior and the possibility of ventricular lead oversensing causing failure of ventricular pacing.
- Careful analysis of the ECG proved that the mode of pacing was set to managed ventricular pacing (MVP) mode.
- The MVP mode should not be used in the setting of a complete atrioventricular conduction block.

CLINICAL PRESENTATION

A 33-year-old woman with rheumatic heart disease had a mitral valve replacement as well as aortic valve replacement 7 years ago. The valvular replacement surgery was done at a different medical center and was complicated by a complete heart block requiring the implantation of a dual-chamber pacemaker system (Medtronic Adapta). The patient was seen at a follow-up visit, and her 12-lead electrocardiogram (ECG) is shown in **Fig. 1**.

CLINICAL QUESTIONS

Is the device behavior appropriate? What does the ECG show?

DISCUSSION

The ECG raises the question of inappropriate device behavior and the possibility of ventricular lead oversensing causing failure of ventricular pacing. Careful analysis of the ECG proved that the mode of pacing was set to managed ventricular pacing (MVP) mode. MVP mode is an atrial-based pacing mode available in Medtronic devices that significantly reduces unnecessary right

ventricular pacing by primarily operating in an AAI(R) pacing mode while providing the safety of a dual-chamber backup mode [AAI(R) ↔ DDD(R)] if necessary. Algorithms such as atrioventricular (AV) search hysteresis and MVP allow the assurance of ventricular activation when needed and avoid unnecessary ventricular pacing.

The patient is in complete heart block and the device was programmed inappropriately at a different medical center in MVP mode. The ECG in **Fig. 1** shows pacing in AAI mode, pacing the atrium and sensing the junctional escape beats. The device considered the junctional escape beats as intrinsic conducted beats (**Fig. 2**). In the MVP mode when the device is in AAI(R), if the device senses that an atrial paced event is not followed by a ventricular sensed event, it follows with backup ventricular pacing at a shortened paced AV delay of 80 milliseconds (see **Fig. 2**). In the absence of a single ventricular sensed event, there is no switching to DDD(R) pacing in MVP mode pacing. The device then stays in AAI(R) mode and allows for an atrial paced event again with no ventricular sensed event. This property led to prolonged inappropriate AAI(R) pacing. If persistent loss of AV conduction is detected, defined as 2 of the most recent 4 A-A intervals with no

Disclosures: None.
Cardiac Electrophysiology Section, Cardiology Division, Department of Internal Medicine, American University of Beirut Medical Center, Beirut, Lebanon
* Corresponding author. Department of Biochemistry and Molecular Genetics, American University of Beirut Faculty of Medicine and Medical Center, PO Box 11-0236, Riad El-Solh, Beirut 1107 2020, Lebanon.
E-mail address: mr48@aub.edu.lb

Card Electrophysiol Clin 8 (2016) 181–183
http://dx.doi.org/10.1016/j.ccep.2015.10.025
1877-9182/16/$ – see front matter © 2016 Elsevier Inc. All rights reserved.

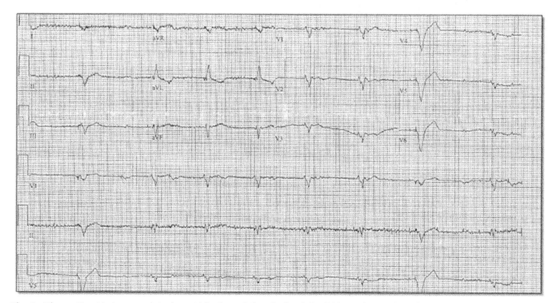

Fig. 1. The patient is in complete heart block and the device is in AAI mode, pacing the atrium, sensing the junctional escape beats, and considering them as conduced beats.

ventricular sensed events (2 consecutive losses of ventricular sensed events), the device switches after the second backup ventricular pacing to AV-sequential pacing DDD(R) mode with ventricular capture or fusion of the ventricular pacing output and intrinsic QRS complex. After 1 minute of DDD(R) mode, the device searches for intrinsic conduction. If there is no intrinsic conduction, the device remains in DDD(R) mode for 2 minutes before rechecking again. This process exponentially increases until the interval reaches 16 hours, at which time the device continues to check every 16 hours until the MVP mode is reprogrammed. The device appropriately paced in DDD(R) mode and searched for intrinsic conduction with a missed beat (**Fig. 3**), showing that the atrial paced beat is not followed by a ventricular sensed event, which led the device to remain in DDD(R) mode.

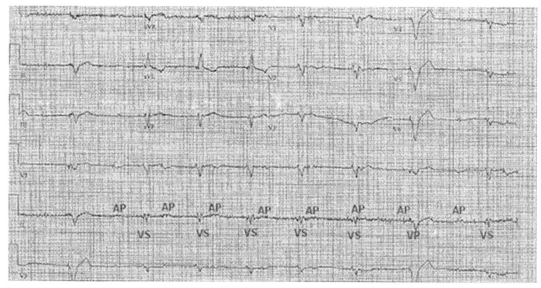

Fig. 2. The patient is in complete heart block and the device is in AAI mode, pacing the atrium, sensing the junctional escape beats, and considering them as conduced beats until the paced AV interval is exceeded, which is when the device paces the ventricle (VP, in red). One dropped beat does not result in switching to DDD pacing in MVP pacing, which led to prolonged inappropriate AAI pacing. VS, ventricular sensed.

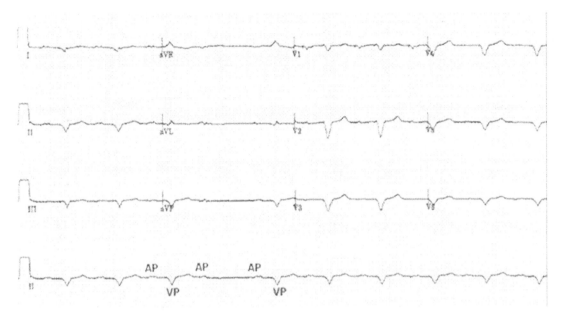

Fig. 3. The device is appropriately pacing in DDD mode and searching for intrinsic conduction with a dropped beat (atrial paced beat not followed by an intrinsic ventricular beat) so dual-chamber sequential pacing (APVP) is resumed.

SUMMARY

The MVP mode should not be used in the setting of a complete AV conduction block.

A Subclavian Arteriovenous Fistula Associated with Implantable Cardioverter-Defibrillator Implantation

Salman Rahman, BS, Adam C. Oesterle, MD, Nitish Badhwar, MD, FHRS*

KEYWORDS

- Implantable cardioverter-defibrillator • Implantation • Arteriovenous fistula

KEY POINTS

- Subclavian arteriovenous fistulas (AVFs) should be considered in the differential diagnosis of a patient presenting with worsening CHF symptoms or unilateral edema immediately after device implantation.
- A palpable thrill may be present or a bruit may be auscultated in the region of the fistula.
- Ultrasonography has limitations in the subclavian region and definitive diagnosis is only made by angiogram.
- Percutaneous occlusion of the AVF is preferred as surgical repair is associated with significant morbidity and mortality.

Implantable cardioverter-defibrillators (ICDs) have been shown to improve mortality in New York Heart Association (NYHA) class II and III patients with heart failure (HF) with left ventricular ejection fractions (LVEF) <35%.[1] Cardiac resynchronization therapy (CRT) reduces HF-related mortality and hospitalizations for patients with advanced HF, a wide QRS, and left ventricular dysfunction.[2] ICD implantation has been associated with procedural complication rates ranging from 3% to 6%, whereas CRT has higher procedural complication rates.[3,4] Subclavian arteriovenous fistula (AVF) associated with ICD implantation has only been reported once in the literature.[5]

CLINICAL PRESENTATION

A 61-year-old man with history of nonischemic dilated cardiomyopathy, LVEF 20% to 25%, NYHA class III HF, chronic kidney disease, hypertension, and diabetes presented with dyspnea on exertion despite medical management. He was on stable doses of carvedilol, spironolactone, and losartan. Baseline electrocardiogram showed prolonged PR interval with QRS duration of 114 milliseconds. He was enrolled in the EchoCRT trial that evaluated the effects of CRT in patients with advanced HF caused by left ventricular systolic dysfunction who have a narrow QRS width (<130 milliseconds) and echocardiographic evidence of ventricular dyssynchrony. The intrathoracic axillary vein approach was used to access the subclavian vein and a Biotronik Lumax 740 HF-T cardiac resynchronization therapy defibrillator (CRT-D) device was implanted. The patient presented a week later with left upper extremity edema.

Section of Cardiac Electrophysiology, Division of Cardiology, Department of Medicine, University of California, San Francisco, 500 Parnassus Avenue, MU East 431, Box 1354, San Francisco, CA 94143, USA
* Corresponding author.
E-mail address: badhwar@medicine.ucsf.edu

Card Electrophysiol Clin 8 (2016) 185–189
http://dx.doi.org/10.1016/j.ccep.2015.10.026

cardiacEP.theclinics.com

CLINICAL QUESTION

What is the cause of left upper extremity swelling after CRT-D implantation?

CLINICAL COURSE

The patient underwent a negative ultrasonography scan on the same day. He returned to clinic 4 days later with continued and progressive edema and was directly admitted for further evaluation. He denied any chest pain, shortness of breath, or symptoms of worsening congestive HF (CHF). Initial physical examination revealed normal heart sounds without detection of a murmur, clear lungs, and no jugular venous distension or lower extremity edema. However, there was significant pitting edema involving the entire left upper extremity with all distal pulses intact. Given the presentation, there was significant concern for acute venous thrombosis and a repeat ultrasonography scan was obtained. The ultrasonography showed a fistula between the subclavian artery and subclavian

vein (**Fig. 1**A). On further examination a bruit was heard over the subclavian vein, providing further evidence for a fistula. The patient's baseline glomerular filtration rate was around 30 mL/min and therefore no further imaging was obtained and vascular surgery was consulted. Perioperative left upper extremity arteriogram showed patent vasculature and a significant subclavian AVF (**Fig. 1**B, C). A Viabahn 5 × 8 cm self-expanding stent graft was placed percutaneously in the left subclavian artery and subsequent selective arteriography showed no further AVF (**Fig. 1**D). He was discharged the next day on aspirin 81 mg and Plavix 75 mg daily. Long-term outpatient follow-up showed resolution of left upper extremity edema.

DISCUSSION

ICDs have been shown to improve mortality in NYHA class II and III patients with HF with LVEFs less than 35%.[1] CRT reduces HF-related mortality and hospitalizations for patients with advanced HF, a wide QRS, and left ventricular dysfunction.[2]

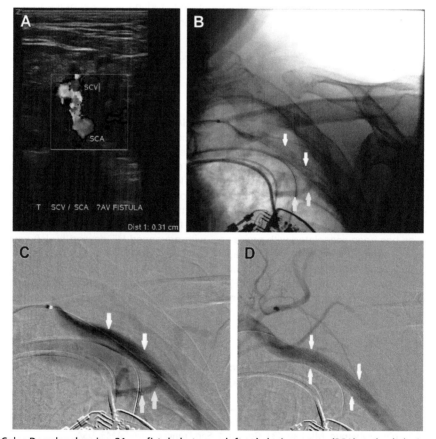

Fig. 1. (*A*) Color Doppler showing 31-cm fistula between left subclavian artery (SCA) and subclavian vein (SCV). (*B, C*) Selective injection of the left subclavian artery (*white arrows*) revealed the presence of a subclavian AVF (*yellow arrows*). (*D*) A 5 × 8 mm self-expanding stent graft was percutaneously placed (*white arrows*) and repeat angiography shows no residual arteriovenous flow. AV, arteriovenous.

ICD implantation has been associated with procedural complication rates ranging from 3% to 6%, whereas CRT has higher procedural complication rates.[3,4] Subclavian AVF associated with ICD implantation has only been reported once in the literature.[5]

This article describes unilateral left arm swelling 1 week after a de novo CRT-D implantation that was caused by subclavian AVF. Our initial concern was for a device-related thrombosis because this is a well-described complication. An initial ultrasonography scan did not reveal evidence of thrombus; however, clots can be masked on ultrasonography because of the clavicular shadow. Further imaging with contrast was deferred as a result of the patient's renal function. We also considered empiric anticoagulation, but a second ultrasonography scan revealed the presence of a subclavian AVF. Anticoagulation carried the risk of exacerbating the underlying fistula.

A search of published reports was conducted in PubMed with the following search terms: implantable cardioverter defibrillator, complications, and fistula. An additional search was performed for all randomized controlled trials (RCTs) involving ICDs or CRT that reported on complications. Subclavian AVF was not mentioned in any major RCT.[6–26] Data from several registries and databases also revealed no mention of AVF as a complication of ICD implantation.[23,27–38] Recently published articles using the National Cardiovascular Data Registry ICD database note that AVF occurred in 11 patients out of 167,000 (0.01%) who underwent ICD implantation.[39–43] We contacted the investigators for more information, but further patient information is not available in the database, so the location or presentation of the AVFs is unclear.

One previous case of a subclavian AVF following ICD implantation has been reported.[5] That case was a 53-year-old woman with nonischemic cardiomyopathy who developed worsening CHF symptoms after ICD generator replacement. Evaluation revealed the presence of a left subclavian AVF in the region of the proximal end of the ICD lead. The patient was successfully treated with percutaneous endovascular repair using an Amplatzer vascular occlusion plug, which led to resolution of her symptoms.

Iatrogenic fistula formation can occur as a complication of any endovascular catheterization. AVF following percutaneous groin access is reported in between 0.006% and 1% of cases.[44–46] AVFs have also been reported in pacemaker and ICD lead extractions. Most AVFs are small, spontaneously heal within a year, and rarely become symptomatic. Management is often expectant.[47–49]

Symptoms of subclavian AVFs include worsening CHF symptoms, limb edema, persistent bleeding from the puncture site, and occasionally death.[5,50,51] Often a palpable thrill is present or a bruit may be auscultated in the region of the fistula. Initial diagnostic imaging is usually duplex ultrasonography.[47] Ultrasonography has some limitations in the subclavian region because the clavicular shadow can obscure the fistula. Computed tomography angiography has sensitivity of 90% to 95% and specificity of 98.7% to 100%.[52] Symptomatic subclavian AVFs often require surgery or percutaneous repair. Surgical repair is associated with significant morbidity and mortality, and percutaneous occlusion of the AVF with coil embolization or stent graft placement is preferred.[47,53–55] Coil embolization and covered stents can occasionally migrate and form clot. Patency rates for stent graft repair of AVF range between 88% and 100% at up to 1 year.[56–59] Subclavian AVF is a rare, but likely underreported, complication of ICD implantation. It should be considered in the differential diagnosis of patients presenting with worsening CHF symptoms or unilateral edema immediately after device implantation.

REFERENCES

1. Bardy GH, Lee KL, Mark DB, et al. Amiodarone or an implantable cardio-defibrillator for congestive heart failure. N Engl J Med 2005;352:225–37.
2. Tang AS, Wells GA, Talajic M, et al. Cardiac-resynchronization therapy for mild-to moderate heart failure. N Engl J Med 2010;363:2385–95.
3. Atwater BD, Daubert JP. Implantable cardioverter defibrillators: risks accompany the life-saving benefits. Heart 2012;98:764–72.
4. Lee DS, Krahn AD, Healey JS, et al. Evaluation of early complications related to de novo cardioverter defibrillator implantation. J Am Coll Cardiol 2010; 55:774–82.
5. Hess CN, Ohman EM, Patel MR. Amplatzer vascular plug closure of a subclavian arteriovenous fistula associated with implantable cardioverter-defibrillator implantation. Catheter Cardiovasc Interv 2011;77: 761–3.
6. Moss AJ, Hall WJ, Cannom DS, et al. Improved survival with an implanted defibrillator in patients with coronary disease at high risk for ventricular arrhythmia. Multicenter Automatic Defibrillator Implantation Trial Investigators. N Engl J Med 1996; 335(26):1933–40.
7. Bigger JT. Prophylactic use of implanted cardiac defibrillators in patients at high risk for ventricular arrhythmias after coronary-artery bypass graft surgery. Coronary Artery Bypass Graft (CABG) Patch

Trial Investigators. N Engl J Med 1997;337(22): 1569–75.

8. Moss AJ, Zareba W, Hall WJ, et al. Prophylactic implantation of a defibrillator in patients with myocardial infarction and reduced ejection fraction. N Engl J Med 2002;346(12):877–83.

9. Bänsch D, Antz M, Boczor S, et al. Primary prevention of sudden cardiac death in idiopathic dilated cardiomyopathy: the Cardiomyopathy Trial (CAT). Circulation 2002;105(12):1453–8.

10. Hohnloser SH, Kuck KH, Dorian P, et al. Prophylactic use of an implantable cardioverter-defibrillator after acute myocardial infarction. N Engl J Med 2004; 351(24):2481–8.

11. Kadish A, Dyer A, Daubert JP, et al. Prophylactic defibrillator implantation in patients with nonischemic dilated cardiomyopathy. N Engl J Med 2004; 350(21):2151–8.

12. Bardy GH, Lee KL, Mark DB, et al. Amiodarone or an implantable cardioverter-defibrillator for congestive heart failure. N Engl J Med 2005;352(3):225–37.

13. Steinbeck G, Andresen D, Seidl K, et al. Defibrillator implantation early after myocardial infarction. N Engl J Med 2009;361(15):1427–36.

14. A comparison of antiarrhythmic-drug therapy with implantable defibrillators in patients resuscitated from near-fatal ventricular arrhythmias. The Antiarrhythmics versus Implantable Defibrillators (AVID) Investigators. N Engl J Med 1997;337(22):1576–83.

15. Connolly SJ, Gent M, Roberts RS, et al. Canadian implantable defibrillator study (CIDS): a randomized trial of the implantable cardioverter defibrillator against amiodarone. Circulation 2000;101(11): 1297–302.

16. Kuck KH, Cappato R, Siebels J, et al. Randomized comparison of antiarrhythmic drug therapy with implantable defibrillators in patients resuscitated from cardiac arrest: the Cardiac Arrest Study Hamburg (CASH). Circulation 2000;102(7):748–54.

17. Abraham WT, Fisher WG, Smith AL, et al. Cardiac resynchronization in chronic heart failure. N Engl J Med 2002;346(24):1845–53.

18. Young JB, Abraham WT, Smith AL, et al. Combined cardiac resynchronization and implantable cardioversion defibrillation in advanced chronic heart failure: the MIRACLE ICD Trial. JAMA 2003;289(20): 2685–94.

19. Bristow MR, Saxon LA, Boehmer J, et al. Cardiac-resynchronization therapy with or without an implantable defibrillator in advanced chronic heart failure. N Engl J Med 2004;350(21):2140–50.

20. Cleland JG, Daubert JC, Erdmann E, et al. The effect of cardiac resynchronization on morbidity and mortality in heart failure. N Engl J Med 2005;352(15): 1539–49.

21. Beshai JF, Grimm RA, Nagueh SF, et al. Cardiac-resynchronization therapy in heart failure with narrow QRS complexes. N Engl J Med 2007; 357(24):2461–71.

22. Linde C, Abraham WT, Gold MR, et al. Randomized trial of cardiac resynchronization in mildly symptomatic heart failure patients and in asymptomatic patients with left ventricular dysfunction and previous heart failure symptoms. J Am Coll Cardiol 2008;52(23):1834–43.

23. Whitson BA, Andrade RS, Mitiek MO, et al. Thoracoscopic thymectomy: technical pearls to a 21st century approach. J Thorac Dis 2013;5(2):129–34.

24. Kron J, Herre J, Renfroe EG, et al. Lead- and device-related complications in the Antiarrhythmics versus Implantable Defibrillators Trial. Am Heart J 2001; 141(1):92–8.

25. Gras D, Böcker D, Lunati M, et al. Implantation of cardiac resynchronization therapy systems in the CARE-HF trial: procedural success rate and safety. Europace 2007;9(7):516–22.

26. León AR, Abraham WT, Curtis AB, et al. Safety of transvenous cardiac resynchronization system implantation in patients with chronic heart failure: combined results of over 2,000 patients from a multicenter study program. J Am Coll Cardiol 2005; 46(12):2348–56.

27. van Rees JB, Borleffs CJ, Thijssen J, et al. Prophylactic implantable cardioverter-defibrillator treatment in the elderly: therapy, adverse events, and survival gain. Europace 2012;14(1):66–73.

28. Sterliński M, Przybylski A, Gepner K, et al. Over 10 years with an implantable cardioverter-defibrillator - a long term follow-up of 60 patients. Kardiol Pol 2010;68(9):1023–9.

29. Al-Khatib SM, Lucas FL, Jollis JG, et al. The relation between patients' outcomes and the volume of cardioverter-defibrillator implantation procedures performed by physicians treating Medicare beneficiaries. J Am Coll Cardiol 2005; 46(8):1536–40.

30. Reynolds MR, Cohen DJ, Kugelmass AD, et al. The frequency and incremental cost of major complications among Medicare beneficiaries receiving implantable cardioverter-defibrillators. J Am Coll Cardiol 2006;47(12):2493–7.

31. Healey JS, Birnie DH, Lee DS, et al. Defibrillation testing at the time of ICD insertion: an analysis from the Ontario ICD Registry. J Cardiovasc Electrophysiol 2010;21(12):1344–8.

32. Gradaus R, Block M, Brachmann J, et al. Mortality, morbidity, and complications in 3,344 patients with implantable cardioverter defibrillators: results from the German ICD Registry EURID. Pacing Clin Electrophysiol 2003;26(7p1):1511–8.

33. Rosenqvist M, Beyer T, Block M, et al. Adverse events with transvenous implantable cardioverter-defibrillators: a prospective multicenter study. Circulation 1998;98(7):663–70.

34. Lee DS, Krahn AD, Healey JS, et al. Evaluation of early complications related to de novo cardioverter defibrillator implantation: insights from the Ontario ICD database. J Am Coll Cardiol 2010;55(8):774–82.

35. Kremers MS, Hammill SC, Berul CI, et al. The National ICD Registry Report: Version 2.1 including leads and pediatrics for years 2010 and 2011. Heart Rhythm 2013;10(4):e59–65.

36. Haines DE, Wang Y, Curtis J. Implantable Cardioverter-Defibrillator Registry risk score models for acute procedural complications or death after implantable cardioverter-defibrillator implantation. Circulation 2011;123(19):2069–76.

37. Freeman JV, Wang Y, Curtis JP, et al. Physician procedure volume and complications of cardioverter-defibrillator implantation. Circulation 2012;125(1):57–64.

38. Freeman JV, Wang Y, Curtis JP, et al. The relation between hospital procedure volume and complications of cardioverter-defibrillator implantation from the Implantable Cardioverter-Defibrillator Registry. J Am Coll Cardiol 2010;56(14):1133–9.

39. Dewland TA, Pellegrini CN, Wang Y, et al. Dual-chamber implantable cardioverter-defibrillator selection is associated with increased complication rates and mortality among patients enrolled in the NCDR implantable cardioverter-defibrillator registry. J Am Coll Cardiol 2011;58(10):1007–13.

40. Peterson PN, Daugherty SL, Wang Y, et al. Gender differences in procedure-related adverse events in patients receiving implantable cardioverter-defibrillator therapy. Circulation 2009;119(8):1078–84.

41. Tsai V, Goldstein MK, Hsia HH, et al. Influence of age on perioperative complications among patients undergoing implantable cardioverter-defibrillators for primary prevention in the United States. Circ Cardiovasc Qual Outcomes 2011;4(5):549–56.

42. Aggarwal A, Wang Y, Rumsfeld JS, et al. Clinical characteristics and in-hospital outcome of patients with end-stage renal disease on dialysis referred for implantable cardioverter-defibrillator implantation. Heart Rhythm 2009;6(11):1565–71.

43. Curtis JP, Luebbert JJ, Wang Y, et al. Association of physician certification and outcomes among patients receiving an implantable cardioverter-defibrillator. JAMA 2009;301(16):1661–70.

44. Oweida SW, Roubin GS, Smith RB, et al. Postcatheterization vascular complications associated with percutaneous transluminal coronary angioplasty. J Vasc Surg 1990;12(3):310–5.

45. Glaser RL, McKellar D, Scher KS. Arteriovenous fistulas after cardiac catheterization. Arch Surg 1989;124(11):1313–5.

46. Kim D, Orron DE, Skillman JJ, et al. Role of superficial femoral artery puncture in the development of pseudoaneurysm and arteriovenous fistula complicating percutaneous transfemoral cardiac catheterization. Cathet Cardiovasc Diagn 1992;25(2):91–7.

47. González SB, Busquets JC, Figueiras RG, et al. Imaging arteriovenous fistulas. AJR Am J Roentgenol 2009;193(5):1425–33.

48. Toursarkissian B, Allen BT, Petrinec D, et al. Spontaneous closure of selected iatrogenic pseudoaneurysms and arteriovenous fistulae. J Vasc Surg 1997;25(5):803–8.

49. Kelm M, Perings SM, Jax T, et al. Incidence and clinical outcome of iatrogenic femoral arteriovenous fistulas: implications for risk stratification and treatment. J Am Coll Cardiol 2002;40(2):291–7.

50. García-Bolao I, Macías A, Moreno J, et al. Fatal left internal mammary artery graft to subclavian vein fistula complicating dual-chamber pacemaker implantation. Europace 2008;10(7):890–1.

51. Kumins NH, Tober JC, Love CJ, et al. Arteriovenous fistulae complicating cardiac pacemaker lead extraction: recognition, evaluation, and management. J Vasc Surg 2000;32(6):1225–8.

52. Miller-Thomas MM, West OC, Cohen AM. Diagnosing traumatic arterial injury in the extremities with CT angiography: pearls and pitfalls. Radiographics 2005;25(Suppl 1):S133–42.

53. Azpurua FE, Dougherty KG, Massumi A, et al. Fistula from right internal mammary artery to superior vena cava after use of a laser sheath to extract a pacemaker lead. Tex Heart Inst J 2012;39(5):727–30.

54. Anguera I, Real I, Morales M, et al. Left internal mammary artery to innominate vein fistula complicating pacemaker insertion. Treatment with endovascular transarterial coil embolization. J Cardiovasc Surg (Torino) 1999;40(4):523–5.

55. Anastacio MM, Castillo-Sang M, Smith TW, et al. Iatrogenic left internal thoracic artery to left subclavian vein fistula after excimer laser pacemaker lead extraction. J Thorac Cardiovasc Surg 2012;143(4):e35–7.

56. Ruebben A, Tettoni S, Muratore P, et al. Arteriovenous fistulas induced by femoral arterial catheterization: percutaneous treatment. Radiology 1998;209(3):729–34.

57. Thalhammer C, Kirchherr AS, Uhlich F, et al. Postcatheterization pseudoaneurysms and arteriovenous fistulas: repair with percutaneous implantation of endovascular covered stents. Radiology 2000;214(1):127–31.

58. Baltacioğlu F, Cimşit NC, Cil B, et al. Endovascular stent-graft applications in iatrogenic vascular injuries. Cardiovasc Intervent Radiol 2003;26(5):434–9.

59. Joffe HV. Upper-extremity deep vein thrombosis. Circulation 2002;106(14):1874–80.

Section 5: Adult Congenital Cardiac Disease

Editor: Ronn Tanel

Slow Pathway Modification in a Patient with D-Transposition of the Great Arteries and Atrial Switch Procedure

Emily Sue Ruckdeschel, MD, Joseph Kay, MD,
Paul Varosy, MD, Duy Thai Nguyen, MD*

KEYWORDS

- Congenital heart disease • Transposition of the great arteries • Supraventricular tachycardia
- Atrioventricular nodal reentrant tachycardia

KEY POINTS

- Patients are often not able to tolerate frequent, rapid, or incessant atrial arrhythmias without developing significant symptoms and ventricular dysfunction.
- Atrial arrhythmias are associated with an increased risk of ventricular arrhythmias and sudden cardiac death.
- Rhythm disturbances must be aggressively addressed in this population with frequent screening, follow-up, and treatment.

CLINICAL PRESENTATION

A 48-year-old man with dextrotranspostion of the great arteries (d-TGA) and atrial switch procedure (Mustard) presented with palpitations. He had a history of atrial arrhythmias and underwent an attempted ablation at another hospital. The ablation was not completed because his presumed atrial tachycardia was in proximity to the atrioventricular (AV) node, he had a pacemaker placed with atrial antitachycardia pacing technology, and he was started on antiarrhythmic medications. However, given continued daily symptoms despite medications, and a decline in systemic ventricular function caused by incessant tachycardia, he was referred to our institution for evaluation and ablation.

CLINICAL COURSE

The patient presented to the electrophysiology (EP) laboratory in supraventricular tachycardia (SVT). Venous access was obtained and a standard EP study was performed. A decapolar catheter was advanced through the patient's Mustard baffle and placed into the left atrial appendage. A quadripolar catheter was advanced through the baffle, across the nonsystemic AV valve (mitral valve), and into the subpulmonary left ventricle. The patient was in an incessant A-on-V tachycardia at a cycle length of 430 milliseconds.

At baseline, the patient's A-on-V SVT had intermittent spontaneous AV block (**Fig. 1**), thus ruling out AV reciprocating tachycardia. Ventricular overdrive pacing accelerated the tachycardia and,

Cardiology Division, University of Colorado, Denver, Aurora, CO, USA
* Corresponding author. University of Colorado, Denver, Anschutz Medical Campus, 12401 East 17th Avenue, B-132, Aurora, CO 80045.
E-mail address: duy.t.nguyen@ucdenver.edu

Card Electrophysiol Clin 8 (2016) 191–196
http://dx.doi.org/10.1016/j.ccep.2015.10.027

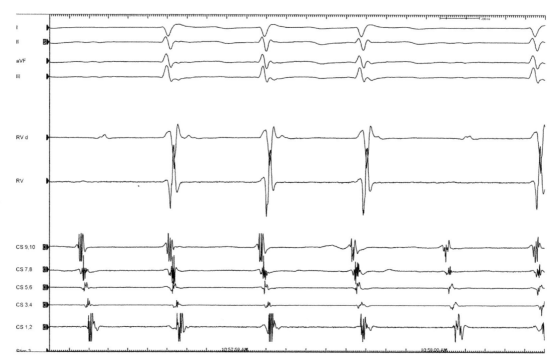

Fig. 1. At baseline, the patient was in an A-on-V tachycardia with intermittent spontaneous AV block, thus ruling out AV reciprocating tachycardia.

after cessation, showed a V-A-V response (**Fig. 2**), thus ruling out atrial tachycardia. The postpacing interval minus tachycardia cycle length and the Stim-A minus VA were long, and both were consistent with typical slow-fast AV nodal reentrant tachycardia (AVNRT) (**Fig. 3**).

CLINICAL QUESTION

How can the slow pathway for AVNRT be modified in patients with d-TGA who have had an atrial switch procedure?

MANAGEMENT AND ABLATION

The His electrogram could not be located within the baffle and good A/V electrogram ratios for slow pathway modification were not possible from within the baffle. Femoral arterial access was obtained, and a standard 4-mm tip radiofrequency ablation catheter was advanced around the aortic arch. The catheter was prolapsed retrograde across the aortic valve into the systemic right ventricle (RV), and then retroflexed through the systemic AV valve (tricuspid valve) annulus. Atrial overdrive pacing accelerated the ventricular electrograms and, after cessation, showed an A-H-A response, consistent with typical slow-fast AVNRT and ruling out junctional tachycardia.

Electroanatomic mapping was performed to define a His cloud. Preprocedure imaging with a computed tomography (CT) scan had defined the patient's anatomy. This imaging was merged with the electroanatomic map to create an image of the tricuspid valve, aorta, and septum, in order to better delineate the slow pathway region for ablation (**Fig. 4**). The ablation catheter was lowered to the inferior portion of the AV annulus, well below the His cloud. The fast pathway was mapped away from this region, and was closer to the His cloud.

A large ventricular and small atrial electrogram was present, and ablation in this region repeatedly initiated SVT (see **Fig. 4**, red lesion tags). Because we could not safely assess ablation efficacy or impending heart block because of tachycardia initiation with ablation, we decided to change to cryoablation. The 4-mm tip radiofrequency ablation catheter was removed. A 5-French pigtail catheter was used to guide a long 8.5-French SL0 sheath across the aortic valve and into the systemic RV. A 4-mm tip cryoablation catheter was placed through the long sheath and retroflexed toward the slow pathway region where the prior radiofrequency lesions were attempted (**Fig. 5**, white arrow). Several cryoablations were applied, without causing initiation of tachycardia during ablation. However, the tachycardia

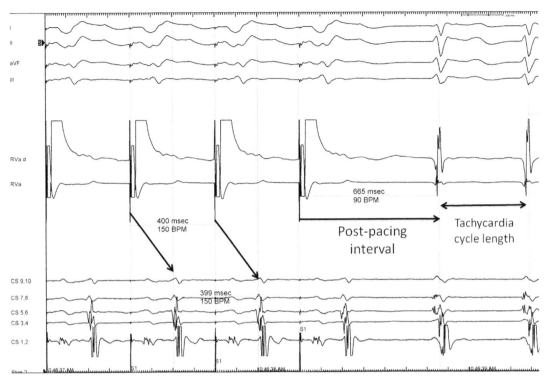

Fig. 2. Ventricular overdrive pacing accelerated the tachycardia, and after cessation, showed a V-A-V response, thus ruling out atrial tachycardia. The postpacing interval minus tachycardia cycle length and the Stim-A minus VA were long. Both of these findings were consistent with typical slow-fast AV nodal reentrant tachycardia. BPM, beats per minute.

remained easily inducible. The tip of the cryoablation catheter was slowly raised, toward the inferior border of the His cloud (see **Fig. 5**, raised orange catheter). With this last cryoablation lesion, there was PR interval prolongation. The delivery of cryothermal energy was immediately stopped, and PR interval prolongation recovered. AVNRT could no longer be induced after this ablation lesion, with or without isoproterenol. There was no inducible tachycardia throughout a 30-minute waiting period.

DISCUSSION

Atrial arrhythmias are common in patients with re-paired congenital heart disease, and patients with d-TGA who are treated with an atrial switch operation are at particularly high risk for atrial arrhythmias.[1] Historically, d-TGA was a fatal condition. Pulmonary venous blood is routed from the left atrium to the left ventricle, and then back to the pulmonary arteries. Systemic venous blood is routed from the right atrium to the RV, and out the aorta to the systemic circulation. This arrangement results in 2 parallel circuits, which is not compatible with life. However, in the 1960s, the atrial switch procedures were developed and were used as the mainstay of surgical palliation for several decades.[2] This procedure is complex and involves rerouting blood from the superior vena cava and inferior vena cava to the left ventricle through a surgically created baffle within the atria, while pulmonary venous blood flow is rerouted to the RV. Patients then have a normal circulatory pattern, although they are left with a systemic RV.

The atrial switch procedure involves extensive suturing by the surgeon. The resulting scar within the atria allows for the formation of multiple reentrant pathways and atrial tachycardias. In addition, because of surgical manipulation and scar development, they are also at risk for developing bradyarrythmias from sinus node injury.[2] The rate of atrial arrhythmias in this population is very high, and estimates range from 30% to 70% over long-term follow-up.[3,4] There is also an increased risk of atrial arrhythmias in patients with systemic right ventricular dysfunction, pulmonary hypertension, and junctional rhythm before 18 years of age.[4]

Ablation of atrial arrhythmias is challenging because the surgically created baffle limits access

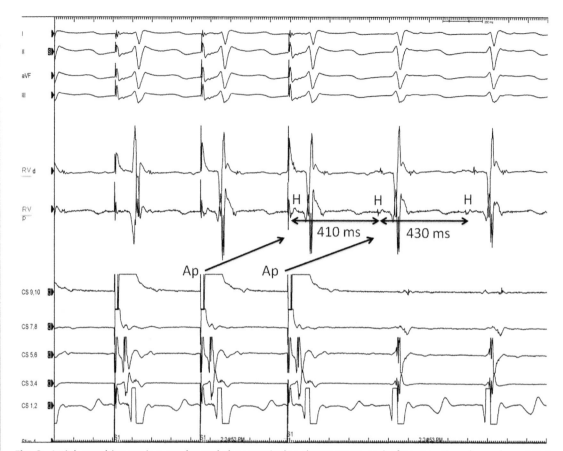

Fig. 3. Atrial overdrive pacing accelerated the ventricular electrograms and after cessation showed an A-H-A response, consistent with typical slow-fast AV nodal reentrant tachycardia and ruling out junctional tachycardia. Ap, atrial pacing; H, His.

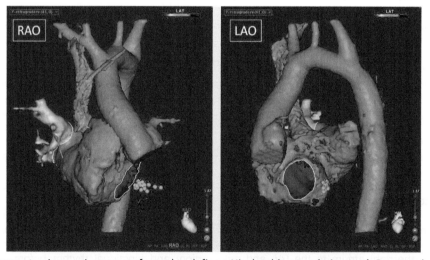

Fig. 4. Electroanatomic mapping was performed to define a His cloud (*orange lesion tags*). Preprocedure imaging with a CT scan had defined the patient's anatomy. This imaging was merged with the electroanatomic mapping to create an image of the tricuspid valve, aorta, and septum, in order to better delineate the slow pathway region for ablation (*red lesion tags*). LAO, left anterior oblique; RAO, right anterior oblique.

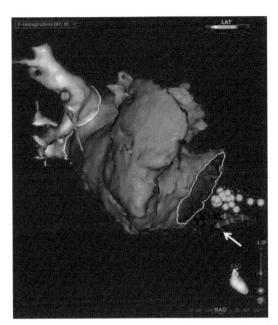

Fig. 5. A 4-mm tip cryoablation catheter was placed through a long sheath across the aortic valve and retro-flexed toward the slow pathway region where the prior radiofrequency lesions were attempted (*white arrow*). When the cryoablation catheter was raised toward the inferior border of the His cloud (*orange lesion tags*), successful cryoablation lesions were delivered.

to some of the atrial tissue. It is difficult to know before an EP study whether arrhythmogenic foci are within the systemic venous baffle or the pulmonary venous baffle. Transbaffle puncture may be required to access atrial tissue on the pulmonary venous side if there is no baffle leak. Small studies have shown this to be a safe and effective option, when necessary.[5] Catheter ablation has been shown to be safe with good short-term outcomes, although there is a high rate of recurrence (as high as 30% for intra-atrial reentry tachycardia).[6,7]

Typical AVNRT is less common than intra-atrial reentry tachycardia in patients with d-TGA and a prior atrial switch procedure. Typical AVNRT may be the result of prior ablation lesions in this patient population, which may alter the properties of the slow pathway into the AV node.[7] The creation of a surgical baffle within the atria may lead to isolation of the AV node, His bundle, and slow pathway to the arterial side and therefore makes ablation of AVNRT challenging. As was seen with this patient, it was not possible to adequately evaluate the triangle of Koch from venous access alone. Retrograde aortic access or transbaffle access is frequently needed to reach the area of interest.

The location of the compact AV node, fast pathway, and slow pathway can be altered by surgery and the underlying anatomy. Mapping the

fast pathway, as well as creating a large His cloud, is prudent when performing ablation in this region. Cryoablation should be considered if there is any concern for AV block, especially when the assessment of safety and efficacy of ablation is limited by tachycardia or anatomy. Maneuvering a cryoablation catheter into this region can be challenging, given the retrograde aortic approach. A long sheath across the aortic valve can improve access to the systemic tricuspid valve. Remote magnetic navigation may also be considered, but does not help if cryoablation is needed.

Systemic right ventricular failure is common in this group, and heart failure is a leading cause of death.[8] Patients are often not able to tolerate frequent, rapid, or incessant atrial arrhythmias without developing significant symptoms and ventricular dysfunction. Atrial arrhythmias are associated with an increased risk of ventricular arrhythmias and sudden cardiac death in this patient population. Thus, rhythm disturbances must be aggressively addressed in this population with frequent screening, follow-up, and treatment.[9]

REFERENCES

1. Khairy P, Van Hare GF, Balaji S, et al. PACES/HRS expert consensus statement on the recognition and management of arrhythmias in adult congenital heart disease: developed in partnership between the Pediatric and Congenital Electrophysiology Society (PACES) and the Heart Rhythm Society (HRS). Endorsed by the governing bodies of PACES, HRS, the American College of Cardiology (ACC), the American Heart Association (AHA), the European Heart Rhythm Association (EHRA), the Canadian Heart Rhythm Society (CHRS), and the International Society for Adult Congenital Heart Disease (ISACHD). Can J Cardiol 2014;30(10):e1–63.
2. Warnes CA. Transposition of the great arteries. Circulation 2006;114(24):2699–709.
3. Khairy P, Landzberg MJ, Lambert J, et al. Long-term outcomes after the atrial switch for surgical correction of transposition: a meta-analysis comparing the Mustard and Senning procedures. Cardiol Young 2004;14(3):284–92.
4. Puley G, Siu S, Connelly M, et al. Arrhythmia and survival in patients >18 years of age after the mustard procedure for complete transposition of the great arteries. Am J Cardiol 1999;83(7):1080–4.
5. Jones DG, Jarman JW, Lyne JC, et al. The safety and efficacy of trans-baffle puncture to enable catheter ablation of atrial tachycardias following the Mustard procedure: a single centre experience and literature review. Int J Cardiol 2013;168(2):1115–20.
6. Wu J, Deisenhofer I, Ammar S, et al. Acute and long-term outcome after catheter ablation of supraventricular

tachycardia in patients after the Mustard or Senning operation for D-transposition of the great arteries. Europace 2013;15(6):886–91.

7. Kanter RJ, Papagiannis J, Carboni MP, et al. Radiofrequency catheter ablation of supraventricular tachycardia substrates after Mustard and Senning operations for d-transposition of the great arteries. J Am Coll Cardiol 2000;35(2):428–41.

8. Verheugt CL, Uiterwaal CS, van der Velde ET, et al. Mortality in adult congenital heart disease. Eur Heart J 2010;31(10):1220–9.

9. Schwerzmann M, Salehian O, Harris L, et al. Ventricular arrhythmias and sudden death in adults after a Mustard operation for transposition of the great arteries. Eur Heart J 2009;30(15):1873–9.

Intra-atrial Reentrant Tachycardia in Complete Transposition of the Great Arteries Without Femoral Venous Access

 CrossMark

Ryan T. Borne, MD, Joseph Kay, MD, Thomas Fagan, MD, Duy Thai Nguyen, MD*

KEYWORDS

- d-TGA • Atrial flutter • Catheter ablation • Hepatic venous access

KEY POINTS

- Catheter ablation for patients with transposition of the great arteries (d-TGA) requires multiple considerations and careful preprocedural planning.
- Knowledge of the patient's anatomy and surgical correction, in addition to electroanatomic mapping and entrainment maneuvers, are important to identify and successfully treat arrhythmias.
- This case was unique in that the lack of femoral venous access required transhepatic venous access and bidirectional block was attained with ablation lesions along the cavotricuspid isthmus on both sides of the baffle.

CLINICAL PRESENTATION

A 49-year-old woman with history of transposition of the great arteries (d-TGA) presented with recurrent episodes of drug-refractory, symptomatic atrial flutter. Her history was notable for surgical atrial septostomy via a right lateral thoracotomy (Blalock-Hanlon septectomy) and a surgical atrial switch (Mustard) procedure at the age of 6 years. In addition, she had a baffle leak and underwent closure with a percutaneous Amplatzer atrial septal occluder device (St Jude Medical, St Paul, MN). She has known bilateral femoral vein occlusions. She was referred for catheter ablation.

CLINICAL QUESTION

What is the approach to catheter ablation for intra-atrial reentrant tachycardia (IART) in a patient with d-TGA?

CLINICAL COURSE

The initial approach to IART in this patient is similar for any patient with atrial flutter. Using entrainment and activation mapping, we identified the circuit involved and the critical isthmus that was required to maintain the IART. Once the circuit was identified, we then considered the specific challenges for this patient, which included her atrial baffle and the lack of femoral venous access.

The patient was brought to the electrophysiology (EP) laboratory, where access was obtained in the right internal jugular vein and the right common femoral artery. A standard EP study was performed. Incremental right atrial pacing induced tachycardia with a cycle length of 290 milliseconds. Entrainment from the systemic venous side of the cavotricuspid isthmus (CTI) showed a postpacing interval (PPI) minus tachycardia cycle length (TCL) of 21 milliseconds, indicating that

Cardiac Electrophysiology, University of Colorado, Denver, 12605 East 16th Avenue, Mailstop B136, Aurora, CO 80045, USA
* Corresponding author.
E-mail address: duy.t.nguyen@ucdenver.edu

Card Electrophysiol Clin 8 (2016) 197–200
http://dx.doi.org/10.1016/j.ccep.2015.10.028
1877-9182/16/$ – see front matter © 2016 Elsevier Inc. All rights reserved.

cardiacEP.theclinics.com

the systemic venous CTI was integral to the arrhythmia circuit (**Fig. 1**A). Entrainment from the left atrium established that it was not part of the circuit (see **Fig. 1**B). The catheter was moved to the anterior portion of the systemic venous atrium (toward the tricuspid valve) and entrainment showed that it was part of the circuit (see **Fig. 1**C). Given the lack of catheter stability from a superior approach, a high suspicion for CTI-dependent IART, and the presence of a significant amount of the CTI on the systemic venous side of the baffle, percutaneous transhepatic venous access was obtained with ultrasonography guidance. An 8.5-French long sheath was placed into the inferior vena cava (IVC) via a hepatic vein before heparin administration for arterial catheter placement (**Fig. 2**).

Access to the tricuspid valve, or the systemic atrioventricular (AV) valve, was performed via a retrograde aortic approach. Entrainment from the pulmonary venous medial and lateral CTI confirmed that the PPI-TCL was less than 30 milliseconds (see **Fig. 1**D). Activation mapping revealed a counterclockwise IART circuit encompassing the full TCL around the tricuspid valve annulus (**Fig. 3**).

Given that the critical isthmus was confirmed to be the CTI for an IART circuit around the systemic AV valve (tricuspid valve), ablation targeted the CTI using an irrigated tip catheter. On the systemic venous side, via the transhepatic access, a series of ablation lesions were delivered in a linear fashion to create a line of block from the baffle along the CTI to the IVC (see **Fig. 3**, *red lesion tags*). IART terminated during ablation along the systemic venous side of the CTI, but bidirectional block was not achieved. Next, the ablation catheter was advanced via a retrograde aortic approach, prolapsed across the aortic valve, and into the systemic right ventricle. The ablation catheter was then advanced into the pulmonary venous atrium, and ablation was performed on that side of the CTI. Bidirectional block was confirmed and persisted after a waiting period. No other arrhythmias were inducible. The hepatic access was occluded with coil embolization to prevent bleeding from the tract. The patient has remained arrhythmia free over a 3-year follow-up period.

DISCUSSION

d-TGA accounts for 5% to 7% of congenital heart defects, with most adults now having had a Mustard or Senning procedure. These surgeries involve extensive atrial reconstruction and predispose to both sinus node dysfunction and atrial tachyarrhythmias. Up to 25% of patients have atrial tachyarrhythmias (IART being the most

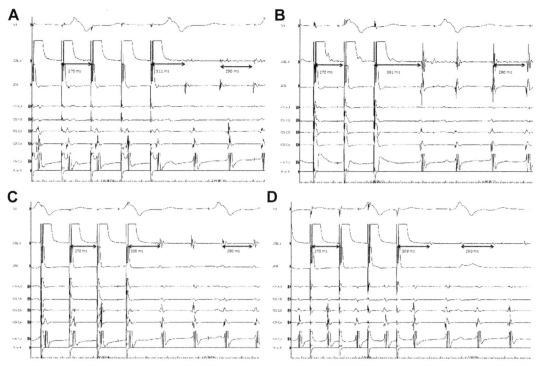

Fig. 1. Entrainment pacing performed in (*A*) venous portion of the CTI, (*B*) left atrium, (*C*) anterior baffle of the systemic venous CTI, (*D*) arterial portion of the CTI from a retrograde aortic approach.

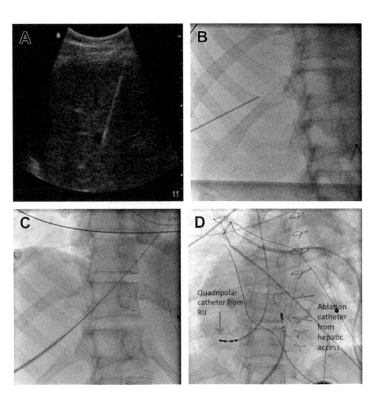

Fig. 2. (*A*) Ultrasonography image showing the 22-gauge needle being advanced into the hepatic vein. (*B–D*) Fluoroscopy images of transhepatic access. (*B*) Needle is advanced through the right midaxillary line into the liver. (*C*) A sheath is advanced over the wire in the hepatic vein and into the systemic venous atrium. (*D*) Ablation catheter is placed through the hepatic sheath and into the systemic venous side of the baffle. A quadripolar catheter is present in the systemic venous atrium from the right internal jugular vein (RIJ).

common) by 20 years after surgery.[1,2] Observational data have suggested an increased risk of death among patients with atrial arrhythmias.[1,3] Because typical atrial flutter rates tend to be slower and 1:1 AV conduction often occurs, hemodynamic compromise may be an important cause of sudden cardiac death.[4] Aggressive management of tachyarrhythmias is recommended by most adult congenital heart disease experts to reduce these dangers.

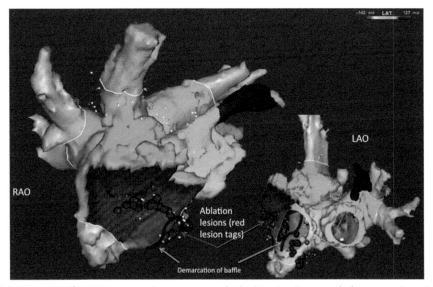

Fig. 3. Activation map of IART representing a counterclockwise circuit around the systemic atrioventricular (tricuspid) valve in the right anterior oblique (RAO) and left anterior oblique (LAO) projections. Red represents earliest, purple represents latest. Red lesion tags are ablation lesions.

The most common form of IART is a circuit that rotates around the systemic AV valve (tricuspid), similar to typical CTI-dependent atrial flutter in the structurally normal heart.[2] However, several characteristics differ from typical flutter. By redirecting venous return, the Mustard and Senning baffles partition the CTI into 2 distinct regions. Surgical techniques vary considerably, and the relative portion of the CTI on each side depends on the specific surgical variant. Furthermore, the tricuspid valve is not directly accessible from the systemic venous circulation and requires a retrograde aortic approach, access through baffle leaks if they are present, or a transbaffle approach. As in this case, successful ablation often needs to be accomplished in both the systemic venous and pulmonary venous atria.

Many patients with congenital heart disease who survive to adulthood either lose conventional venous access (occluded femoral access from prior procedures) or have anatomy (interrupted IVC) that makes cardiac catheterization procedures difficult. Percutaneous transhepatic venous access has been shown to be a safe and effective way of accessing the systemic venous system.[5] The procedure generally includes using a small-gauge needle and stylet to puncture through the right midaxillary line midway between the diaphragm and the lower margin of the liver (see **Fig. 2**). The stylet is removed and the needle withdrawn slowly as a small volume of contrast is infused gently until the needle is positioned in a hepatic vein. A wire is advanced through the needle into the hepatic vein and into the right atrium. The needle is exchanged for a sheath, which is then exchanged over a second wire for a standard hemostatic vascular sheath. At the termination of the procedure, the sheath is withdrawn from the hepatic vein into the liver parenchyma where a vascular coil is placed to minimize the risk of bleeding.

Catheter ablation for patients with d-TGA requires multiple considerations and careful preprocedural planning. Knowledge of the patient's anatomy and surgical correction, in addition to electroanatomic mapping and entrainment maneuvers, is important to identify and successfully treat arrhythmias. This case was unique in that the lack of femoral venous access required transhepatic venous access and bidirectional block was attained with ablation lesions along the CTI on both sides of the baffle.

REFERENCES

1. Gelatt M, Hamilton RM, McCrindle BW, et al. Arrhythmia and mortality after the Mustard procedure: a 30-year single-center experience. J Am Coll Cardiol 1997;29:194–201.

2. Khairy P, Landzberg MJ, Lambert J, et al. Long-term outcomes after the atrial switch for surgical correction of transposition: a meta-analysis comparing the Mustard and Senning procedures. Cardiol Young 2004;14:284–92.

3. Sarkar D, Bull C, Yates R, et al. Comparison of long-term outcomes of atrial repair of simple transposition with implications for a late arterial switch strategy. Circulation 1999;100:II176–81.

4. Khairy P, Harris L, Landzberg MJ, et al. Sudden death and defibrillators in transposition of the great arteries with intra-atrial baffles: a multicenter study. Circ Arrhythm Electrophysiol 2008;1:250–7.

5. Nguyen DT, Gupta R, Kay J, et al. Percutaneous transhepatic access for catheter ablation of cardiac arrhythmias. Europace 2013;15:494–500.

Ventricular Tachycardia Following Surgical Repair of Complex Congenital Heart Disease

CrossMark

Sherrie Joy Baysa, MD, Ronald J. Kanter, MD*

KEYWORDS

- Congenital heart disease • Tetralogy of Fallot • Double-outlet right ventricle • Pulmonary atresia
- Ventricular tachycardia • Sudden cardiac death • Implantable cardioverter-defibrillator
- Antiarrhythmic drugs

KEY POINTS

- Although uncommon, ventricular tachycardia can occur even in children following complex right ventricular outflow tract surgery.
- Programmed ventricular stimulation has reasonably high predictive value in patients having undergone right ventricular outflow tract surgery for complex congenital heart disease.
- Antiarrhythmic drug therapy still has a role in the management of the occasional youngster with congenital heart disease and ventricular tachycardia, although it does not provide the same level of protection of that provided by an implantable cardioverter-defibrillator.
- Cardiac MRI has an increasingly important role in surgical planning for patients having congenital heart disease. Even as MRI compatible implantable cardioverter-defibrillators are becoming available, the effect that these device components have on data acquisition may make their implantation problematic.

CLINICAL PRESENTATION

A 9-year old boy with surgically repaired complex congenital heart disease (CHD) presented with a 1-year history of self-limited palpitations, unassociated with syncope, light-headedness, shortness of breath, or chest pain. He was born with double-outlet RV, pulmonary atresia, subaortic ventricular septal defect (VSD), and normal-sized branch pulmonary arteries. Interventions included placement of 3.0-mm right modified Blalock-Taussig shunt as a neonate; shunt takedown, VSD closure, and right ventricle (RV) to pulmonary artery homograft conduit at 8 months; surgical revision of the stenotic conduit at 5 years; and complex interventional catheterization at 7 years because of distal conduit stenosis (dilation with stent), right pulmonary artery stenosis (dilation with stent), and severe pulmonary valve insufficiency (Melody valve placement [Medtronic; St Paul, MN]). Because attempts at documenting the rhythm during clinical episodes using an attached event recorder were unsuccessful, the patient underwent cardiac catheterization. The procedure was performed under propofol-based general anesthesia. He was found to have two-thirds systemic RV pressure, mild pulmonary valve insufficiency, moderate stenosis of both stents, and left ventricular end-diastolic pressure of 10 mm Hg. After balloon angioplasty of the stents, electrophysiologic study (EPS) was performed.

Division of Cardiology, The Heart Program, Nicklaus Children's Hospital, Miami Children's Hospital Health System, 3100 Southwest 62nd Avenue, Miami, FL 33155, USA
* Corresponding author.
E-mail address: Ronald.Kanter@mch.com

Card Electrophysiol Clin 8 (2016) 201–204
http://dx.doi.org/10.1016/j.ccep.2015.10.029
1877-9182/16/$ – see front matter © 2016 Elsevier Inc. All rights reserved.

ELECTROPHYSIOLOGY STUDY

Baseline intervals showed incomplete right bundle branch block (RBBB) with a QRS duration of 132 milliseconds (**Fig. 1**), normal AH (atrium-to-His) and HV (His-to-ventricle) intervals, and absent VA (ventriculoatrial) conduction. Atrial flutter of 2-second duration was inducible at baseline, and no supraventricular tachyarrhythmias were inducible under the influence of isoproterenol. During ventricular programmed stimulation at baseline and using an output twice diastolic pacing threshold at 2 milliseconds pulse width, sustained rapid ventricular tachycardia (VT) (cycle length 200 milliseconds) was induced and reinduced by a drivetrain cycle length of 400 milliseconds and coupling intervals of 260, 210, and 190 milliseconds from the RV apex (**Fig. 2**). Ventricular diastole was difficult to discern, but the best estimation was that this had left bundle branch block morphology with superior QRS axis. It generated no blood pressure by arterial line, requiring cardioversion at 50 J.

MANAGEMENT AND CLINICAL COURSE

The patient was treated with enteral phenytoin and, with a therapeutic plasma level, programmed ventricular stimulation was repeated. The study was negative for inducible VT using an aggressive pacing protocol: 2 drivetrains (600 and 400 milliseconds), 3 premature beats down to cycle length

180 milliseconds, and from 2 RV sites (apex and outflow tract). An insertable loop recorder (Reveal LINQ; Medtronic; St Paul, MN) was implanted for documentation of the patient's rhythm during subsequent symptoms, and the patient was discharged with an automated external defibrillator (AED).

CLINICAL CONSIDERATIONS

This patient's cardiac anatomy and subsequent interventions can logically be viewed from the perspective of a patient with tetralogy of Fallot (TOF), a condition for which far more experience has been accrued. Several key questions influenced this patient's management. What is the relationship between this patient's symptoms and the results of electrophysiologic testing? What is the risk of sudden cardiac death (SCD) or clinical VT in this patient? What is the positive predictive value of inducible VT in this disease? In addition, what are the risks and benefits of implantable cardioverter-defibrillators (ICDs) in this population?

DISCUSSION

It was not thought that the induced rapid VT could account for the patient's more mild symptoms. Although atrioventricular (AV) reciprocating tachycardia could not exist in the absence of VA

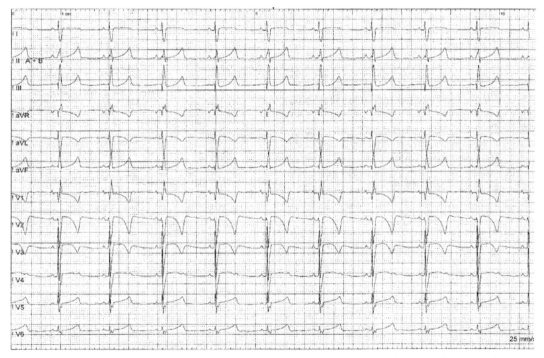

Fig. 1. Baseline surface electrocardiogram (ECG). Baseline intervals were normal, except for incomplete RBBB with QRS duration of 132 milliseconds.

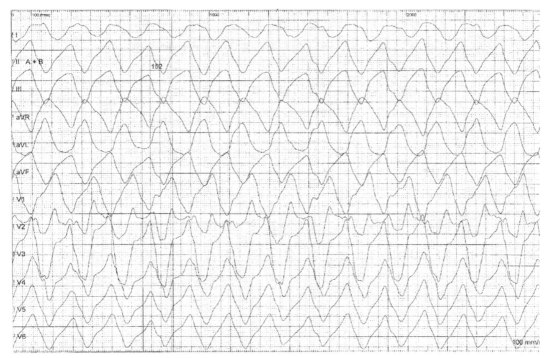

Fig. 2. Twelve-lead ECG of induced rapid VT (100 mm/s).

conduction and AV nodal reentrant tachycardia is unlikely, but still possible, in the absence of VA conduction, atrial flutter does remain a possibility, despite the inability to induce sustained atrial flutter. For these reasons, because supraventricular tachycardias may be treated with catheter ablation, and because programming of a future ICD would be affected by coexisting supraventricular tachycardias, an insertable loop recorder was implanted.

Ventricular arrhythmias are common in patients with TOF. SCD is the most common cause of death years after repair, with an estimated incidence of 1.2% to 3.0% per decade of follow-up.[1–4] SCD is most commonly attributed to VT, although rapidly conducted atrial flutter or AV block has also been implicated.[5] Thus, reliably identifying patients at risk for SCD has been a subject of much investigation. Studies have shown that SCD risk factors include history of initial palliative shunt, older age at the time of corrective surgery, abnormal hemodynamics (especially increased left ventricular end-diastolic pressure), induced or spontaneous VT, and QRS duration (in the presence of RBBB) longer than 180 milliseconds.[3–8] By virtue of the prior palliative shunt and the inducible VT, our patient would be considered at intermediate risk of having a shockable tachycardia (3.8%/y), according to one risk stratification schema.[9]

Among patients with TOF, inducible VT during EPS may identify patients at higher risk of sudden death.[8,10,11] In a study by Khairy and colleagues[8] of 252 patients with repaired TOF, monomorphic VT was inducible in 30% and polymorphic VT was inducible in 4%. With a mean follow-up of nearly 18 years after corrective surgery, a positive EPS had good diagnostic accuracy for predicting cardiac events, with a sensitivity and specificity of almost 80%. The positive predictive value was 55% in the absence of symptoms and 67% in their presence, with a 3-fold increase in the odds of having clinical VT or SCD after positive EPS. This study excluded patients like ours with double-outlet RV or pulmonary atresia, but a similar study that analyzed the utility of EPS in various patients with CHD also found an increased risk of future VT or SCD in those with inducible VT.[12] Among adults with TOF and inducible sustained VT, implantation of an ICD is considered a reasonable option and is a class IIa recommendation.[13]

The efficacy of ICDs in preventing SCD in children and adults with CHD is well established. However, the complication rates in children and in those with CHD are higher than in adults and those not having CHD. In the multicenter retrospective review by Berul and colleagues[14] of 443 patients, inappropriate shocks occurred in more than 20%, primarily caused by lead failure (14%), sinus or atrial tachycardia (9%), and/or oversensing (4%). The current contraindication to perform an MRI study in a patient with an in situ ICD should also be considered an undesirable consequence of ICD implantation, especially in patients having complex CHD. The decision to not place an ICD in our patient at that time was influenced by the likelihood that he will benefit from serial cardiac MRIs to evaluate RV function and outflow tract regurgitation over the next several years. Full-body MRI-compatible ICDs are currently in clinical trials, meaning that our patient, and others who could safely undergo transvenous device implantation, may soon be candidates for ICD implantation and cardiac MRI studies.

As an alternative to ICD implantation in our patient, we currently are using antiarrhythmic drug therapy with AED backup. The data on the use of antiarrhythmic drugs to prevent VT in CHD are limited and, before the ICD era, most information was generated from adults with ischemic and nonischemic cardiomyopathy. In a randomized study by Mitchell and colleagues,[15] individualizing therapy based on the ability to suppress VT inducibility by serial EPS prevented recurrence better than selection based on Holter results. Based entirely on anecdotal experience and the known sodium channel kinetics effect of class Ib antiarrhythmic drugs (with respect to its short inactivation time constant and theoretic efficacy for fast VT), we chose phenytoin. We emphasize that this approach is temporizing in this particular patient, because all adult studies have shown ICD superiority to antiarrhythmic drugs in increasing overall survival in patients having ischemic and nonischemic cardiomyopathy.[16,17]

In addition, another future option for our patient is ablation of the VT substrate. This option could only be performed with substrate mapping (intraoperatively or transcatheter), because the very rapid rate was not hemodynamically tolerated. Alternatively, the critical zones of slow conduction could be mapped during VT, provided that there is mechanical assistance of cardiac output.

REFERENCES

1. Gillette PC, Garson A Jr. Sudden cardiac death in the pediatric population. Circulation 1992;85:I64–9.
2. Murphy JG, Gersh BJ, Mair DD, et al. Long-term outcome in patients undergoing surgical repair of tetralogy of Fallot. N Engl J Med 1993;329:593–9.
3. Nollert G, Fischlein T, Bouterwek S, et al. Long-term survival in patients with repair of tetralogy of Fallot: 36-year follow-up of 490 survivors of the first year after surgical repair. J Am Coll Cardiol 1997;30:1374–83.
4. Gatzoulis MA, Balaji S, Webber SA, et al. Risk factors for arrhythmia and sudden cardiac death late after repair of tetralogy of Fallot: a multicentre study. Lancet 2000;356:975–81.
5. Warnes CA, Williams RG, Bashore TM, et al. ACC/AHA 2008 guidelines for the management of adults with congenital heart disease: a report of the American College of Cardiology/American Heart Association. J Am Coll Cardiol 2008;52:e143–263.
6. Chandar JS, Wolff GS, Garson A, et al. Ventricular arrhythmias in postoperative tetralogy of Fallot. Am J Cardiol 1990;65:655–61.
7. Gatzoulis MA, Till JA, Somerville J, et al. Mechanoelectrical interaction in tetralogy of Fallot. QRS prolongation relates to right ventricular size and predicts malignant ventricular arrhythmias and sudden death. Circulation 1995;92:231–7.
8. Khairy P, Landzberg MJ, Gatzoulis MA, et al. Value of programmed ventricular stimulation after tetralogy of Fallot repair: a multicenter study. Circulation 2004;109:1994–2000.
9. Khairy P, Harris L, Landzberg MJ, et al. Implantable cardioverter-defibrillators in tetralogy of Fallot. Circulation 2008;117:363–70.
10. Garson A, Porter CJ, Gillette PC, et al. Induction of ventricular tachycardia during electrophysiologic study after repair of tetralogy of Fallot. J Am Coll Cardiol 1983;1:1493–502.
11. Lucron H, Marçon F, Bosser G, et al. Induction of sustained ventricular tachycardia after surgical repair of tetralogy of Fallot. Am J Cardiol 1999;83:1369–73.
12. Alexander ME, Walsh EP, Saul JP, et al. Value of programmed ventricular stimulation in patients with congenital heart disease. J Cardiovasc Electrophysiol 1999;10:1033–44.
13. Khairy P, Van Hare GF, Balaji S, et al. PACES/HRS expert consensus statement on the recognition and management of arrhythmias in adult congenital heart disease. Heart Rhythm 2014;11:e102–65.
14. Berul CI, Van Hare GF, Kertesz NJ, et al. Results of a multicenter retrospective implantable cardioverter-defibrillator registry of pediatric and congenital heart disease patients. J Am Coll Cardiol 2008;51:1685–91.
15. Mitchell LB, Duff HJ, Gillis AM, et al. A randomized clinical trial of the noninvasive and invasive approaches to drug therapy for ventricular tachycardia: long-term follow-up of the Calgary trial. Prog Cardiovasc Dis 1996;38:377–84.
16. A comparison of antiarrhythmic-drug therapy with implantable defibrillators in patients resuscitated from near-fatal ventricular arrhythmias. The Antiarrhythmics Versus Implantable Defibrillators (AVID) Investigators. N Engl J Med 1997;337:1576–83.
17. Prystowsky EN, Nisam S. Prophylactic implantable cardioverter defibrillator trials: MUSTT, MADIT, and beyond. Am J Cardiol 2000;86:1214–5.

Ventricular Tachycardia in Congenital Pulmonary Stenosis

Emily Sue Ruckdeschel, MD, Joseph Schuller, MD,
Duy Thai Nguyen, MD*

KEYWORDS

• Congenital heart disease • Congenital pulmonary stenosis • Ventricular tachycardia

KEY POINTS

• With modern surgical techniques, there is significantly increased life expectancy for those with congenital heart disease.
• Although congenital pulmonary valve (PV) stenosis is not as complex as tetralogy of Fallot, there are many similarities between the 2 lesions, such that patients with either of these conditions are at risk for ventricular arrhythmias and sudden cardiac death.
• Those patients who have undergone surgical palliation for congenital pulmonary stenosis are at an increased risk for development of ventricular arrhythmias and may benefit from a more aggressive evaluation for symptoms of palpitations or syncope.

CLINICAL PRESENTATION

A 53-year-old woman with history of congenital PV stenosis, status post–surgical valvotomy and transannular patch at the age of 13 years, presented with left bundle branch block morphology ventricular tachycardia (VT), inferior axis, and transition at leads V_3 to V_4 (**Fig. 1**), which was treated with amiodarone. Further evaluation was significant for severe pulmonary insufficiency, a dilated right ventricle (RV), and an RV outflow tract aneurysm. She ultimately underwent PV replacement with a #29 bovine Carpentier-Edwards valve and aneurysm imbrication. At the time of her valve replacement, she underwent surgical cryoablation of the RV outflow tract. Cryoablation was performed from the RV outflow tract to the PV, from below the PV annulus and around either side of the transannular patch, and from the tricuspid valve to the PV. After her surgery, she underwent an electrophysiology (EP) study and was not inducible for either atrial or ventricular

arrhythmias. One year later, she presented with recurrent episodes of the same VT requiring cardioversion. She was referred to the EP laboratory for evaluation.

CLINICAL QUESTION

What is the approach to VT ablation in a patient with congenital pulmonary stenosis?

CLINICAL COURSE

The initial approach to VT in this patient was similar for any patient with VT. The authors considered the presenting electrocardiogram and the underlying substrate that was predisposing to VT. This included the congenital cardiac lesion, the surgical history, and the prior surgical cryoablation. Although VT in patients with isolated pulmonary stenosis is rare, this patient's history of a transannular patch and subsequent ventricular surgeries confer features that are similar to those

Cardiology Division, University of Colorado, Denver, Aurora, CO, USA
* Corresponding author. University of Colorado, Denver, Anschutz Medical Campus, 12401 East, 17th Avenue, B-132, Aurora, CO 80045.
E-mail address: duy.t.nguyen@ucdenver.edu

Card Electrophysiol Clin 8 (2016) 205–209
http://dx.doi.org/10.1016/j.ccep.2015.10.030

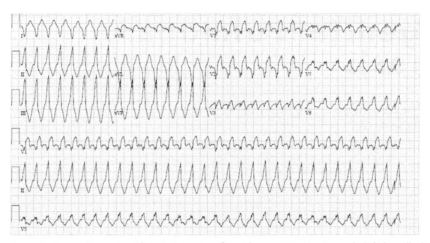

Fig. 1. Presenting electrocardiogram with VT at a rate of 160 beats per minute with left bundle branch block morphology.

in patients with tetralogy of Fallot, who are at higher risk of ventricular arrhythmias.

Hence, the authors anticipated that the VT would have an RV origin. The patient presented to the EP laboratory in sinus rhythm, and delayed RV activation was noted at baseline (**Fig. 2**). A voltage map was performed in sinus rhythm, and she was found to have extensive scar in the RV outflow tract, anterior RV, RV apex, and around the tricuspid valve (**Fig. 3**). A potential isthmus was identified between the PV annulus and the region of scar extending from the RV outflow tract to the anterior RV (corresponding to the site of aneurysm imbrication). The ablation catheter was placed near this isthmus in preparation for entrainment and activation mapping, and programmed stimulation was performed to induce VT.

Two separate VTs were induced, and the second VT was consistent with her clinical presentation (**Fig. 4**). Using entrainment and activation

mapping, the authors identified the circuit involved and the critical isthmus that was required to maintain the VT. Entrainment mapping at this site demonstrated concealed fusion with a post–pacing interval minus tachycardia cycle length (PPI − TCL) of 0 ms (**Fig. 5**). Mid-diastolic potentials were present (**Fig. 6**), and pace mapping at the same site in sinus rhythm demonstrated a near-perfect pace map to the clinical VT (see **Fig. 6**). Ablation during VT at this isthmus terminated the VT, and further ablation was performed to eliminate the isthmus and to connect the dense scar in the RV outflow tract to the PV annulus (see **Fig. 3**). At the close of the procedure, she was no longer inducible for any VT, and the authors believe that the first VT was likely using the same isthmus, but in the counterclockwise direction, given that both VTs had similar cycle lengths. The patient also underwent placement of an implantable cardioverter-defibrillator for secondary prevention.

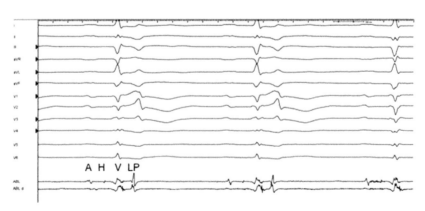

Fig. 2. Baseline sinus rhythm intracardiac electrograms with delayed RV activation at baseline. A, atrial electrogram; H, His electrogram; LP, late potential consistent with delayed RV conduction; V, ventricular electrogram.

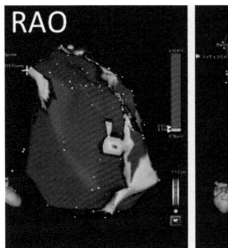
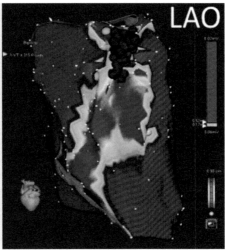

Fig. 3. Electroanatomic voltage map (CARTO, Biosense Webster) in sinus rhythm. Extensive scar was found in the RV outflow tract, anterior RV, RV apex, and around the tricuspid valve. Red lesion tags are ablation lesions within critical isthmus connecting the dense RV outflow tract scar with the PV annulus. RAO, right anterior oblique; LAO, left anterior oblique.

DISCUSSION

With modern surgical techniques, there is significantly increased life expectancy for those with congenital heart disease. Surgical palliation is not a definitive cure, however. There are typically residual anatomic lesions, as well as consequences of the surgical repair, that cause long-term sequelae. Congenital pulmonary stenosis is a common congenital heart defect with a range of severity. It occurs in an isolated form in 8% to

10% of congenital heart disease and 25% to 30% in association with other lesions.[1] It may not require any intervention, or it can be treated initially with either balloon valvuloplasty or surgical valvotomy and RV outflow tract augmentation. Historically, surgery was the only option until the advent of percutaneous techniques in the 1980s. In the early years of surgical palliation, there was thought to be little consequence of long-standing pulmonary insufficiency, and surgical techniques were geared toward opening the outflow tract without

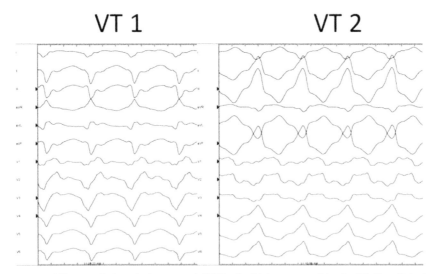

Fig. 4. Two separate VTs were induced, the second (VT2) of which was consistent with the clinical presentation (left bundle branch block morphology, inferior axis, and transition at V_4). The first VT (VT1) was likely using the same critical isthmus as the second VT, but in a counterclockwise direction, because both had similar cycle lengths and were noninducible after ablation of the same critical isthmus.

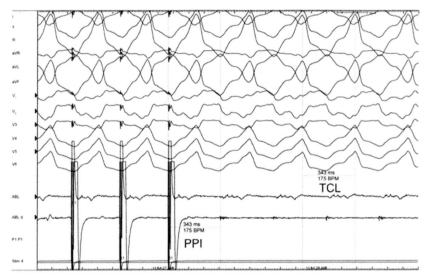

Fig. 5. Entrainment mapping near the critical isthmus demonstrated concealed fusion with a PPI – TCL of 0 ms.

thought to preserving the PV. Consequently, many patients were left with severe pulmonary insufficiency.

On its own, congenital PV stenosis is not often associated with significant arrhythmias.[2] Surgical repair of congenital PV stenosis, however, results in similar RV fibrosis and scar, as may be seen with more complex congenital heart diseases, such as tetralogy of Fallot. In tetralogy of Fallot, there is subpulmonary and PV obstruction, which may require surgical resection of subvalvular and valvular tissue as well as possible use of a transannular patch. Additionally, patients with tetralogy of Fallot require closure of a ventricular septal defect. Any site of surgical repair can predispose to future arrhythmias. If relief of PV obstruction results in long-standing pulmonary insufficiency, RV dilation and dysfunction may occur. This is important because RV dilation can be associated with inducible ventricular arrhythmias.[3,4]

Much attention has been paid to patients with tetralogy of Fallot and their risk for sudden cardiac death due to ventricular arrhythmias as well as

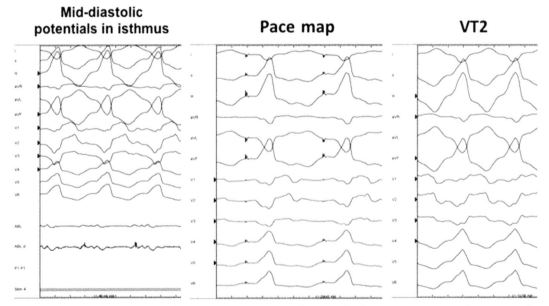

Fig. 6. Mid-diastolic potentials (*left panel*) were present in the critical isthmus. Pace mapping (*center panel*) at the same site in sinus rhythm demonstrated a near-perfect pace map to the clinical VT (*right panel*).

predictors for sudden cardiac death. Adult patients with repaired tetralogy of Fallot are at risk for sudden cardiac death at a rate of 6% to 10% per decade of follow-up.[5,6] Many factors have been implicated as increasing the risk for sudden cardiac death in these patients. Some of the risk factors associated with sustained ventricular arrhythmias in patients with tetralogy of Fallot include ventricular dysfunction, RV enlargement, atrial arrhythmias, and QRS duration greater than 180 ms.[7,8] In those patients with known risk factors, there is evidence that inducible VT at the time of EP study is associated with increased 5-year mortality.[9] Targeted cryoablation at the time of surgical PV replacement in patients with tetralogy of Fallot has been shown to decrease the rate of ventricular and atrial arrhythmias postoperatively.[10]

Although there are few data, catheter ablation can be attempted for ventricular arrhythmias in patients with congenital heart disease. Small studies with short-term follow-up suggest reasonable outcomes.[11,12] Nevertheless, challenges exist, including anatomic obstruction, unstable ventricular arrhythmias, and high-risk location near the His bundle or coronary artery.[13]

SUMMARY

Although congenital PV stenosis is not as complex as tetralogy of Fallot, there are many similarities between the 2 lesions, such that patients with either of these conditions are at risk for ventricular arrhythmias and sudden cardiac death. Those patients who have undergone surgical palliation for congenital pulmonary stenosis are at an increased risk for development of ventricular arrhythmias and may benefit from a more aggressive evaluation for symptoms of palpitations or syncope.

REFERENCES

1. Moss AJ, Allen HD. Moss and Adams' heart disease in infants, children, and adolescents: including the fetus and young adult. Philadelphia: Wolters Kluwer Health/Lippincott Williams & Wilkins; 2008.
2. Khairy P, Van Hare GF, Balaji S, et al. PACES/HRS expert consensus statement on the recognition and management of arrhythmias in adult congenital heart disease: developed in partnership between the Pediatric and Congenital Electrophysiology Society (PACES) and the Heart Rhythm Society (HRS). Endorsed by the governing bodies of PACES, HRS, the American College of Cardiology (ACC), the American Heart Association (AHA), the European Heart Rhythm Association (EHRA), the Canadian Heart Rhythm Society (CHRS), and the International Society for Adult Congenital Heart Disease (ISACHD). Can J Cardiol 2014;30(10):e1–63.
3. Daliento L, Rizzoli G, Menti L, et al. Accuracy of electrocardiographic and echocardiographic indices in predicting life threatening ventricular arrhythmias in patients operated for tetralogy of Fallot. Heart 1999;81(6):650–5.
4. Marie PY, Marçon F, Brunotte F, et al. Right ventricular overload and induced sustained ventricular tachycardia in operatively "repaired" tetralogy of Fallot. Am J Cardiol 1992;69(8):785–9.
5. Nollert G, Fischlein T, Bouterwek S, et al. Long-term survival in patients with repair of tetralogy of Fallot: 36-year follow-up of 490 survivors of the first year after surgical repair. J Am Coll Cardiol 1997;30(5): 1374–83.
6. Gatzoulis MA, Balaji S, Webber SA, et al. Gillette PC and others. Risk factors for arrhythmia and sudden cardiac death late after repair of tetralogy of Fallot: a multicentre study. Lancet 2000;356(9234):975–81.
7. Valente AM, Gauvreau K, Assenza GE, et al. Contemporary predictors of death and sustained ventricular tachycardia in patients with repaired tetralogy of fallot enrolled in the indicator cohort. Heart 2014;100(3):247–53.
8. Walsh EP. Sudden death in adult congenital heart disease: risk stratification in 2014. Heart Rhythm 2014;11(10):1735–42.
9. Khairy P, Landzberg MJ, Gatzoulis MA, et al. Value of programmed ventricular stimulation after tetralogy of fallot repair: a multicenter study. Circulation 2004; 109(16):1994–2000.
10. Therrien J, Siu SC, Harris L, et al. Impact of pulmonary valve replacement on arrhythmia propensity late after repair of tetralogy of Fallot. Circulation 2001;103(20):2489–94.
11. Gonska BD, Cao K, Raab J, et al. Radiofrequency catheter ablation of right ventricular tachycardia late after repair of congenital heart defects. Circulation 1996;94(8):1902–8.
12. Furushima H, Chinushi M, Sugiura H, et al. Ventricular tachycardia late after repair of congenital heart disease: efficacy of combination therapy with radiofrequency catheter ablation and class III antiarrhythmic agents and long-term outcome. J Electrocardiol 2006;39(2):219–24.
13. Morwood JG, Triedman JK, Berul CI, et al. Radiofrequency catheter ablation of ventricular tachycardia in children and young adults with congenital heart disease. Heart Rhythm 2004;1(3):301–8.

Section 6: Arrhythmias in Patients with Genetic Arrhythmia Syndromes

Editor: Marwan M. Refaat

Twin Atrioventricular Nodal Reentrant Tachycardia Associated with Heterotaxy Syndrome with Malaligned Atrioventricular Canal Defect and Atrioventricular Discordance

Akash Patel, MD*, Ronn Tanel, MD

KEYWORDS

• Congenital heart disease • Heterotaxy syndrome • Twin atrioventricular nodes

KEY POINTS

- Pre-procedural planning should include an understanding of the cardiac anatomy, location of the conduction system, and prior surgical interventions in patients with congenital heart disease.
- Vascular access and approach for ablation in patients with Fontan palliation may be limited and require collaboration with an interventional congenital cardiologist.
- Supraventricular tachycardia in the setting of Fontan palliation can be due to a variety of mechanisms that depend on the underlying cardiac and/or acquired post-surgical anatomy.
- In the setting of heterotaxy syndrome with atrioventricular discordance and atrioventricular canal defect, presence of twin atrioventricular nodes should be considered as a mechanism for supraventricular tachycardia.
- For twin atrioventricular nodal reentrant tachycardia, careful assessment of both atrioventricular nodes should be undertaken to determine which AV node should be targeted for ablation.

CLINICAL VIGNETTE

A 29-year-old woman with a history of heterotaxy syndrome and complex congenital heart disease consisting of unbalanced atrioventricular (AV) canal defect with right ventricular hypoplasia, L-malposed great vessels with pulmonary atresia, and right atrial isomerism with bilateral superior vena cavae underwent staged single-ventricle palliation with an extracardiac Fontan operation and mechanical mitral valve replacement. She presented at the age of 17 years with episodes of paroxysmal supraventricular tachycardia (Fig. 1), which were responsive to vagal maneuvers and controlled with digoxin and atenolol. At 25 years of age, she developed more frequent episodes, which were acutely responsive to adenosine, but proved to be refractory to chronic medical therapy, including sotalol and digoxin. She was referred to the electrophysiology laboratory for further evaluation and management.

Department of Pediatrics, Electrophysiologist, Pediatric and Congenital Arrhythmia Center, UCSF Benioff Children's Hospital, University of California–San Francisco, Box 0544, 550 16th Street, Floor 5, San Francisco, CA 94158, USA
* Corresponding author.
E-mail address: Akash.Patel@ucsf.edu

Card Electrophysiol Clin 8 (2016) 211–216
http://dx.doi.org/10.1016/j.ccep.2015.12.001
1877-9182/16/$ – see front matter © 2016 Elsevier Inc. All rights reserved.

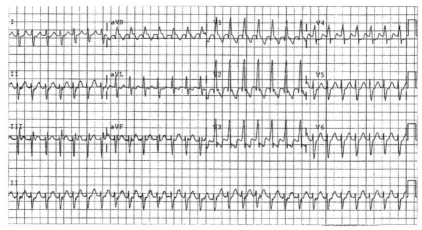

Fig. 1. Electrocardiogram of supraventricular tachycardia at a rate of 170 bpm with baseline incomplete right bundle branch block morphology.

PREPROCEDURE PREPARATION

What forms of paroxysmal supraventricular tachycardia can be seen in this patient with heterotaxy syndrome and Fontan palliation, and how does this unique anatomy of AV discordance with L-malposed great vessels and complete AV canal defect play a role?

The evaluation of supraventricular tachycardia is based on clinical history and electrocardiographic findings, which can result in a broad differential diagnosis. In this case, the patient had a narrow complex tachycardia that was responsive to vagal maneuvers and adenosine, which suggests an AV nodal-dependent reentrant tachycardia, such as AV reciprocating tachycardia or AV nodal reentrant tachycardia. In addition, because of the history of complex atrial surgeries performed as part of single-ventricle palliation in the setting of right atrial isomerism, an adenosine-sensitive atrial tachycardia should be considered. An understanding of the underlying congenital heart disease offers additional information as to the likely arrhythmia mechanism. First, patients with AV discordance with L-malposed great vessels and an Ebsteinoid tricuspid valve are more likely to have an accessory pathway.[1] Second, patients with heterotaxy syndrome and a complete AV canal defect may have twin or dual AV nodes; this may provide the substrate for an AV reciprocating tachycardia involving 2 distinct AV nodes or AV nodal reentrant tachycardia using a single AV node.[2] Based on these possibilities, the diagnostic electrophysiology study should focus on maneuvers that will help to identify a specific mechanism.

Finally, vascular access for procedures in patients with complex anatomy and multiple prior surgeries can be complicated and limited. Therefore, careful planning for an interventional procedure should include an understanding of the underlying anatomy and prior surgical procedures. Additional 3-dimensional imaging, such as cardiac MRI or computed tomography, can be helpful. In addition, these images can potentially be integrated with electroanatomic mapping systems and/or fluoroscopy. The location of suspected targets for mapping and ablation might also impact the desired approach for access via the femoral vein and artery and jugular vein. In the case of femoral and jugular venous occlusion, transhepatic access may be indicated. In patients who have had a Fontan operation, it may be necessary to cross a prosthetic surgically created baffle by either a residual leak or a created transbaffle puncture. For some of these unusual approaches for access, it may be helpful to collaborate with an interventional congenital cardiologist.

ELECTROPHYSIOLOGY STUDY AND ABLATION

This patient underwent a standard diagnostic electrophysiology study. During atrial overdrive pacing, there was an abrupt shift to an alternate QRS complex morphology (**Fig. 2**). Adenosine administered during sinus rhythm resulted in transition from the baseline QRS complex to the alternate QRS complex before AV block (**Fig. 3**). There was decremental ventriculoatrial conduction during ventricular overdrive pacing. Adenosine administered during ventricular pacing resulted in ventriculoatrial block. Dual AV node physiology was not observed, but twin AV nodes were

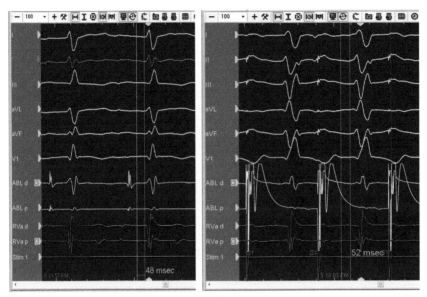

Fig. 2. Atrial overdrive pacing resulting in an abrupt shift to an alternate QRS morphology and axis.

suspected based on the change in QRS complex morphology and axis.

Because of the described underlying anatomy, an anteriorly displaced AV node was suspected due to its association with AV discordance with L-malposed great vessels, and a posteriorly and inferiorly displaced AV node was suspected due to its association with common AV canal defects. Electroanatomic mapping was performed, which demonstrated 2 anatomically distinct AV nodes, each with its own His bundle electrogram (**Fig. 4**). Atrial overdrive pacing performed in the region of each AV node demonstrated a distinct QRS complex with a different His bundle electrogram, confirming the presence of 2 AV nodes. Finally, evaluation of the

conduction properties of each AV node determined that the posterior AV node was the dominant AV node with more robust antegrade conduction properties.

Programmed stimulation from both the atrium and the ventricle during an isoproterenol infusion resulted in a narrow complex tachycardia similar to the clinical tachycardia. The tachycardia cycle length was 324 ms with a VA interval of 135 ms. The QRS complex morphology was the same as the baseline atrial paced rhythm QRS complex morphology, which represented conduction down the posterior AV node (see **Fig. 1**). Diagnostic maneuvers were performed during tachycardia. His-refractory premature ventricular complexes delivered during supraventricular

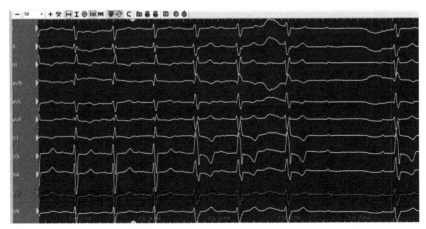

Fig. 3. Adenosine results in change in QRS morphology before AV block without evidence of pre-excitation.

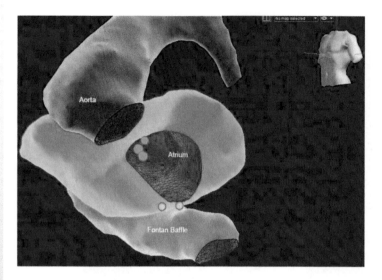

Fig. 4. Electroanatomic map (NavX; St. Jude Medical, St. Paul, MN, USA) in sinus rhythm. His bundle locations are marked: anterior His bundle (*green*) and posterior/inferior His bundle (*yellow*).

tachycardia resulted in a premature subsequent atrial electrogram. There was a V-A-V response to ventricular overdrive pacing during supraventricular tachycardia with a postpacing interval minus tachycardia cycle length (PPI – TCL) of 100 ms. Adenosine administered during supraventricular tachycardia result in prolongation of the AV interval and no change in the ventriculoatrial interval. In addition, the earliest retrograde atrial activation during tachycardia was mapped to the region of the anterior AV node. Based on these data, it was determined that the arrhythmia occurred on the basis of twin AV nodes.

Because the anterior AV node was thought to be less dominant, and this AV node position historically has an increased likelihood of spontaneous AV block,[3] this was targeted for ablation. During attempts at cryothermal catheter ablation, there was an abrupt change in QRS complex morphology and prolongation of the AV interval (**Fig. 5**). Immediately following completion of the cryoablation lesions, testing revealed the absence of ventriculoatrial conduction. However, during further postablation testing, there was recurrence of ventriculoatrial conduction. Therefore, the same site was targeted with nonirrigated radiofrequency catheter ablation. There was successful elimination of anterior node antegrade conduction, and there was no ventriculoatrial conduction following these lesions. All antegrade conduction observed at the end of the procedure was via the posterior AV node.

In addition, there are several technical aspects of the procedure that are important to highlight. There was no direct access to any atrial tissue

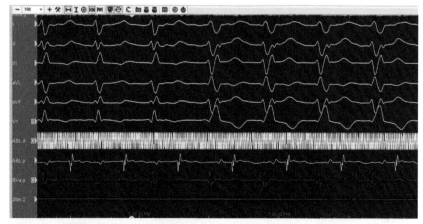

Fig. 5. Abrupt change in QRS morphology with mild and stable prolongation of the PR interval during cryoablation of the anterior AV node.

due to the type of Fontan operation (extracardiac type) that was performed. In addition, retrograde arterial access to the atrium was limited by the presence of a prosthetic common AV valve. For these reasons, a transbaffle puncture was performed across the wall of the extracardiac conduit in order to access the atrium. In addition, His bundle mapping of the anterior AV node was facilitated by a retrograde approach after an antegrade approach was unsuccessful. Difficulty mapping the anterior His bundle from an antegrade approach was attributed to the presence of the prosthetic common AV valve ring. The anterior His bundle electrogram was ultimately identified under the posterior facing aortic valve cusp.

DISCUSSION

AV reciprocating tachycardia involving twin AV nodes is a rare form of AV reentrant tachycardia, typically seen in the unique setting of complex congenital heart disease with AV discordance and a complete AV canal defect.[2,4] As mentioned, these 2 unique congenital cardiac malformations are associated with displacement of the normal conduction system. In combination, these lesions may be associated with persistence of both an anterior and a posterior AV node. L-malposed great vessels are most often seen in the setting of congenitally corrected transposition of the great arteries and have been shown to result in anterior displacement of the compact AV node outside the triangle of Koch with the His bundle penetrating to the upper ventricular septum through the fibrous continuity of the right-sided mitral valve and the pulmonary artery.[5] The complete AV canal defect has been shown to result in posterior and inferior displacement of the compact AV node, anterior to the coronary sinus and along the continuity between the atrium and ventricle. The His bundle runs along the posterior course of the ventricular septal defect.[6] In the setting of twin AV nodes, there is speculation of a sling of specialized conduction tissue, a "Monckeberg sling," that bridges between the 2 conductions systems and thus allows for the potential of AV reciprocating tachycardia (**Fig. 6**).[7]

There are several notable findings that should raise suspicion for this type of supraventricular tachycardia: (1) the presence of 2 distinct non-pre-excited QRS complex morphologies associated with independent His-bundle electrograms, (2) decremental antegrade and retrograde conduction, (3) adenosine resulting in AV and ventriculoatrial block if ventriculoatrial conduction is present, (4) inducible AV reciprocating tachycardia

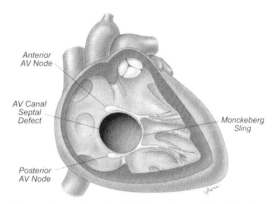

Fig. 6. Illustration of twin AV nodes and the Monckeberg sling. (*From* Walsh EP, Cecchin F. Congenital heart disease for the adult cardiologist: arrhythmias in adult patients with congenital heart disease. Circulation 2007;115:534–5; with permission.)

with anterograde conduction using one AV node and retrograde conduction using the other, and (5) accelerated junctional rhythm seen during radiofrequency catheter ablation with the same QRS morphology as during antegrade conduction over the ablated AV node.[2]

In addition to the unusual form of supraventricular tachycardia, the complex cardiac anatomy and its effect on the vascular access and technical approach is equally important to appreciate. Fontan palliation surgery can be performed with several technical variations (atriopulmonary, lateral tunnel, extracardiac), and understanding how each variation affects systemic venous drainage to the heart and which cardiac chambers are accessible is critically important to the interventionalist. In this patient, who had an extracardiac Fontan operation, the pulmonary and systemic venous atria were disconnected from the systemic venous circulation, which required a transbaffle puncture to gain access to the atrial muscle. Access to the atrial muscle may not always be achievable and depends on the type of Fontan operation, the materials used by the surgeon to construct the Fontan pathway, a lack of continuity between cardiac structures, and the presence of calcification. This patient had a fenestrated Fontan operation, which would generally imply that there was no significant extracardiac space between the Fontan baffle and the atrium. This was confirmed by cardiac MRI and allowed for a transbaffle puncture across the extracardiac conduit and into the atrium. Consequences of the transbaffle puncture may not be recognized until the transbaffle sheath is removed. Therefore, close observation is required, because extracardiac bleeding, hemopericardium, and cardiac tamponade may require interventional or surgical backup. This patient was monitored with transesophageal echocardiography, and no significant extracardiac bleeding was observed.

There are limited data on the experience of transbaffle access for catheter ablation in patients who have undergone a Fontan palliation for complex congenital heart.[8,9] Nevertheless, these issues will be encountered more frequently, because patients who have undergone Fontan palliation continue to survive into adulthood and develop a variety of arrhythmias that may be refractory to medical therapy.

REFERENCES

1. Attenhofer Jost CH, Connolly HM, Edwards WD, et al. Ebstein's anomaly: review of a multifaceted congenital cardiac condition. Swiss Med Wkly 2005;135: 269–81.

2. Epstein MR, Saul JP, Weindling SN, et al. Atrioventricular reciprocating tachycardia involving twin atrioventricular nodes in patients with complex congenital heart disease. J Cardiovasc Electrophysiol 2001; 12(6):671–9.

3. Huhta JC, Maloney JD, Ritter DG, et al. Complete atrioventricular block in patients with atrioventricular discordance. Circulation 1983;67: 1374–7.

4. Wu MH, Wang JK, Lin JL, et al. Supraventricular tachycardia in patients with right atrial isomerism. J Am Coll Cardiol 1998;32:773–9.

5. Anderson RH, Becker AE, Arnold R, et al. The conducting tissues in congenitally corrected transposition. Circulation 1974;50:911–23.

6. Thiene G, Wenick ACG, Frescura C, et al. Surgical anatomy and pathology of the conduction tissues in atrioventricular defects. J Thorac Cardiovasc Surg 1981;82:928–37.

7. Walsh EP, Cecchin F. Congenital heart disease for the adult cardiologist: arrhythmias in adult patients with congenital heart disease. Circulation 2007;115:534–45.

8. Correa R, Sherwin ED, Kovach J, et al. Mechanism and ablation of arrhythmia following total cavopulmonary connection. Circ Arrhythm Electrophysiol 2015; 8(2):318–25.

9. Correa R, Walsh EP, Alexander ME, et al. Transbaffle mapping and ablation for atrial tachycardias after mustard, senning, or Fontan operations. J Am Heart Assoc 2013;2(5):e000325.

Arrhythmogenic Right Ventricular Cardiomyopathy Caused by a Novel Frameshift Mutation

Marwan M. Refaat, MD, FHRS, FESC[a,b,c,*], Paul Tang, PhD[d],
Nassier Harfouch, BS[e], Julianne Wojciak, MS[f],
Pui-Yan Kwok, MD, PhD[d], Melvin Scheinman, MD[f]

KEYWORDS

- Arrhythmogenic right ventricular cardiomyopathy • PKP2 gene • Syncope • Palpitations

KEY POINTS

- ARVC is a rare cardiomyopathy that might be asymptomatic or symptomatic, causing palpations or syncope, and might lead to sudden cardiac death.
- It is recommended that physical exertion be reduced.
- It is also recommended that those with syncope and ventricular tachycardia/ventricular fibrillation have an ICD placed.
- β-Blockers, antiarrhythmic drugs, and radiofrequency ablation should be used to control the ventricular arrhythmia burden in ARVC.

CASE PRESENTATION

A middle-aged man whose brother had arrhythmogenic right ventricular cardiomyopathy (ARVC) presented for genetic evaluation because he met the 2010 Revised Task force criteria for ARVC. The patient had dilatation of his right ventricle on echocardiography and he had ventricular arrhythmias. A 12-lead electrocardiogram (ECG) of a patient with ARVC with inverted T waves (V1, V2, V3) and ventricular tachycardia (VT) with left bundle branch block morphology in the same patient are shown in **Fig. 1** and two-dimensional echocardiogram of the same patient shows right ventricular enlargement in the apical four-chamber view (**Fig. 2**). Our patient was found to be heterozygous for a novel frameshift mutation H91fsX94 on the exon 2 of plakophilin 2 gene (*PKP2*), which led to a truncated PKP2 protein.

DISCUSSION

ARVC is characterized by the loss of cardiomyocytes and replacement by fibrofatty tissue. Patients with ARVC can be asymptomatic or can complain from symptoms related to palpitations

Disclosure: None.
[a] Division of Cardiology, Department of Internal Medicine, American University of Beirut Medical Center, PO Box 11-0236, Riad el Solh, Beirut 1107.2020, Lebanon; [b] Department of Biochemistry and Molecular Genetics, American University of Beirut, Beirut, Lebanon; [c] Cardiac Electrophysiology, Cardiology, Department of Internal Medicine, American University of Beirut Faculty of Medicine and Medical Center, 3 Dag Hammarskjold Plaza, 8th Floor, New York, NY 10017, USA; [d] Institute for Human Genetics, University of California, San Francisco, CA, USA; [e] University of South Florida College of Medicine, Tampa, FL, USA; [f] Division of Cardiology, Department of Medicine, University of California San Francisco Medical Center, San Francisco, CA, USA
* Corresponding author. Department of Internal Medicine, Division of Cardiology, American University of Beirut Medical Center, PO Box 11-0236, Riad el Solh, Beirut 1107.2020, Lebanon.
E-mail address: mr48@aub.edu.lb

Card Electrophysiol Clin 8 (2016) 217–221
http://dx.doi.org/10.1016/j.ccep.2015.10.033
1877-9182/16/$ – see front matter Crown Copyright © 2016 Published by Elsevier Inc. All rights reserved.

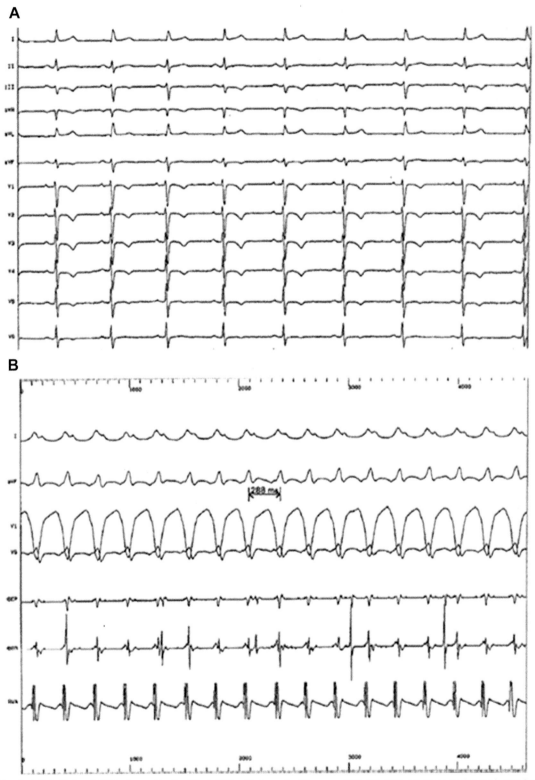

Fig. 1. (*A*) A 12-lead ECG of a patient with ARVC with inverted T waves (V1, V2, V3). (*B*) Ventricular tachycardia with left bundle branch block morphology in the same patient.

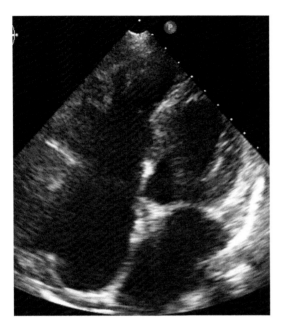

Fig. 2. Two-dimensional echocardiography of a patient with ARVC showing right ventricular enlargement in the apical four-chamber view.

from arrhythmias (that commonly precede structural changes, might be life threatening, and cause sudden cardiac death) or to right heart failure from right ventricular structural changes. ARVC occurs with an incidence of 1:2000 to 1:5000. It is mostly caused by a genetic background; however, about 50% of the time there is no familial pattern to inheritance. ARVC is seen to affect men more than women, with a ratio of about 3:1. The genetics of ARVC has been attributed in 40% to 50% of the cases to malfunction in desmosomal proteins. PKP2 is a main component of the desmosome and truncated PKP2 proteins have been shown to be associated with ARVC in the past.[1-4] PKP2 is made up of two main parts: the N-terminus head region and the C-terminal armadillo repeat (arm) regions.

We identified in our patient a novel frameshift mutation H91fsX94 on the second exon. This mutation deletes four basepairs at position 268 and inserts another 16 basepairs (268_272delACAC and 268_284InsTGGTTGTAGATGATTT). It creates a frameshift at amino acid position 91, and a stop codon at position 94, and results in a truncated PKP2 protein in the head region. Previously identified mutations on the head region (first 352 amino acids of PKP2) that would also result in a truncated PKP2 in the head region are listed in **Table 1**. It has been shown that this head region of PKP2 is responsible for targeting to points of cell-cell adhesion at the cell membrane, whereas the arm repeat region is responsible for interacting with other desmosomal proteins, such as plakoglobin and desmoplakin, and gap junction proteins, such as connexin 43.[5,6] As a linker protein and an integral component to the formation of the desmosome complex, a truncated PKP2 would result in an abnormal desmosomal complex and affect the linking of the desmoglein/desmocollin adhesion molecules (desmosomal cadherins) at the cell membrane of the intercalated disk to desmin (intermediate filament) and cytoskeletal fibers, which lead to altered myocardial biomechanical properties especially during exercise.

GENETICS

One of the most common genetic mutations found in ARVC is the plakophilin-2 mutation. The PKP2 gene is responsible for the desmosomal protein plakophilin-2, which maintains cell-cell adherence. Plakophilin-2 mutations make the cell more prone to damage specifically in areas of high mechanical stress, such as the right ventricle. Knockout of the mouse *PKP2* gene induced myocardial architecture instability and proved to be fatal. Some other genes also encoding desmosomal proteins were also found in ARVC cases, such as JUP (junction plakoglobin), DSP (desmoplakin), DSG2 (desmoglein-2), and DSC2 (desmocollin-2) (**Table 2**).[2]

Table 1 Closely related mutations in the PKP2 head region				
Exon	Nucleotide Change	Amino Acid Change	Type of Mutation	Reference
2	268_272delACAC 268_284InsTGGTTGTAGATGATTT	H91fsX94	Frameshift	Our Study
1	145_148delCAGA	S50fsX110	Frameshift	[1,2]
1	216insG	Q74fsX85	Frameshift	[2]
2	235C → T	R79X	Nonsense	[2-4]
3	534_535insCT	C179fsX190	Frameshift	[2]
3	983_984insGG	E329fsX352	Frameshift	[3,4]

Table 2
Genetic mutations found in ARVC cases

Name	Chromosomal Location
Plakophilin-2 (PKP2)	12q11
Desmoplakin (DSP)	6p24
Desmoglein-2 (DSG2)	18q12
Plakoglobin (JUP)	17q21
Desmocollin-2 (DSC2)	18q12
Transmembrane protein 43 (TMEM43)	3p25
Desmin (DES)	2q35
Titin (TTN)	2q31
Lamin A/C (LMNA)	1q22
T-catenin (CTNNA3)	10q22.2
Phospholamban (PLN)	6q22.1

Other genes include DSC1/DSC3 (desmocollin 1 and 3), PLEC1 (plectin 1), DSG1/DSG3/DSG4 (desmoglein 1, 2 and 4), PKP4 (plakophilin 4), DMPK (dystrophia myotonica protein kinase), RPSA (ribosomal protein SA), LAMR1 (laminin receptor 1), GJA1 (gap junction alpha 1), TGFβ3, RyR2, PTPLA (protein tyrosine phophatase-like, member A), DES, ZASP (Z-band alternatively spliced PDZ-motif protein), and CSN6 (COP9 signalosome subunit 6 that controls ubiquitin proteolysis).

Some nondesmosomal genes that cause ARVC include transforming growth factor-β (TGFβ), transmembrane protein 43 (TMEM43), desmin (DES), titin (TTN), lamin A/C (LMNA), T-catenin (CTNNA3), and phospholamban (PLN; which was described in families with Dutch ancestry).[2] The PKP2 mutations may create shorter or longer versions of the protein, depending on the mutation. Once acquired, the myocardial cells usually cannot adhere to one another, displace from one another, and die as a result. As more myocardial cells in the right ventricle die, scar and fatty tissue begin to build up, limiting the myocardial contractility because of structural changes. A recessive mutation in the C-terminus of plakoglobin leads to Naxos disease, which is a cardiocutaneous syndrome (palmoplantar keratoderma, wooly hairs, and ARVC). A recessive truncation of the C-terminus of desmoplakin leads to Carvajal syndrome, which is an overlap disease of ARVC with dilated cardiomyopathy with penetrance close to 100%.

CLINICAL PRESENTATION

ARVC might remain asymptomatic or might present itself as several symptoms, such as syncope, palpations, and lightheadedness, most likely in middle life (20–40 years). The ventricular arrhythmias in patients with ARVC usually have a left bundle branch morphology. ARVC might be the first presentation of a sudden cardiac arrest. Regarding penetrance of the disease into first-degree relatives, probands with an identified gene mutation showed a 28.9% penetrance into first-degree relatives and those without an identified gene mutation had a 20% penetrance.

The ECG usually shows a delay in the depolarization of the right ventricle, which is detected by a prolonged terminal activation (S-wave) duration in V1 to V3 ECG finding in patients with ARVC.[7] Another key finding that occurred in up to 87% was the inversion of the T-wave in right precordial leads in the absence of a bundle branch block (see **Fig. 1**).[8] Epsilon waves might be identified in the ECG leads V1 to V3 and in the right precordial leads by doubling the sensitivity of the record, and use of filter setting 40 Hz (instead of 150 Hz) to lower the noise level. The bipolar Fontaine precordial electrocardiographic leads I to III may enhance the recording of epsilon waves by applying placement of the right arm electrode on the manubrium, of the left arm electrode on the xiphoid, and of the left leg lead in V4.

Other notable findings are fibrofatty replacement of myocardium, dilation and reduction in right ventricular ejection fraction (see **Fig. 2**), and right ventricular aneurysms as a result of dilation and progressive pathology.[8] In some patients, the left ventricle is involved (left dominant arrhythmogenic cardiomyopathy) and biventricular involvement might also be seen. The left and biventricle involvements may lead to left heart failure and biventricular failure, respectively, in patients with this form of ARVC. Reduced plakoglobin (γ-catenin) staining on immunohistochemical analysis of conventional endomyocardial biopsy sample has been reported in myocardial samples with ARVC (sensitivity 91%, specificity 82%, positive predictive value 83%, and negative predictive value 90%).[9] The diagnosis of ARVC is also helped by signal averaged ECG in patients with right VTs, cardiac MRI with late gadolinium enhancement, and voltage mapping of the right ventricle for scar detection.

RISK CLASSIFICATION AND MANAGEMENT

Patients who have had cardiac arrest, hemodynamically unstable VT, or ventricular fibrillation should have an implantable cardioverter-defibrillator (ICD) placed. Asymptomatic individuals may not benefit from ICD (regardless of family history of sudden cardiac death or inducibility at electrophysiology study) and should be evaluated on a regular basis for early identification of alarming symptoms and disease progression. In patients with heart failure, medical therapy for ARVC includes diuretics, angiotensin-converting enzyme inhibitors/angiotensin receptor blocker and digitalis, and anticoagulants. Antiarrhythmic therapy is the first-line management in patients with ARVC with hemodynamically stable ventricular arrhythmias. Sotalol, a β receptor blocker that inhibits potassium channels, was shown to benefit patients with ARVC. Amiodarone alone or with β-blocker has been reported as an alternative approach.

In patients with ARVC with VT despite medical therapy or frequent VT requiring ICD shocks, radiofrequency catheter ablation of VT should be used to control the ventricular arrhythmias and reduce appropriate ICD shocks. Recently, plasma BIN1 was shown to predict arrhythmia in patients with ARVC.[10] Isthmus ablation via irrigated catheters is achieved using activation mapping (if stable) or substrate mapping (if unstable or not inducible) guided by an isolated delayed component, defined as a ventricular electrogram after the QRS separated by greater than or equal to 40 milliseconds or low-amplitude signal of less than 0.1 mV. VT can recur because of the progressive nature of the disease and the epicardial location of arrhythmogenic substrate if only an endocardial mapping is pursued.

One of the more common differential diagnoses for ARVC is right VT. Other conditions that are considered in the differential diagnosis of ARVC include giant cell and lymphocytic myocarditis, dilated cardiomyopathy, Brugada syndrome, cardiac sarcoidosis with confluence of noncaseating granulomas especially in the setting of AV block, Uhl anomaly, Ebstein anomaly, atrial-septal defects, right ventricular infarctions, and pulmonary hypertension.[11]

SUMMARY

ARVC is a rare cardiomyopathy that might be asymptomatic or symptomatic, causing palpations or syncope, and might lead to sudden cardiac death. It is recommended that physical exertion be reduced. It is also recommended that those with syncope and VT/ventricular fibrillation have an ICD placed. β-Blockers, antiarrhythmic drugs, and radiofrequency ablation should be used to control the ventricular arrhythmia burden in ARVC.

REFERENCES

1. Syrris P, Ward D, Asimaki A, et al. Clinical expression of plakophilin-2 mutations in familial arrhythmogenic right ventricular cardiomyopathy. Circulation 2006; 113(3):356–64.

2. Gerull B, Heuser A, Wichter T, et al. Mutations in the desmosomal protein plakophilin-2 are common in arrhythmogenic right ventricular cardiomyopathy. Nat Genet 2004;36(11):1162–4.

3. Christensen AH, Benn M, Tybjaerg-Hansen A, et al. Missense variants in plakophilin-2 in arrhythmogenic right ventricular cardiomyopathy patients: disease-causing or innocent bystanders? Cardiology 2010; 115(2):148–54.

4. Christensen AH, Benn M, Bundgaard H, et al. Wide spectrum of desmosomal mutations in Danish patients with arrhythmogenic right ventricular cardiomyopathy. J Med Genet 2010;47(11):736–44.

5. Chen X, Bonne S, Hatzfeld M, et al. Protein binding and functional characterization of plakophilin 2. Evidence for its diverse roles in desmosomes and beta -catenin signaling. J Biol Chem 2002;277(12): 10512–22.

6. Joshi-Mukherjee R, Coombs W, Musa H, et al. Characterization of the molecular phenotype of two arrhythmogenic right ventricular cardiomyopathy (ARVC)-related plakophilin-2 (PKP2) mutations. Heart Rhythm 2008;5(12):1715–23.

7. Nasir K, Bomma C, Tandri H, et al. Electrocardiographic features of arrhythmogenic right ventricular dysplasia/cardiomyopathy according to disease severity: a need to broaden diagnostic criteria. Circulation 2004;110(12):1527–34.

8. Quarta G, Muir A, Pantazis A, et al. Familial evaluation in arrhythmogenic right ventricular cardiomyopathy: impact of genetics and revised task force criteria. Circulation 2011;123(23):2701–9.

9. Asimaki A, Tandri H, Huang H, et al. A new diagnostic test for arrhythmogenic right ventricular cardiomyopathy. N Engl J Med 2009;360(11):1075–84.

10. Hong TT, Cogswell R, James CA, et al. Plasma BIN1 correlates with heart failure and predicts arrhythmia in patients with arrhythmogenic right ventricular cardiomyopathy. Heart Rhythm 2012;9(6):961–7.

11. Vasaiwala SC, Finn C, Delpriore J, et al. Prospective study of cardiac sarcoid mimicking arrhythmogenic right ventricular dysplasia. J Cardiovasc Electrophysiol 2009;20(5):473–6.

The Muscle-Bound Heart

Marwan M. Refaat, MD, FHRS, FESC[a,b,c,d,*], Akl C. Fahed, MD[e,f],
Sylvana Hassanieh, BS[c], Mostafa Hotait, MD[d], Mariam Arabi, MD[g], Hadi Skouri, MD[d],
Jonathan G. Seidman, PhD[e], Christine E. Seidman, MD[e,h], Fadi F. Bitar, MD[g],
Georges Nemer, PhD[c]

KEYWORDS

- Hypertrophic cardiomyopathy • Muscle-bound heart • Left ventricle • Phenotype • Genotype

KEY POINTS

- Hypertrophic cardiomyopathy (HCM) is a familial cardiac disease manifested in a wide phenotype and diverse genotype, thus, presenting unpredictable risks mainly on young adults.
- Extensive studies are being conducted to categorize patients and link phenotype with genotype for a better management and control of the disease with all its complications.
- Because the full mechanisms behind HCM are still not revealed, therapeutics are not definitive.
- Further research is to be conducted for the generation of a complete picture and directed therapy for HCM.

INTRODUCTION

Case Presentation

A healthy 40-year-old man presents for evaluation of exertional dyspnea. A murmur is noted, and a transthoracic echocardiography reveals a hypertrophic nonobstructive cardiomyopathy. His mother had hypertrophic cardiomyopathy (HCM) and is asymptomatic at 70 years of age (**Fig. 1**). He had frequent palpitations and was found to have atrial fibrillation (AF) refractory to antiarrhythmic medication as well as an atypical atrial flutter. He underwent catheter ablation for AF as well as for the atypical atrial flutter. After discussing his medical condition, he asks: What will happen to my children? Will I be able to feel well?

BACKGROUND

Back in the 1950s, the disease was first described by Teare who reported the death of young adults with no prior symptoms. He stated the presence of hypertrophied heart involving the basal and midpart of the interventricular septum and the left ventricular (LV) wall. All patients had a similar pathologic picture, and it was then that HCM was defined.[1–3]

HCM is an autosomal dominant cardiac disease and the most prevalent type of inherited cardiomyopathy. The most common way of diagnosing HCM is through echocardiography. Cardiac MRI and Doppler tissue velocity measurements are novel modalities of phenotyping that could detect

Disclosures: none.
This work is supported by a grant from the Dubai Harvard Foundation for Medical Research (DHFMR).
[a] Cardiac Electrophysiology, Cardiology, Department of Internal Medicine, American University of Beirut Faculty of Medicine and Medical Center, PO Box 11-0236, Riad El-Solh, Beirut 1107 2020, Lebanon; [b] Department of Biochemistry and Molecular Genetics, American University of Beirut Faculty of Medicine and Medical Center, PO Box 11-0236, Riad El-Solh, Beirut 1107 2020, Lebanon; [c] Department of Biochemistry and Molecular Genetics, American University of Beirut, Beirut, Lebanon; [d] Department of Internal Medicine, American University of Beirut, Beirut, Lebanon; [e] Department of Genetics, Harvard Medical School, Boston, MA, USA; [f] Department of Medicine, Massachusetts General Hospital, Boston, MA, USA; [g] Department of Pediatrics and Adolescent Medicine, American University of Beirut, Beirut, Lebanon; [h] Division of Cardiology, Howard Hughes Medical Institute, Brigham and Women's Hospital, Boston, MA, USA
* Corresponding author. Cardiac Electrophysiology, Cardiology, Department of Internal Medicine, American University of Beirut Faculty of Medicine and Medical Center, PO Box 11-0236, Riad El-Solh, Beirut 1107 2020, Lebanon.
E-mail address: mr48@aub.edu.lb

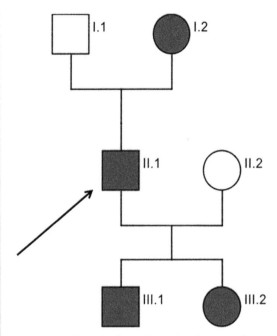

Fig. 1. Pedigree for the family is shown (*circles = females; squares = males*) with affected subjects shown as shaded circles and squares. The arrow marks the proband with HCM.

early disease that is not see on echocardiography. Morphologically, HCM is diagnosed when other cardiac diseases are ruled out in the presence of a hypertrophied septum or lateral wall of the LV.[4] Thus, when the clinical profile or any family history is accompanied with wall thickening of the LV, suspicion of HCM is high.

The complexity of the disease lies in its genetic heterogeneity, broad-spectrum phenotypic presentation, and the difficulty of finding a genotype-phenotype correlation. HCM affects 1 in 500 in the general population and 2 in 1000 of the young adults (<30 years of age) and has a 10 to 50 fold greater occurrence than other familial cardiovascular diseases.[4] The peril of this disease is in its strong association with sudden cardiac death (SCD) in young especially athletes.[5–7] It has a higher incidence in men than in women (0.26%:0.09%) and in blacks than whites (0.24%:0.10%).[8] The authors review the HCM symptoms and diagnosis, the genetics behind this disease, and its variability, complications, and potential available treatments.

SYMPTOMS AND DIAGNOSIS

Most patients with HCM remain asymptomatic and have a normal life expectancy. However, some patients might show symptoms of palpitations, exertional dyspnea, chest pain, systemic thromboembolism, and diminished consciousness. Those symptoms might be accompanied by intolerance to continuous exercise and heart failure symptoms.

The most common phenotypic expression of HCM is asymmetric hypertrophy of the interventricular septum, with or without LV outflow tract obstruction (LVOTO). The highest percentage of patients present with LV obstruction of around 70%, mild to moderate left atrium dilation, microvascular dysfunction, and myocardial bridging.[4,9] Although LV hypertrophy is a hallmark for the diagnosis of the disease, the phenotype includes myocyte disarray, fibrosis, microvascular remodeling, abnormalities of papillary muscles and mitral apparatus, and myocardial crypts.[4,10–12] Thus, the pathophysiology of HCM is varied and complicated, and it manifests itself in diverse ways to include LVOTO, diastolic dysfunction, myocardial ischemia, and arrhythmias.[13] LVOTOs might be triggered by day-to-day activities or strenuous exercise.[14]

Historically the diagnosis of HCM was made through the incorporation of examination with electrocardiogram and invasive angiographic procedures.[15] Today, the diagnosis of HCM is traditionally made noninvasively by echocardiography and more conventionally with MRI. The latter is the most accurate method to get a precise size measurement of the wall thickness of the LV region. HCM is diagnosed when the wall thickness measures 15 mm or more. Borderline wall thickness (12–15 mm) is difficult to diagnose and should be accompanied with family history and other factors to increase the likelihood of HCM diagnosis.[4] Combining exercise with echocardiography is an essential tool for revealing HCM, especially in patients with no LV hypertrophy when at rest.[16]

Furthermore, genetic testing has become a key tool for HCM diagnosis; after being commercially present, it is now considered a confirmative test and a useful test for the identification of affected relatives in families with known genetic mutations.[17] HCM mimickers or cardiomyopathies with apparent hypertrophy should be excluded before making the diagnosis of HCM, and these are due to nonsarcomere gene mutations. These HCM mimickers include storage and metabolic cardiomyopathies (glycogen storage disorders, such as Pompe disease, and lysosomal storage diseases, such as Anderson-Fabry disease and Danon disease), syndromes (such as Noonan, LEOPARD, and Costello), and other conditions, such as cardiac sarcoidosis or cardiac amyloidosis. Many of these HCM mimickers have a poor prognosis if not identified and treated early.

THE GENETICS BEHIND HYPERTROPHIC CARDIOMYOPATHY

DNA methodology studies and molecular analysis back in early 1990 revealed that HCM is caused by a dominant missense mutation in the β-myosin heavy chain gene (MYH7Arg 403 Gln) on chromosome 14.[18,19] Extensive research in the field to date revealed the involvement of 11 or more genes with greater than 1400 mutations encoding sarcomere proteins, Z-disc, or intracellular calcium modulators proteins responsible for the cause of HCM (**Table 1**). Among these genes are

Table 1
Genes involved in HCM

Gene	Protein Translated	Function
MYH7	Cardiac beta-myosin heavy chain	Major component of the thick filament in sarcomeres
MYBPC3	Cardiac myosin binding protein	Associates with the thick filament providing structural support and helping to regulate muscle contractions
TNNT2 TNNI3	Cardiac troponin T Cardiac troponin I	Makes troponin protein complex, which associates with thin filaments of sarcomeres
ACTC1	Alpha cardiac muscle 1	Found in muscle tissue and are a major constituent of the contractile apparatus
ACTN2	Actinin alpha 2	Localized to the Z-disc and dense bodies helping anchor the myofibrillar actin filaments
TPM1	Tropomyosin alpha-1 chain	Forms the predominant tropomyosin of striated muscle, where it also functions in association with the troponin complex to regulate the calcium-dependent interaction of actin and myosin during muscle contraction
TTN	Titin/connectin	Helps in contraction of striated muscle tissues, connects the Z line to the M line in the sarcomere, contributes to the passive stiffness of muscle
MYL2	Myosin regulatory light chain 2	Triggers contraction when phosphorylated
MYL3	Myosin light chain 3	Makes ventricular isoform and the slow skeletal muscle isoform
CSRP3	Cysteine and glycine-rich protein 3	Shares the LIM/double zinc finger motif which have critical function in gene regulation, cell growth, and somatic differentiation
NEXN	New F-actin–associated protein	Stimulates Hela cell migration and adhesion
TCAP	Telethonin	Interacts with titin, which regulates sarcomere assembly
VCL	Vinculin	Links of integrin adhesion molecules to the actin cytoskeleton
CALR 3	Calreticulin 3	Binds to misfolded proteins and prevents them from being exported from the endoplasmic reticulum to the Golgi apparatus
JPH2	Junctophilin 2	Plays a critical role in maintaining the spacing a geometry of the cardiac dyad—the space between the plasma membrane and sarcoplasmic reticulum
MYOZ2	Myozenin 2	Tethers calcineurin to alpha-actinin at the z-line of the sarcomere of cardiac and skeletal muscle cells
PLN	Phospholamban	Inhibiting cardiac muscle sarcoplasmic reticulum Ca^{++}-ATPase in the unphosphorylated state
PRKAG2	5′-AMP–activated protein kinase subunit gamma-2	Energy-sensing enzyme that monitors cellular energy status and functions by inactivating key enzymes involved in regulating de novo biosynthesis of fatty acid and cholesterol

the genes encoding for the β-myosin heavy chain, cardiac myosin binding protein C, troponin T, troponin I, alpha tropomyosin, actin, regulatory light chain, and essential light chain. The 2 most common genetic mutations, accounting for 70% of the mutations, are genes encoding for the β-myosin heavy chain (MYH7) and myosin-binding protein C (MYBPC3), whereas the percentage of patients with the other gene mutations is less, accounting for less than 1% to 5%.[20,21] Most mutations in the MYH7 are missense; however, deletions and premature termination codons have also been identified. Mutations in the MYBPC3 are insertions, deletions, or frameshift mutations that result in truncation of the cMyBP-C protein with loss of function.[22] Some studies are investigating whether harboring of more than one mutation can increase the severity of prognosis of the disease. Data compared between patients with homozygous, compound heterozygous, and double heterozygous compound mutations revealed that the clinical features of patients with more than one mutation led to an increase in phenotype severity of the HCM manifested in greater risk of sudden death and LV hypertrophy.[23] The consequences of mutations in the genes of the sarcomere result in proteins that activate myofilament drastically leading to myocyte hypercontractility and higher energy usage. These defects in the mitochondria of the myocytes lead to hypertrophic phenotypes. Furthermore, mutations in the intracellular calcium cycling proteins would alter the energetics of the myocyte resulting in decreased myocyte relaxation, myofibril disarray, and myocardial fibrosis.[24] Mouse models of HCM show that the increased calcium concentration during diastole is likely to lead to signaling pathways that alter the physiologic state leads to arrhythmias.[25,26] A study has showed the association of a polymorphism in the 3′ untranslated region of angiotensin II type 2 receptor with LV hypertrophy.[27] Another study has revealed that resistin, a novel cytokine that was previously suspected to induce hypertrophy in rat cardiomyocytes, is increased with patients with HCM compared with controls.[28] Moreover, polymorphism in the calmodulin III gene was suspected to be a modifier gene in HCM.[29] Other gene mutations include ACTN2, which encodes alpha actin 2[30]; ANKRD1, which encodes cardiac ankyrin repeat protein[31]; and PRKGA2, which encodes the gamma subunit of AMP-activated protein kinase.[32] All this evidence shows that there are different mechanisms and pathways involved in HCM. These pathways potentially affect signals common to the downstream consequences of the myofilaments mutations.[24]

Genetic screening, family history, and pedigree analysis are essential to detect family members with no phenotypic expression of HCM. Identifying those carrying a mutation will facilitate their management and counseling. Most mutations are private and arise de novo, although some have a founder effect in genetically homogeneous populations, such as the MYBPC3 c.927-2A>G mutation identified in 58% of patients with HCM in Iceland.[33] Rare variations in sarcomere genes are also present in the general population and might be associated with an increased risk of cardiovascular disease, as suggested in the Framingham and Jackson Heart Study cohorts.[34]

HYPERTROPHIC CARDIOMYOPATHY COMPLICATIONS

Because HCM is a heterogeneous hereditary disease with a broad-spectrum phenotype, its implications and manifestations differ widely in patients. Some patients progress to have serious complications, mainly SCD,[5–7,33,34] heart failure with exertional dyspnea and chest pain, and AF with embolic stroke.[35,36]

One of the most unpredictable and serious complications of HCM is SCD, with 1% to 2% annual mortality rate in children and 0.5% to 1.0% in adults. Its risk lies in the fact that it could be the primary manifestation of the disease with mild or no prior symptoms.[37] SCD mainly occurs in children and young adults, but it is not particularly restricted to an age group.[6] The highest risk in SCD of patients with HCM has been associated with specific markers: prior cardiac arrest or VT, prior family history of HCM causative death, exertional syncope, and hypotensive blood pressure on physical effort[37]; the magnitude of the hypertrophy has shown to be directly related to increased risk of SCD.[38] There has been a proposed correlation between the inherited genetic mutation of a patient and increased risk of SCD. Patients with mutations in the beta myosin heavy chain and troponin T mutations have been documented to have a higher premature death than patients with other mutations.[19,36,39]

Shortness of breath during exercise or exertional dyspnea, attacks of severe shortness of breath and coughing mainly occurring at night or paroxysmal nocturnal dyspnea, and extreme fatigue are another set of complications caused by HCM. These symptoms are signals of heart failure that can occur at any age of affected patients. The main cause behind heart failure is the dynamic LV outflow obstruction or systolic dysfunction in the absence of obstruction. Other causes might be myocardial ischemia, outflow obstruction, and AF.[37,40,41]

Another common arrhythmia and consequent complication seen in HCM is AF. It has an occurrence rate of 20% to 25% in patients with HCM and is mainly accompanied by embolic stroke and, thus, accounting for 1% of the annual death rate and disability.[35,36] AF may be the cause of heart failure, especially when manifested before 50 years of age, accompanied by basal outflow obstruction.[41] Studies on HCM correlation with AF revealed that patients with AF had worse symptoms, worse exercise capacity, and a significantly higher risk of death from any cause compared with patients without AF, even after accounting for known risk factors of mortality in HCM or the use of antithrombotic, antiarrhythmic, and septal reduction therapies.[42]

THERAPY AND PREVENTION

Patients with HCM can be clinically classified into subgroups for treatment and management, yet those groups are not mutually exclusive and overlap between groups might occur. Patients who are genotype positive phenotype negative should always be followed up because they might undergo a conversion to phenotype positive with LV hypertrophy.[43–47] Early diagnostic tools are helpful in this population, such as cardiac magnetic resonance and Doppler tissue imaging on echocardiography. The use of diltiazem showed a benefit in this population.[48]

Patients with none or mild symptoms should follow a drug therapy of beta-blockers, calcium channel blockers, disopyramide, and/or diuretic agents. Patients with progressive heart failure symptoms should also be on beta-blockers, disopyramide, and/or diuretic. Patients with none or mild symptoms might develop AF with time or become at high risk for sudden death.[39]

The decision for implantable cardioverter-defibrillator (ICD) implantation for primary prevention is based on the HCM Risk-SCD score, which depends on the maximal LV wall thickness, left atrial diameter, maximal (rest/Valsalva but not exercise induced) LV outflow pressure gradient, family history of SCD, nonsustained VT, unexplained syncope, and age.[49] An ICD should be considered with a 5-year SCD risk of 6% or greater, and an ICD may be considered with 5-year SCD risk of 4% or greater and 6% or less. The HCM Risk-SCD score should not be used in patients less than 16 years of age, elite athletes, in individuals with metabolic/infiltrative diseases (eg, Anderson-Fabry disease) and syndromes (eg, Noonan syndrome), or before and after myectomy or alcohol septal ablation. The HCM Risk-SCD score should be used cautiously in patients with a maximum thickness of 35 mm or greater.[49]

An ICD is recommended for secondary prevention of patients with HCM in the setting of cardiac arrest due to VT or ventricular fibrillation (VF) and spontaneous sustained VT causing syncope or hemodynamic compromise and a life expectancy greater than 1 year.

It is recommended that patients be assessed for SCD at presentation and monitored continuously every 1 to 2 years or on clinical episodes.[50] Those with sustained tachycardia or prior cardiac arrest should have an ICD. Studies show that ICD interventions appropriately terminated VT/VF in 20% of patients.[51] Yet the dilemma in decision, especially with patients aged 17 ± 5 years, lies in the increased risk (40%) of ICD complications, typically inappropriate shocks and device malfunction.[52]

Patients with heart failure with exertional symptoms are conventionally treated with beta-adrenergic blockers with or without obstruction (**Fig. 2**). Patients with outflow pressure gradient at rest, severe heart failure, and obstruction are recommended to be on disopyramide with a beta-blocker and not verapamil, which should be avoided with those patients. Exercise echocardiography is the preferred method for provoking outflow-tract gradients in patients with hypertrophic cardiomyopathy. On the other hand, patients with severe symptoms of heart failure accompanied by systolic dysfunction should be on diuretics, vasodilators, and digitalis. Whenever pharmacologic treatment fails with those patients and a life-threatening condition is at stake, surgical intervention should be assessed whenever the outflow gradient is 50 mm Hg and more.[2,36,40,53,54]

The third protuberant complication of HCM is AF and is mainly associated with age and left atrial enlargement. Paroxysmal or chronic AF can affect the quality of life with multiple hospital visits and lower quality of life.[55] Patients with episodes of AF are managed by anticoagulation along with electrical cardioversion. Recurrences of AF are managed by amiodarone.[56,57] New therapeutic strategies for patients with HCM with AF are emerging, like radiofrequency catheter ablation. A successful sinus rhythm restoration is achieved with a decrease of AF recurrence in two-thirds of the tested patients, illustrating hope of a better management. The role of genetics in clinical management remains minimal in the absence of genotype-phenotype correlations, which will always be challenging because of the many private mutations. The role of genetics is to screen family members for HCM and attempt earlier diagnosis to prevent complications. However, genetic screening does not affect any other clinical decision making, including treatment and ICD implantation.

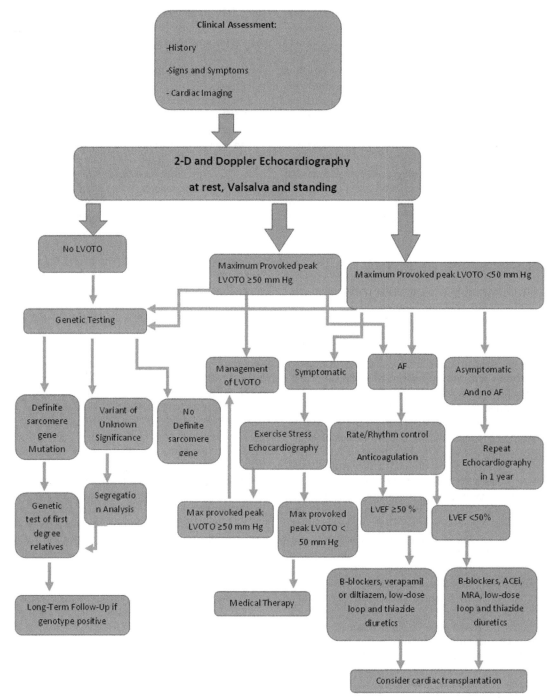

Fig. 2. Management algorithm of patients with HCM. 2-D, 2 dimensional; ACEi, angiotensin-converting enzyme inhibitor; LVEF, LV ejection fraction; MRA, magnetic resonance angiography.

SUMMARY

HCM is a familial cardiac disease manifested in a wide phenotype and diverse genotype, thus, presenting unpredictable risks mainly on young adults. Extensive studies are being conducted to categorize patients and link phenotype with genotype for a better management and control of the disease with all its complications. Because the full mechanisms behind HCM are still not revealed, therapeutics are not definitive. Further research is to be conducted for the generation of a complete picture and directed therapy for HCM.

CASE PRESENTATION: FOLLOW-UP

The patient's symptoms improved with bisoprolol. An ICD was implanted given an exertional unexplained syncope. Genetic testing identified a missense mutation in Myosin Heavy Chain 7 (*MYH7*) in exon 14:p.R453C (Arg453Cys) by next-generation sequencing. This pathogenic mutation in *MYH7* is also confirmed to be present in his mother and his 2 children (see **Fig. 1**). Arg453Cys was one of the first discovered myosin missense mutations in HCM.[58] Arg-453 is in a conserved surface loop of the upper 50-kDa domain of the myosin motor domain; the mutation at this site results in one of the more severe HCM forms, reduced ATP binding to the motor domain as well as reduced ATP hydrolysis step/recovery stroke.[59–64]

The patient's systolic function worsened; he had an upgrade to an ICD with cardiac resynchronization in the setting a left bundle branch block. He had multiple heart failure hospitalizations, and a LV assist device was recently implanted. Serial follow-up is planned for his children who inherited the mutation and have echocardiographic evidence of HCM.

REFERENCES

1. Richardson P, McKenna W, Bristow M, et al. Report of the 1995 World Health Organization/International Society and Federation of Cardiology task force on the definition and classification of cardiomyopathies. Circulation 1996;93(5):841–2.
2. Maron B, Towbin J, Thiene G, et al. Contemporary definitions and classification of the cardiomyopathies: an American Heart Association scientific statement from the Council on Clinical Cardiology, Heart Failure and Transplantation Committee; Quality of Care and Outcomes Research and Functional Genomics and Translational Biology Interdisciplinary Working Groups; and Council on Epidemiology and Prevention. Circulation 2006;113:1807–16.
3. Teare D. Asymmetrical hypertrophy of the heart in young adults. Br Heart J 1958;20(1):1–8.
4. Bogaert J, Olivotto I. MR imaging in hypertrophic cardiomyopathy: from magnet to bedside. Radiology 2014;273:329–48.
5. Maron BJ, Haas TS, Murphy CJ, et al. Incidence and causes of sudden death in U.S. college athletes. J Am Coll Cardiol 2014;63(16):1636–43.
6. McKenna WJ, Camm AJ. Sudden death in hypertrophic cardiomyopathy: assessment of patients at high risk. Circulation 1989;80:1489–92.
7. Maron BJ, Shirani J, Mueller FO, et al. Cardiovascular causes of 'athletic field' deaths: analysis of sudden death in 84 competitive athletes. Circulation 1993;88:I-50.
8. Maron BJ, Gardin J, Flack J, et al. Prevalence of hypertrophic cardiomyopathy in a general population of young adults. Circulation 1995;92(4):785–9.
9. Keren A, Syrris P, McKenna WJ. Hypertrophic cardiomyopathy: the genetic determinants of clinical disease expression. Nat Clin Pract Cardiovasc Med 2008;5(3):158–68.
10. Harris KM, Spirito P, Maron MS, et al. Prevalence, clinical profile, and significance of left ventricular remodeling in the end-stage phase of hypertrophic cardiomyopathy. Circulation 2006;114(3):216–25.
11. Thaman R, Gimeno JR, Reith S, et al. Progressive left ventricular remodeling in patients with hypertrophic cardiomyopathy and severe left ventricular hypertrophy. J Am Coll Cardiol 2004;44(2):398–405.
12. Olivotto I, Cecchi F, Poggesi C, et al. Patterns of disease progression in hypertrophic cardiomyopathy: an individualized approach to clinical staging. Circ Heart Fail 2012;5(4):535–46.
13. Wigle ED, Rakowski H, Kimball BP, et al. Hypertrophic cardiomyopathy: clinical spectrum and treatment. Circulation 1995;92:1680–92.
14. Geske JB, Sorajja P, Ommen SR, et al. Left ventricular outflow tract gradient variability in hypertrophic cardiomyopathy. Clin Cardiol 2009;32:397–402.
15. Braunwald E, Lambrew CT, Rockoff SD, et al. Morrow idiopathic hypertrophic subaortic stenosis: I. A description of the disease based on an analysis of 64 patients. Circulation 1964;30:3–119.
16. Gersh BJ, Maron BJ, Bonow RO, et al. ACCF/AHA guideline for the diagnosis and treatment of hypertrophic cardiomyopathy: executive summary— a report of the American College of Cardiology Foundation/ American Heart Association Task Force on Practice Guidelines. Circulation 2011;124(24):2761–96.
17. Christiaans I, van Langen IM, Birnie E, et al. Quality of life and psychological distress in hypertrophic cardiomyopathy mutation carriers: a cross-sectional cohort study. Am J Med 2009;149A:602–12.
18. Jarcho J, McKenna W, Pare J, et al. Mapping a gene for familial hypertrophic cardiomyopathy to chromosome 14q1. N Engl J Med 1989;321:1372–8.
19. Geisterfer-Lowrance A, Kass S, Tanigawa G, et al. A molecular basis for familial hypertrophic cardiomyopathy: a beta cardiac myosin heavy chain gene missense mutation. Cell 1990;62:999–1006.
20. Maron BJ, Maron MS, Semsarian C. Genetics of hypertrophic cardiomyopathy after 20 years: clinical perspectives. J Am Coll Cardiol 2012;60(8):705–15.
21. Bowles NE, Bowles KR, Towbin JA. The "final common pathway" hypothesis and inherited cardiovascular disease. The role of cytoskeletal proteins in dilated cardiomyopathy. Herz 2000;25:168–75.

22. Fatkin D, Graham RM. Molecular mechanisms of inherited cardiomyopathies. Physiol Rev 2002;82(4): 945–80.

23. Kelly M, Semsarian C. Multiple mutations in genetic cardiovascular disease: a marker of disease severity? Circ Cardiovasc Genet 2009;2(2):182–90.

24. Watkins H, Ashrafian H, Redwood C. Inherited cardiomyopathies. N Engl J Med 2011;364:1643–56.

25. Knollmann BC, Kirchhof P, Sirenko SG, et al. Familial hypertrophic cardiomyopathy-linked mutant troponin T causes stress induced ventricular tachycardia and Ca2+ dependent action potential remodeling. Circ Res 2003;92:428–36.

26. Huke S, Knollmann BC. Increased myofilament Ca2+ sensitivity and arrhythmia susceptibility. J Mol Cell Cardiol 2010;48:824–33.

27. Carstens N, van der Merwe L, Revera M, et al. Genetic variation in angiotensin II type 2 receptor gene influences extent of left ventricular hypertrophy in hypertrophic cardiomyopathy independent of blood pressure. J Renin Angiotensin Aldosterone Syst 2011;12(3):274–80.

28. Hussain S, Asghar M, Javed Q. Resistin gene promoter region polymorphism and the risk of hypertrophic cardiomyopathy in patients. Transl Res 2010; 155(3):142–7.

29. Friedrich FW, Bausero P, Sun Y, et al, EUROGENE Heart Failure Project. A new polymorphism in human calmodulin III gene promoter is a potential modifier gene for familial hypertrophic cardiomyopathy. Eur Heart J 2009;30(13):1648–55.

30. Chiu C, Bagnall RD, Ingles J, et al. Mutations in alpha actinin-2 cause hypertrophic cardiomyopathy: a genome wide analysis. J Am Coll Cardiol 2010;55: 1127–35.

31. Arimura T, Bos JM, Sato A, et al. Cardiac ankyrin repeat protein gene (ANKRD1) mutations in hypertrophic cardiomyopathy. J Am Coll Cardiol 2009; 54:334–42.

32. Blair E, Redwood C, Ashrafian H, et al. Mutations in the gamma (2) subunit of AMP-activated protein kinase cause familial hypertrophic cardiomyopathy: evidence for the central role of energy compromise in disease pathogenesis. Hum Mol genet 2001;10:1215–20.

33. Adalsteinsdottir B, Teekakirikul P, Maron BJ, et al. Nationwide study on hypertrophic cardiomyopathy in Iceland: evidence of a MYBPC3 founder mutation. Circulation 2014;130(14):1158–67.

34. Bick AG, Flannick J, Ito K, et al. Burden of rare sarcomere gene variants in the Framingham and Jackson Heart Study cohorts. Am J Hum Genet 2012;91(3):513–9.

35. Moolman J, Corfield VA, Posen B, et al. Sudden death due to troponin T mutations. J Am Coll Cardiol 1997;29:549–55.

36. Spirito P, Bellone P, Harris KM, et al. Magnitude of left ventricular hypertrophy and risk of sudden death in hypertrophic cardiomyopathy. N Engl J Med 2000; 342(24):1778–85.

37. Maron BJ, Casey SA, Poliac LC, et al. Clinical course of hypertrophic cardiomyopathy in a regional United States cohort. JAMA 1999;281(7):650–5.

38. Maron BJ, Olivotto I, Bellone P, et al. Clinical profile of stroke in 900 patients with hypertrophic cardiomyopathy. J Am Coll Cardiol 2002;39(2):301–7.

39. Maron BJ, Maron S. Hypertrophic cardiomyopathy. Lancet 2013;381:242–55.

40. Niimura H, Bachinski LL, Sangwatanaroj S, et al. Mutations in the gene for cardiac myosin-binding protein C and late-onset familial hypertrophic cardiomyopathy. N Engl J Med 1998;338(18): 1248–57.

41. Watkins H, McKenna WJ, Thierfelder L, et al. The role of cardiac troponin T and alfa tropomyosin mutations in hypertrophic cardiomyopathy. N Engl J Med 1995;332:1058–64.

42. Nihoyannopoulos P, Karatasakis G, Frenneaux M, et al. Diastolic function in hypertrophic cardiomyopathy. J Am Coll Cardiol 1992;19:536–40.

43. Ho CY. Hypertrophic cardiomyopathy: preclinical and early phenotype. J Cardiovasc Transl Res 2009;2(4):462–70.

44. Maron BJ, Ho CY. Hypertrophic cardiomyopathy without hypertrophy: an emerging pre-clinical subgroup composed of genetically affected family members. JACC Cardiovasc Imaging 2009;2(1): 65–8.

45. Ho CY, Sweitzer NK, McDonough B, et al. Assessment of diastolic function with Doppler tissue imaging to predict genotype in preclinical hypertrophic cardiomyopathy. Circulation 2002;105(25): 2992–7.

46. Valente AM, Lakdawala NK, Powell AJ, et al. Comparison of echocardiographic and cardiac magnetic resonance imaging in hypertrophic cardiomyopathy sarcomere mutation carriers without left ventricular hypertrophy. Circ Cardiovasc Genet 2013;6(3): 230–7.

47. Ho CY, Carlsen C, Thune JJ, et al. Echocardiographic strain imaging to assess early and late consequences of sarcomere mutations in hypertrophic cardiomyopathy. Circ Cardiovasc Genet 2009;2(4): 314–21.

48. Ho CY, Lakdawala NK, Cirino AL, et al. Diltiazem treatment for pre-clinical hypertrophic cardiomyopathy sarcomere mutation carriers: a pilot randomized trial to modify disease expression. JACC Heart Fail 2015;3(2):180–8.

49. Elliott PM, Anastasakis A, Borger MA, et al. 2014 ESC guidelines on diagnosis and management of hypertrophic cardiomyopathy: the Task Force for the Diagnosis and Management of Hypertrophic Cardiomyopathy of the European Society of Cardiology (ESC). Eur Heart J 2014;35(39):2733–79.

50. Muramatsu T, Ozaki Y. European Society of Cardiology (ESC) congress report from Barcelona 2014. Circ J 2014;78(11):2610–8.

51. Maron BJ, Spirito P, Shen WK, et al. Implantable cardioverter-defibrillators and prevention of sudden cardiac death in hypertrophic cardiomyopathy. JAMA 2007;298(4):405–12.

52. Maron BJ, Spirito P, Ackerman MJ, et al. Prevention of sudden cardiac death with implantable cardioverter-defibrillators in children and adolescents with hypertrophic cardiomyopathy. J Am Coll Cardiol 2013;61(14):1527–35.

53. Maron BJ. Hypertrophic cardiomyopathy: an important global disease. Am J Med 2004;116(1):63–5.

54. Maron MS, Olivotto I, Zenovich AG. Hypertrophic cardiomyopathy is predominantly a disease of left ventricular outflow tract obstruction. Circulation 2006;114:2232–9.

55. Sherrid MV, Barac I, McKenna WJ. Multicenter study of the efficacy and safety of disopyramide in obstructive hypertrophic cardiomyopathy. J Am Coll Cardiol 2005;45:1251–8.

56. Olivotto I, Cecchi F, Casey SA, et al. Impact of atrial fibrillation on the clinical course of hypertrophic cardiomyopathy. Circulation 2001;104:2517–24.

57. Siontis K, Geske J, Ong K, et al. Atrial fibrillation in hypertrophic cardiomyopathy: prevalence, clinical correlations, and mortality in a large high-risk population. J Am Heart Assoc 2014;3(3):e001002.

58. Watkins H, Rosenzweig A, Hwang DS, et al. Characteristics and prognostic implications of myosin missense mutations in familial hypertrophic cardiomyopathy. N Engl J Med 1992;326(17):1108–14.

59. Palmer BM, Fishbaugher DE, Schmitt JP, et al. Differential cross-bridge kinetics of FHC myosin mutations R403Q and R453C in heterozygous mouse myocardium. Am J Physiol Heart Circ Physiol 2004;287(1):H91–9.

60. Debold EP, Schmitt JP, Patlak JB, et al. Hypertrophic and dilated cardiomyopathy mutations differentially affect the molecular force generation of mouse alpha-cardiac myosin in the laser trap assay. Am J Physiol Heart Circ Physiol 2007;293(1):H284–91.

61. Zou Y, Wang J, Liu X, et al. Multiple gene mutations, not the type of mutation, are the modifier of left ventricle hypertrophy in patients with hypertrophic cardiomyopathy. Mol Biol Rep 2013;40(6):3969–76.

62. van Spaendonck-Zwarts KY, van Rijsingen IA, van den Berg MP, et al. Genetic analysis in 418 index patients with idiopathic dilated cardiomyopathy: overview of 10 years' experience. Eur J Heart Fail 2013;15(6):628–36.

63. Sommese RF, Sung J, Nag S, et al. Molecular consequences of the R453C hypertrophic cardiomyopathy mutation on human β-cardiac myosin motor function. Proc Natl Acad Sci U S A 2013;110(31):12607–12.

64. Bloemink M, Deacon J, Langer S, et al. The hypertrophic cardiomyopathy myosin mutation R453C alters ATP binding and hydrolysis of human cardiac β-myosin. J Biol Chem 2014;289(8):5158–67.

Catecholaminergic Polymorphic Ventricular Tachycardia

Marwan M. Refaat, MD, FHRS, FESC[a,b,*],
Sylvana Hassanieh, BS[b], Melvin Scheinman, MD[c]

KEYWORDS

• Cardiac • Catecholaminergic • Polymorphic • Ventricular tachycardia

KEY POINTS

• Catecholaminergic polymorphic ventricular tachycardia (CPVT) is a challenging and serious disease with a high incidence of sudden cardiac deaths.
• Patients with CPVT should not be exposed to physical or emotional exertion that might induce ventricular tachycardia.
• This article presents a case with CPVT and discusses the clinical features of the disease, its genetic background, and the management of CPVT.

CASE PRESENTATION

A 25-year-old woman presented for evaluation in 2005 in the cardiac electrophysiology clinic after several episodes of exercise-induced syncope. Syncope can sometimes be aborted with cessation of activity and rest. The patient's first episode occurred at the age of 18 years in 1998. From 1998 to 2005, she had 1 episode per year, each with strenuous exercise. Her baseline electrocardiogram (ECG) shows a normal sinus rhythm. An exercise treadmill test showed a normal QT response to exercise and in recovery, singlet PVCs, and occasional couplets that occurred with exercise with multifocal non–short-coupled PVCs (predominantly right bundle branch block, inferior axis) **Fig. 1**. A β-blocker was initiated for empiric suppression of the PVCs. The patient had several additional episodes of syncope after she stopped the β-blocker. Genetic testing identified a novel RYR2 mutation. The patient refused transvenous implantable cardioverter-defibrillator (ICD) placement. She was started on flecainide, which controlled the ventricular arrhythmias and her syncopal episodes. She was not eligible for the subcutaneous ICD after failing the screening test designed to identify susceptibility to T-wave oversensing during stress but not rest.

DISCUSSION

The patient had catecholaminergic polymorphic ventricular tachycardia (CPVT).

The disease was first described in 1975 and it was termed CPVT by Coumel in 1978. CPVT is characterized by polymorphic premature ventricular contractions or polymorphic ventricular tachyarrhythmias in genetically predisposed

Disclosure: None.
[a] Cardiology, Department of Internal Medicine, American University of Beirut Faculty of Medicine and Medical Center, PO Box 11-0236, Riad El-Solh, Beirut 1107 2020, Lebanon; [b] Department of Biochemistry and Molecular Genetics, American University of Beirut Medical Center, Beirut, Lebanon; [c] Division of Cardiology, Department of Medicine, University of California San Francisco Medical Center, San Francisco, CA, USA
* Corresponding author. Cardiology, Department of Internal Medicine, American University of Beirut Faculty of Medicine and Medical Center, PO Box 11-0236, Riad El-Solh, Beirut 1107 2020, Lebanon.
E-mail address: mr48@aub.edu.lb

Card Electrophysiol Clin 8 (2016) 233–237
http://dx.doi.org/10.1016/j.ccep.2015.10.035
1877-9182/16/$ – see front matter © 2016 Elsevier Inc. All rights reserved.

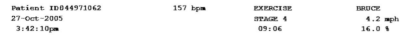

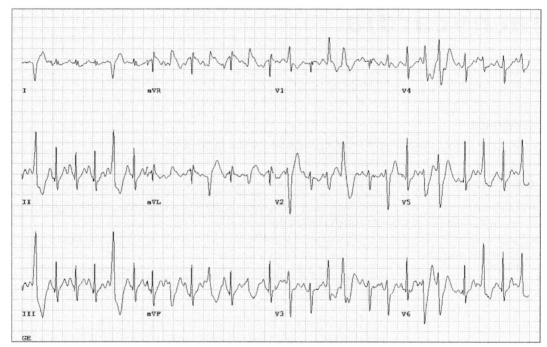

Fig. 1. Electrocardiogram of the patient with catecholaminergic polymorphic ventricular tachycardia after treadmill stress test (Bruce protocol). The recording shows sinus tachycardia with polymorphic ventricular beats.

individuals on physical or emotional stress.[1] Most of the CPVT mutations are in the gene encoding the ryanodine receptor (*RyR2*).[2] Also, researchers have shown mutations in cardiac calsequestrin (*CASQ2*) to result in CPVT.[3] Recently alterations in triadin[4,5] and calmodulin,[6] which regulate RyR2 channel openings, were found to cause CPVT. Classic CPVT is manifested in dysregulated calcium handling. On exercise or emotional stress, the release of catecholamines increases diastolic calcium leak from the sarcoplasmic reticulum and causes intracellular calcium overload, which triggers the sodium/calcium pumps to restore homeostasis by importing sodium inside the cell and extruding calcium ions.[7] The sodium current induces depolarization of the cell membrane in the myocyte, which is visualized at late diastole (transient inward current) and is responsible for delayed afterdepolarization (DAD).[7–9]

CLINICAL CHARACTERISTICS AND DIAGNOSIS

The first clinical manifestation of CPVT is syncope induced by physical or emotional stress.[1] Less prevalent signs and symptoms are dizziness or palpitations. There is generally a 2-year delay between the first and second syncope episode

observed in patients with CPVT. In some cases the first incidence is sudden cardiac arrest or death. The age at presentation is between 7 and 11 years.[10] The prevalence of the disease is not exactly reported but is estimated to be 1:10,000.[11]

Exercise ECG unmasks features diagnostic of CPVT.[12] This develops at a heart rate of 110 to 130 beats per minute.[10] On continuation of exercise, premature ventricular complexes progress to polymorphic ventricular tachyarrhythmia.[13] Patients with CPVT might present with bidirectional ventricular tachycardia (VT), which is evident in an alternating QRS axis morphology with a rotation of 180° on a beat-to-beat basis.

RyR2 mutation was associated with postpacing abnormal repolarization in CPVT. An RyR2 mutation in the C-terminal channel-forming domain has an increased risk of nonsustained VT compared with N-terminal domain. The first VT complex in CPVT commonly originates from the right ventricular outflow tract.

GENETICS OF CATECHOLAMINERGIC POLYMORPHIC VENTRICULAR TACHYCARDIA

The dominant mutation in cardiac ryanodine receptor (*RyR2*) accounts for CPVT type 1[2,10] and for most cases (55%–65%), with the CPVT locus linked to the long arm of chromosome 1 (1q42–q43) for this mutation.[14] The *RyR2* is a channel located in the membrane of the sarcoplasmic reticulum that is responsible for the control of calcium release. The other type of CPVT is confined to the autosomal recessive mutation in the cardiac calsequestrin (*CASQ2*)[15] and this variant is linked to chromosome 1 (1p13–p21),[16] accounting to 3% to 5% of cases[17] (**Table 1**). Calsequestrin is the major calcium storage protein in the sarcoplasmic reticulum and forms, along with *RyR2*, triadin, and junctin, a major regulatory unit that strictly regulates intracellular calcium.[18]

More than 100 mutations in *RyR2* have been documented in CPVT1. These mutations are single base pair substitutions with many of them affecting the *FKBP12.6*-binding domain.[19,20] Most of the RyR2 mutations are in the transmembrane segments (cluster IV). One of the proposed mechanism of the most common mutation reported (*R4497C-RyR2*) to cause CPVT is by reducing the binding affinity of RyR2 to the regulatory protein *FKBP12.6* (calstabin 2) under basal conditions, and such reduced binding is further exaggerated after protein kinase A phosphorylation of RyR2 during adrenergic activation.[21] Mice knockout for *FKBP12.6* develop arrhythmias that are typical for CPVT. On administration of a derivative of 1.4-benzothiazepine called K201, which enhances the binding of FKBP12.6 to *RyR2*, the arrhythmias disappear.[21] Another proposed mechanism is that RyR2 mutations that cause CPVT increase the sensitivity of RyR2 to luminal calcium activation, which causes spontaneous calcium release from the sarcoplasmic reticulum. Those events caused by store overload–induced Ca^{2+} release lead to DADs that consequently induce arrhythmias and thus explain how the mutations increase the susceptibility to adrenergically mediated arrhythmias on exercise or emotional stress.[22,23] A third proposed mechanism is that RyR2 mutations impair the interdomain interactions and the proper folding

controlling channel gating and thus lead to unzipping of the 2 domains and sarcoplasmic reticulum calcium leakage.

Only 12 CPVT mutations and 3 nonsynonymous polymorphisms pertaining to calsequestrin have been reported.[17] The major recessive mutation in this group is *D307H* mutation.[15] Another mutation that has been reported, and shows the possibility of interaction of *CASQ2* with *RyR2*, is *R33Q*. Adult rat myocytes carrying this mutation showed an increase in excitation-contraction coupling gain along with repetitive consecutive spontaneous propagating calcium waves and local calcium signals compared with cells expressing wild-type *CASQ2*. It was concluded that the *R33Q* mutation disrupts interactions of *CASQ2* with the *RyR2* channel complex and impairs regulation of RyR2 by luminal calcium.[24] *CASQ2* has a recessive mode of inheritance but some investigators have reported heterozygosity cases in nonconsanguineous families.[25]

Genetic testing for patients with CPVT with clinical diagnosis aids in identifying mutations in 65% of cases.[26] The high incidence of sudden cardiac death as the primary outcome makes CPVT a serious cardiac channelopathy disorder (30% of cases).[10] Thus genetic testing for patients showing a clinical picture (such as bidirectional VT) is cost-effective, whereas, in patients with no clinical correlation, genetic testing is less often performed.[26] Because of the large size of the RyR2 gene, critical exons have been selected for screening; typically a set of 105 translated exons is available for the purpose of the test.[17] Because *CASQ2* inheritance is still suspected, recommendations are to screen *CASQ2* in *RyR2*-negative index cases.

Other genes have been reported to cause CPVT-like phenotype. These genes include *KCNJ2* encoding the Kir2.1 potassium channel[27] and *ANK2* encoding for ankyrin-B,[28] a cytoskeletal protein. No genetic tests are performed for the genes mentioned earlier except when there is a clinical diagnosis linked to negative *RyR2* mutation.

Table 1
Causative genes in CPVT

Gene	Protein	Frequency (%)	Transmission Mode	Chromosome
RYR2	Ryanodine receptor	60	Autosomal dominant	1q42.1
CASQ2	Calsequestrin isoform 2	1–3	Autosomal recessive	1p13.3-p11
KCNJ2	Inward rectifier (I_{K1}) K+ channel, Kir 2.1	5–10	Autosomal dominant	17q24.3
CALM1	Calmodulin 1	Rare	Autosomal dominant	14q32.11
TRDN	Triadin	Rare	Autosomal recessive	6q22.31
ANK2	Ankyrin-B	Rare	Autosomal dominant	4q25

Because CPVT is a genetic disease, first-degree family screening is required whenever a mutation is identified in an affected patient for *RyR2* and *CASQ2* genes. First-degree and second-degree families are to be evaluated clinically and genetically in identified cases of CPVT mutation.[17]

MANAGEMENT

Because sudden cardiac death might be the first manifestation in patients with CPVT, genetic screening of relatives is crucial. This presymptomatic diagnosis with proper counseling and medication administration is important in CPVT management.[29] Patients with a previous episode of ventricular fibrillation, those with unstable VT while they are on β-blockers, and those with a younger age at diagnosis are all considered at high risk.[10]

Patients with CPVT should not be exposed to physical or emotional exertion that might induce VT. Thus no vigorous physical activity is allowed, along with control of emotional challenges and triggers.[30] Usually, β-blockers are indicated then increased until an appropriate dose has been achieved, on exercise testing and Holter monitoring.[31,32] Targeted therapy to *RyR2*-mediated calcium release has been promising with flecainide in combination with β-blockers.[33] Alpha-blockade has been shown to potentiate CPVT therapy in a calsequestrin-mutant mice model of CPVT.[34] Ongoing studies are assessing the protection from cardiac arrhythmia through ryanodine receptor–stabilizing protein calstabin 2 (Rycals). CaMKII (Ca^{2+}/calmodulin-dependent protein kinase II) inhibition has been shown to rectify arrhythmic phenotype in a patient-specific induced pluripotent stem cell model of CPVT.[35]

ICD implantation is indicated for patients with CPVT who have survived a cardiac arrest (class I indication).[31] ICD might also be the selected choice in high-risk patients having a strong family history of sudden death.

SUMMARY

CPVT is a challenging and serious disease with a high incidence of sudden cardiac deaths. This article presents a case with CPVT and discusses the clinical features of the disease, its genetic background, and the management of CPVT.

REFERENCES

1. Leenhardt A, Lucet V, Denjoy I, et al. Catecholaminergic polymorphic ventricular tachycardia in children. A 7-year follow-up of 21 patients. Circulation 1995;91(5):1512–9.

2. Priori SG, Napolitano C, Tiso N, et al. Mutations in the cardiac ryanodine receptor gene (hRyR2) underlie catecholaminergic polymorphic ventricular tachycardia. Circulation 2001;103(2):196–200.

3. Postma AV, Denjoy I, Hoorntje TM, et al. Absence of calsequestrin 2 causes severe forms of catecholaminergic polymorphic ventricular tachycardia. Circ Res 2002;91(8):e21–6.

4. Chopra N, Knollmann BC. Triadin regulates cardiac muscle couplon structure and microdomain ca(2+) signalling: a path towards ventricular arrhythmias. Cardiovasc Res 2013;98(2):187–91.

5. Roux-Buisson N, Cacheux M, Fourest-Lieuvin A, et al. Absence of triadin, a protein of the calcium release complex, is responsible for cardiac arrhythmia with sudden death in human. Hum Mol Genet 2012;21:2759–67.

6. Nyegaard M, Overgaard MT, Sondergaard MT, et al. Mutations in calmodulin cause ventricular tachycardia and sudden cardiac death. Am J Hum Genet 2012;91:703–12.

7. Faggioni M, van der Werf C, Knollmann BC. Sinus node dysfunction in catecholaminergic polymorphic ventricular tachycardia: risk factor and potential therapeutic target? Trends Cardiovasc Med 2014;24(7):273–8.

8. Fabiato A. Time and calcium dependence of activation and inactivation of calcium-induced release of calcium from the sarcoplasmic reticulum of a skinned canine cardiac Purkinje cell. J Gen Physiol 1985;85:247–89.

9. Liu N, Colombi B, Memmi M, et al. Arrhythmogenesis in catecholaminergic polymorphic ventricular tachycardia: Insights from a RyR2 R4496C knock-in mouse model. Circ Res 2006;99:292–8.

10. Priori SG, Napolitano C, Memmi M, et al. Clinical and molecular characterization of patients with catecholaminergic polymorphic ventricular tachycardia. Circulation 2002;106:69–74.

11. Napolitano C, Priori SG. Diagnosis and treatment of catecholaminergic polymorphic ventricular tachycardia. Heart Rhythm 2007;4:675–8.

12. Refaat MM, Hotait M, Tseng ZH. Utility of the exercise electrocardiogram testing in sudden cardiac death risk stratification. Ann Noninvasive Electrocardiol 2014;19(4):311–8.

13. Liu N, Ruan Y, Priori SG. Catecholaminergic polymorphic ventricular tachycardia. Prog Cardiovasc Disease 2008;51(1):23–30.

14. Swan H, Piippo K, Viitasalo M, et al. Arrhythmic disorder mapped to chromosome 1q42-q43 causes malignant polymorphic ventricular tachycardia in structurally normal hearts. J Am Coll Cardiol 1999;34:2035–42.

15. Lahat H, Pras E, Olender T, et al. A missense mutation in a highly conserved region of CASQ2 is associated with autosomal recessive catecholamine-induced

polymorphic ventricular tachycardia in Bedouin families from Israel. Am J Hum Genet 2001;69:1378–84.

16. Lahat H, Eldar M, Levy-Nissenbaum E, et al. Autosomal recessive catecholamine- or exercise-induced polymorphic ventricular tachycardia: clinical features and assignment of the disease gene to chromosome 1p13-21. Circulation 2001;103:2822–7.

17. Ackerman MJ, Priori SG, Willems S, et al. HRS/EHRA expert consensus statement on the state of genetic testing for the channelopathies and cardiomyopathies: this document was developed as a partnership between the Heart Rhythm Society (HRS) and the European Heart Rhythm Association (EHRA). Heart Rhythm 2011;8:1308–39.

18. Mohamed U, Napolitano C, Priori SG. Molecular and electrophysiological bases of catecholaminergic polymorphic ventricular tachycardia. J Cardiovasc Electrophysiol 2007;18(7):791–7.

19. Medeiros-Domingo A, Bhuiyan ZA, Tester DJ, et al. The RYR2-encoded ryanodine receptor/calcium release channel in patients diagnosed previously with either catecholaminergic polymorphic ventricular tachycardia or genotype negative, exercise-induced long QT syndrome: a comprehensive open reading frame mutational analysis. J Am Coll Cardiol 2009;54:2065–74.

20. Priori SG, Napolitano C. Cardiac and skeletal muscle disorders caused by mutations in the intracellular Ca2+ release channels. J Clin Invest 2005;115:2033–8.

21. Wehrens XH, Lehnart SE, Huang F, et al. FKBP12.6 deficiency and defective calcium release channel (ryanodine receptor) function linked to exercise-induced sudden cardiac death. Cell 2003;113:829–40.

22. Jiang D, Wang R, Xiao B, et al. Enhanced store overload-induced Ca2+ release and channel sensitivity to luminal Ca2+ activation are common defects of RyR2 mutations linked to ventricular tachycardia and sudden death. Circ Res 2005;97:1173–81.

23. Jiang D, Xiao B, Yang D, et al. RyR2 mutations linked to ventricular tachycardia and sudden death reduce the threshold for store-overload-induced Ca2+ release (SOICR). Proc Natl Acad Sci U S A 2004;101:13062–7.

24. Terentyev D, Nori A, Santoro M, et al. Abnormal interactions of calsequestrin with the ryanodine receptor calcium release channel complex linked to exercise-induced sudden cardiac death. Circ Res 2006;98:1151–8.

25. Raffaele di Barletta M, Viatchenko-Karpinski S, Nori A, et al. Clinical phenotype and functional characterization of CASQ2 mutations associated with

catecholaminergic polymorphic ventricular tachycardia. Circulation 2006;114:1012–9.

26. Bai R, Napolitano C, Bloise R, et al. Yield of genetic screening in inherited cardiac channelopathies: how to prioritize access to genetic testing. Circ Arrhythm Electrophysiol 2009;2:6–15.

27. Tristani-Firouzi M, Jensen JL, Donaldson MR, et al. Functional and clinical characterization of KCNJ2 mutations associated with LQT7 (Andersen syndrome). J Clin Invest 2002;110(3):381–8.

28. Mohler PJ, Splawski I, Napolitano C, et al. A cardiac arrhythmia syndrome caused by loss of ankyrin-B function. Proc Natl Acad Sci U S A 2004;101:9137–42.

29. Pflaumer A, Davis AM. Guidelines for the diagnosis and management of catecholaminergic polymorphic ventricular tachycardia. Heart Lung Circ 2012;21(2):96–100.

30. Maron BJ, Chaitman BR, Ackerman MJ, et al. Recommendations for physical activity and recreational sports participation for young patients with genetic cardiovascular diseases. Circulation 2004;109:2807–16.

31. Zipes DP, Camm AJ, Borggrefe M, et al. ACC/AHA/ESC 2006 guidelines for management of patients with ventricular arrhythmias and the prevention of sudden cardiac death: a report of the American College of Cardiology/American Heart Association Task Force and the European Society of Cardiology Committee for Practice Guidelines (Writing Committee to Develop Guidelines for Management of Patients with Ventricular Arrhythmias and the Prevention of Sudden Cardiac Death): developed in collaboration with the European Heart Rhythm Association and the Heart Rhythm Society. Circulation 2006;114:e385–484.

32. Hayashi M, Denjoy I, Extramiana F, et al. Incidence and risk factors of arrhythmic events in catecholaminergic polymorphic ventricular tachycardia. Circulation 2009;119:2426–34.

33. Watanabe N, Chopra D, Laver HS, et al. Flecainide prevents catecholaminergic polymorphic ventricular tachycardia in mice and humans. Nat Med 2009;15:380–3.

34. Kurtzwald-Josefson E, Hochhauser E, Bogachenko K, et al. Alpha blockade potentiates CPVT therapy in calsequestrin-mutant mice. Heart Rhythm 2014;11:1471–9.

35. Di Pasquale E, Lodola F, Miragoli M, et al. CaMKII inhibition rectifies arrhythmic phenotype in a patient-specific model of catecholaminergic polymorphic ventricular tachycardia. Cell Death Dis 2013;4:e843.

Brugada Syndrome

Marwan M. Refaat, MD, FHRS, FESC[a,b,c,d],*, Mostafa Hotait, MD[d],
Melvin Scheinman, MD[e]

KEYWORDS

- Brugada syndrome • Diagnosis • Implantable cardioverter defibrillator • Sudden cardiac death

KEY POINTS

- Brugada syndrome might stay undetected in patients until surviving cardiac arrest.
- Despite the prominent advances in exploring the disease in the past 2 decades, many questions remain unanswered and the controversies continue.
- Despite all mutations identified to be associated with the disease, two-thirds of cases have a negative genetic test.
- Future studies should be directed toward modulating factors to help physicians in risk stratification and optimally implementing an implantable cardioverter defibrillator to prevent sudden cardiac death.

CASE PRESENTATION

A 26-year-old man presented for evaluation after several episodes of palpitations over the last year. During these episodes that commonly happen at night, his lips turn purple and he has difficulty breathing. He had recurrent episodes of syncope. His electrocardiogram (ECG) showed interventricular conduction delay and underwent a procainamide challenge that did not show the Brugada pattern. However, his genetic test showed an SCN5A mutation c.5219 C>T (p. Ser1710Leu) and was diagnosed with Brugada syndrome. His daughter was diagnosed with Brugada syndrome owing to compound heterozygosity with 2 mutations in the SCN5A gene: Arg1512Trp and Ser1710Leu. His wife had the SCN5A Arg1512Trp mutation. He had another daughter that carries the SCN5A Ser1710Leu mutation. The patient was to have an electrophysiology study and an implantable cardioverter defibrillator (ICD) implantation.

DISCUSSION

The Brugada syndrome affects predominantly middle-aged men with mean age of diagnosis around 40 years old and is mostly diagnosed by incidental ECG findings. Although previous reports showed disease prevalence ranging from 1:2000 to 1:100,000 in different parts of the world, these remain rough estimates owing to its incidental finding, dynamic ECG pattern, and masked characteristic.[1] It is inherited in an autosomal-dominant manner with incomplete penetrance. It has been highly associated with high risk of

Disclosure: None.
[a] Cardiac Electrophysiology, Cardiology, Department of Internal Medicine, American University of Beirut Faculty of Medicine and Medical Center, 3 Dag Hammarskjold Plaza, 8th Floor, New York, NY 10017, USA; [b] Department of Biochemistry and Molecular Genetics, American University of Beirut Faculty of Medicine and Medical Center, 3 Dag Hammarskjold Plaza, 8th Floor, New York, NY 10017, USA; [c] Department of Biochemistry and Molecular Genetics, American University of Beirut Medical Center, Beirut, Lebanon; [d] Cardiology Division, Department of Internal Medicine, American University of Beirut Medical Center, Beirut, Lebanon; [e] Division of Cardiology, Department of Medicine, University of California San Francisco Medical Center, San Francisco, CA, USA
* Corresponding author. Cardiology Division, Department of Internal Medicine, American University of Beirut Medical Center, PO Box 11-0236, Riad El-Solh, Beirut 1107 2020, Lebanon.
E-mail address: mr48@aub.edu.lb

Card Electrophysiol Clin 8 (2016) 239–245
http://dx.doi.org/10.1016/j.ccep.2015.10.036
1877-9182/16/$ – see front matter © 2016 Elsevier Inc. All rights reserved.

sudden cardiac death. Patients are at high risk for sudden cardiac death with the cardiac event rate per year being 0.5% in asymptomatic patients, 1.9% in patients with syncope, and 7.7% in patients with aborted sudden cardiac death.[1–4] The syndrome is estimated to be responsible for 4% of all sudden cardiac deaths and 20% of sudden cardiac deaths among patients with structurally normal hearts.[1,3–5]

The Brugada syndrome is typically characterized by a right bundle branch block–like morphology along with 1 of 3 distinctive patterns of ST-segment elevation in the right precordial leads (V1–V3) on ECG in structurally normal hearts. Several Brugada syndrome cases with ST-segment elevation in inferior leads as well as the high lateral leads (I and avL) have been reported and showed a worse prognosis. According to these ST-segment patterns, the 2 Brugada consensus reports classified the disease into 3 types. Type 1 pattern has ST elevation of greater than 2 mm, giving rise to a coved-type ST segment, in electrical continuity with a negative T-wave and without a separating isoelectric (**Fig. 1**). Type 2 has a high take-off ST-segment elevation. In this variant, the J-point elevation (>2 mm) gives rise to a gradually descending elevated ST-segment (remaining >1 mm above the baseline) and a positive or biphasic T-wave. This ST-T segment morphology is referred to as the saddleback type. Type 3 is the coved- or saddleback-type with less than 1 mm ST-segment elevation. The Brugada pattern can be spontaneous or induced by procainamide, ajmaline, flecainide, or pilsicainide. Only type 1 pattern is pathognomonic of the Brugada syndrome; the other patterns are less significant. As for the definite diagnosis of Brugada syndrome, the ECG pattern should be combined with any of following clinical conditions: polymorphic ventricular tachycardia, ventricular fibrillation (VF), syncope, and early sudden cardiac death in the family (<45 years old). In addition to the ECG signs and clinical presentation, the diagnostic workup must exclude the following medical conditions that might mimic Brugada syndrome in ST segment elevation: acute pericarditis, Prinzmetal angina, acute pericarditis, and arrhythmogenic right ventricular cardiomyopathy.

Theories have emerged to explain the link between these ECG signs, possible underlying mechanisms and the increased susceptibility for ventricular arrhythmia.

Repolarization Versus Depolarization Theory

Although Brugada emerged as an exclusively cardiac channel dysfunction affecting the action potential (AP), other studies and even the first consensus report in 2002 included the possibility of underlying structural abnormality and recently investigators reported prevention of VF episodes in Brugada syndrome by catheter ablation over the anterior right ventricular outflow tract epicardium.

The repolarization theory is based on the transmural dispersion of repolarization and the unequal

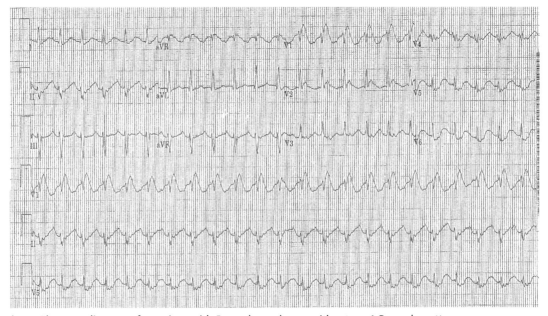

Fig. 1. Electrocardiogram of a patient with Brugada syndrome with a type 1 Brugada pattern.

expression of outward potassium current (I_{to}) between the epicardium and the rest transmural layers. Knowing that RV epicardium has abundant I_{to} channels, a more prominent transmembrane voltage gradient between the right ventricle (RV) epicardium and the endocardium results in early repolarization and responsible for the observed ECG patterns. Using sodium channel blockers to arterial perfused wedge preparations makes the opposing potassium currents more dominant and, thus, showed a notch and dome of epicardial AP. This loss of AP dome in epicardium but not in endocardium further accentuates the heterogeneity and dispersion of repolarization. Unequal shortening of the AP gives rise to development of a phase 2 reentry loop and premature beats that might trigger ventricular tachycardia/VF.

On the other side, depolarization theory explains Brugada syndrome based on a conduction delay in the RV outflow tract (RVOT). It was first shown by Nagase and colleagues[6] as the result of a late potential after the QRS in the free wall of the RVOT. This activation slowing and the delay in the AP of the RVOT causes the electrical gradient from the more positive RV to the RVOT, leading to ST-elevation in the right precordial leads and, as the RVOT depolarizes later (during repolarization of the RV), this gradient is reversed and the net current flows toward the RV, resulting in a negative T-wave in the same right precordial leads.[2,7] In support of this theory, focal fibrosis, myocarditis, apoptosis, and fibrofatty replacement of the RV free wall with RV enlargement, dilation, and RVOT enlargement were shown in Brugada patients.[2,7]

Genetic Component

Sodium channels

The syndrome has a genetic basis, and several mutations have been identified in genes encoding subunits of cardiac sodium, potassium, and calcium channels, as well as in genes involved in the trafficking or regulation of these channels (**Table 1**). Hundreds of variants in various genes have been associated with the Brugada syndrome; however, approximately 65% of Brugada syndrome cases could not be explained genetically. The first gene linked to Brugada syndrome is SCN5A, which encodes the α-subunit of the cardiac sodium channel and estimated to account for 30% of all Brugada cases and more than 75% of genotyped positive cases.[8] This channel is responsible for the inward current rapid initial phase of AP and mutations in SCN5A lead to its reduction. More than 300 mutations have been reported in this gene and linked to Brugada

syndrome type I; one-third of these mutations consist of frameshift mutations, splice site, and insertions/deletions. Meregalli and colleagues[9] showed that carriers of such mutations are more likely to be symptomatic, having history of syncope owing to severe protein defect and the resulting reduction of inward sodium current. These patients, when evaluated, demonstrate a longer baseline PR interval and QRS prolongation.[9] Other SCN5A missense mutations carriers experience symptoms only when febrile, as shown in a study on T1620M mutation, which demonstrated current impairment only when incubated at temperatures representing febrile status.[10,11] In addition to SCN5A encoding the α-subunit of sodium channel, genes encoding the β-subunits and genes affecting trafficking of the channel have been reported. Glycerol-3-phosphate dehydrogenase 1-like gene (GPD1L), linked to Brugada syndrome type II, was shown to affect expression of sodium channel on cell surface.[12] Mutations in GPD1L caused a 50% decrease in the inward current through abnormal trafficking.[12] SCN1B, encoding β1 and β1b subunits, is another gene involved in the sodium channel function and mutations reported have been linked to the disease and shown to decrease channel expression on cell membrane.[13] SCN3B, encoding β3 subunit, and MOG1 mutations also lead to inward current reduction through channel trafficking impairment.[14] Moreover, the voltage-gated sodium channel $Na_v1.8$, encoded by SCN10A, was recently shown to be also involved in Brugada syndrome. In a study done by Hu and colleagues,[15] 3 novel variants were identified in addition to other mutations, most of which were involving the transmembrane-spanning region. Interestingly, 16.7% of Brugada syndrome probands were positive for SCN10A mutations.[15] In addition, subjects carrying SCN10A mutations experienced more symptoms and ECG displayed longer PR and QRS intervals compared with other Brugada syndrome patients not exhibiting this specific gene mutation.[15] Functional studies using the most common SCN10A mutants, R14L and R1268Q, with wild types of SCN5A and SCN3B genes could demonstrate a tremendous reduction/loss of sodium channel function. These 2 mutants solely could reduce the peak density of the channel and caused a major shift of half-activation voltage.[15]

Calcium channels

Voltage-gated calcium channel, Cav1.2, is responsible for maintaining the plateau phase of AP (phase 2) through the influx of calcium ions. In 2007, Antzelevitch and colleagues[16] were the first

Table 1
Causative genes in Brugada syndrome

Channel	Brugada syndrome Subtype	Gene	Protein	Functional Effect
Sodium	BrS 1	SCN5A	α subunit of Na_v1.5	Loss of function
	BrS 2	GPD1-L	G3PD1L, interacts with Na_v1.5 α subunit	Loss of function
	BrS 5	SCN1B/ SCN1Bb1	β1 subunit of Na_v1.5	Loss of function
	BrS 7	SCN3B	β3 subunit of Na_v1.5	Loss of function
	BrS 11	RANGRF	MOG1 protein: Na_v1.5 cofactor	Loss of function
	BrS 15	SLMAP	Sarcolemmal membrane-associated protein	Loss of function
	BrS 17	SCN2B	β2 subunit of Na_v1.5	Loss of function
	[a]	SCN10A	Na_v1.8 channel	Loss of function
Calcium	BrS 3	CACNA1C	α subunit of Ca_v1.2 (L-type voltage gated)	Loss of function
	BrS 4	CACNB2b	β2 of Ca_v1.2	Loss of function
	BrS 10	CACNA2D1	$\alpha2\delta$ subunit of Ca_v1.2	Not Available
Potassium	BrS 6	KCNE3	MiRP2: β-subunit	Gain of function: I_{to}/I_{Ks}
	BrS 8	KCNH2	hERG1	Loss of function: I_{Kr} current
	BrS 9	KCNJ8	Kir6.1/K_{ATP}	Gain of function: I_{KATP} current
	BrS 12	KCNE5	MiRP4: β-subunit	Gain of function: I_{to}/I_{Ks}
	BrS 13	KCND3	α-Subunit of K_v4.3	Gain of function: I_{to} current
	[a]	KCND2	α-Subunit of K_v4.3	Gain of function: I_{to} current
	[a]	ABCC9	ATP binding cassette transporter of K_{ATP} channel	Gain of function: I_{K-ATP} current
Miscellaneous	BrS14	HCN4	Hyperpolarization-activated cyclic nucleotide-gated channel 4	Not available
	BrS 16	TRMP4	Transient receptor potential melastatin protein 4 (TRMP4)	Loss or Gain of function OF NSC_{Ca}
	[a]	FGF12	Fibroblast growth factor homologous factor 12	Loss of function of voltage gated Na^+ and Ca^{2+} channels
	[a]	PKP-2	Plakophilin-2	Reduced I_{Na}
	[a]	PXDNL	Peroxidasin homolog (Drosophila)-like	Unknown
	[a]	IRX5	Iroquois homeobox 5	Upregulation of KCND3 channels
	[a]	DPPX	Dipeptidyl-peptidase-like protein 6	Unknown

Abbreviations: ABCC9 (codes for the cardiac specific sulfonyl urea receptor 2A (SUR2A) subunit of the K_{ATP} potassium channel); *FGF12*, fibroblast growth factor homologous factor 12; *GPD1L*, glycerol-3-phosphate dehydrogenase 1-like; *HCN4*, hyperpolarization-activated cyclic nucleotide-gated channel 4 (responsible for I_f current); IRX5, Iroquois homeobox 5 (missense mutations were described in Hamamy syndrome with severe hypertelorism with midface prominence, myopia, mental retardation and bone fragility); NSC_{Ca}, calcium-activated nonselective cation channel (NSC_{Ca}) function (mediates monovalent cations across membrane and contributes to the transient inward current I_{ti} initiated by Ca^{2+} waves); *RANGRF*, RAN guanine nucleotide release factor; *SLMAP*, sarcolemmal membrane-associated protein; *TRMP4*, transient receptor potential melastatin protein 4.

[a] Novel genes identified and not linked to any Brugada syndrome subtype yet.

to establish the association between voltage-gated calcium channels and the Brugada syndrome by studying the CACNA1C and CACNB2b genes, which encode the α- and β-subunits of the L-type calcium channel, respectively. Mutations in CACNA1C have demonstrated major loss of channel activity and, because the β-subunit are involved in regulating gating process, mutations in *CACNB2b* showed channel trafficking impairment.[16] *CACNAD1* is another gene encoding α2δ subunit of this channel. In 2010, Burashnikov and colleagues[17] identified mutations that were associated with the Brugada syndrome, but the mechanism not well-understood and not investigated thoroughly to date.

Potassium channels

In addition to sodium and calcium channels, potassium channel defects have demonstrated a prominent role in the pathophysiology of Brugada syndrome phenotype in a significant number of cases. KCNE gene plays an important role in modulating various types of cardiac potassium channels. Delpon and colleagues[18] were the first to link KCNE gene mutations to Brugada syndrome.[18] KCNE3 encodes the MiRP2, one of the voltage-gated potassium channel subunits. Mutations in this gene led to increase in peak current and thus, early inactivation of I_{to}. As voltage-gated potassium channel consists of 5 homologous subunits, KCNE5 encodes another one of these β-subunits (MiRP4). Variants in this gene identified by Ohno and colleagues[19] also demonstrated a gain of function effect altering the peak current of I_{to}. More of gain-of-function gene mutations were identified in KCND3 gene, encoding the α-subunit of the channel, which resulted in I_{to} density increase and AP dome loss.[20] Moreover, the KCNH2 gene that encodes rapid delayed rectifier channel and is associated with the long QT syndrome, has been also linked to Brugada syndrome. Verkerk and colleagues[21] were the first to identify mutations of this gene in Brugada syndrome. Variants of this gene were shown to augment the initial upstroke of ventricular AP and Itoh and colleagues[22] confirmed later the gain-of-function effect of these mutations. K_{ATP} channel, encoded by KCNJ8, helps in stopping the inward rectifying potassium current and thus shortening the AP duration. KCNJ8 mutations led to augmented channel function with a reduced sensitivity to adenosine triphosphate. Likewise, the sulfonylurea receptor type 2A SUR2A or ABCC9 gene encodes the adenosine triphosphate binding cassette transporter of the channel and Hu and colleagues[23] could recently show its impact on channel sensitivity to adenosine triphosphate; they uncovered 8 mutations in Brugada syndrome patients.

Clinical Presentation

Clinical manifestations of the Brugada syndrome are heterogeneous and range from being asymptomatic throughout the lifetime to sudden cardiac death. Although most patients remain asymptomatic, palpitations, syncope, seizures, and even aborted sudden cardiac death can occur at all ages and the peak has been reported to be around the fourth decade of life.[2,24] Ventricular arrhythmias/VF represent the main underlying cause of sudden cardiac death and other symptoms. Symptoms might be triggered or augmented in the predominance of vagal activity such as during sleep. Around 40% of Brugada syndrome patients experience syncope; 23% of patients presenting with sudden cardiac death are reported to have history of syncopal episodes. Spontaneous atrial fibrillation has been shown to be high in Brugada patients, with up to 39% of cases in 1 study.[11]

Risk Stratification

Most Brugada syndrome patients are identified incidentally or when they survive aborted sudden cardiac death. It is important to establish guidelines for risk stratifying Brugada patients to receive the appropriate primary management. Many clinical markers and modulating factors have been studied as potential risk parameters, such as a family history of sudden cardiac death, syncope, history of supraventricular tachycardia, a history of atrial fibrillation, and genetic markers. To date, there is no well-established combination of these markers that would help the physician in identifying patients at high, moderate, or mild risk of sudden cardiac death. Although it is clear for patients experiencing recurrent serious symptoms as syncope, seizures, or agonal respiration, it is debatable with respect to the majority of subjects.[25] The preponderance of evidence suggests that inducibility of VF during electrophysiology study alone as a risk factor is not an important predictor for sudden cardiac death. The Japanese guidelines, in 2011, emerged and focused on 3 main "risk" factors: syncope, a family history of sudden cardiac death, and a positive electrophysiology study.[26] The Heart Rhythm Society (HRS), the European Heart Rhythm Association (EHRA), and the Asia Pacific Heart Rhythm Society (APHRS) consensus document focused on spontaneous type 1 Brugada ECG (coved), syncope and electrophysiology study to recommend for primary preventive ICD therapy.[27] Recently, Okamura and colleagues[26] studied these risk factors and provided the significance of combining these factors in risk stratifying patients. These 3 risk factors included spontaneous type 1 Brugada ECG, a positive electrophysiology study (defined as VF or polymorphic ventricular tachycardia lasting >30 s or requiring direct current shock induced at a coupling interval of ≥200 ms) and syncope (judged as likely caused by ventricular arrhythmia and excluding likely neurocardiogenic). Patients with 2 or more of these 3 risk factors were found to be at a higher risk of fatal arrhythmia and sudden cardiac death. A family history of sudden cardiac death was not an independent risk factor for fatal arrhythmia and sudden cardiac death.[26] Priori and colleagues[28] showed from the PRELUDE (PRogrammed ELectrical stimUlation preDictive valuE) registry that the presence of a spontaneous type I ECG, history of syncope, ventricular effective refractory period less than 200 ms and QRS fragmentation favor primary prevention ICD implantation candidacy.

MANAGEMENT

Brugada syndrome patients should avoid medications that might induce a Brugada pattern on ECG (www.brugadadrugs.org), avoid alcohol consumption, and be advised to treat fever aggressively. The ICD is the only effective therapeutic strategy to prevent sudden cardiac death in Brugada syndrome. The eligibility of young patients needs to be assessed for the subcutaneous ICD with screening test designed to identify susceptibility to T-wave oversensing during rest and stress. Isoproterenol (which increases I_{ca} current) is useful for management of electrical storm in Brugada syndrome. Quinidine (which blocks I_{to}) prevents VF induction, and suppresses ventricular arrhythmias in Brugada syndrome patients. Radiofrequency ablation of the PVCs triggering VF as well as a low-voltage substrate over the anterior right ventricular outflow tract epicardium prevented VF episodes in Brugada syndrome patients who were refractory to pharmacologic treatment. Family screening for the Brugada syndrome is recommended in first-degree relatives.

CASE PRESENTATION: FOLLOW-UP

The patient's SCN5A mutation c.5219 C>T (p. Ser1710Leu) is predicted to be deleterious by SIFT and probably damaging by Polyphen-2. His daughter had compound heterozygosity mutations in the SCN5A gene: Arg1512Trp and Ser1710Leu (trans mode). Previous studies showed worse phenotype for compound heterozygosity compared with single allele heterozygosity for the Brugada syndrome.[29]

SUMMARY

The Brugada syndrome might stay undetected in patients until surviving cardiac arrest. Despite the prominent advances in exploring the disease in the past 2 decades, many questions remain unanswered and the controversies continue. Moreover, despite all mutations identified to be associated with the disease, two-thirds of cases have a negative genetic test. Future studies should be directed toward modulating factors and their impact on patients' risk for sudden death to help physicians in risk stratifying their patients and optimally implementing ICD to prevent sudden cardiac death.

REFERENCES

1. Nielsen MW, Holst AG, Olesen SP, et al. The genetic component of Brugada syndrome. Front Physiol 2013;4:179.
2. Jellins J, Milanovic M, Taitz DJ, et al. Brugada syndrome. Hong Kong Med J 2013;19(2):159–67.
3. Letsas KP, Gavrielatos G, Efremidis M, et al. Prevalence of Brugada sign in a Greek tertiary hospital population. Europace 2007;9(11):1077–80.
4. Sinner MF, Pfeufer A, Perz S, et al. Spontaneous Brugada electrocardiogram patterns are rare in the German general population: results from the KORA study. Europace 2009;11(10):1338–44.
5. Holst AG, Jensen HK, Eschen O, et al. Low disease prevalence and inappropriate implantable cardioverter defibrillator shock rate in Brugada syndrome: a nationwide study. Europace 2012;14(7): 1025–9.
6. Nagase S, Kusano KF, Morita H, et al. Epicardial electrogram of the right ventricular outflow tract in patients with the Brugada syndrome: using the epicardial lead. J Am Coll Cardiol 2002;39(12): 1992–5.
7. Veerakul G, Nademanee K. Brugada syndrome: two decades of progress. Circ J 2012;76(12):2713–22.
8. Chen Q, Kirsch GE, Zhang D, et al. Genetic basis and molecular mechanism for idiopathic ventricular fibrillation. Nature 1998;392(6673):293–6.
9. Meregalli PG, Tan HL, Probst V, et al. Type of SCN5A mutation determines clinical severity and degree of conduction slowing in loss-of-function sodium channelopathies. Heart Rhythm 2009;6(3):341–8.
10. Dumaine R, Towbin JA, Brugada P, et al. Ionic mechanisms responsible for the electrocardiographic phenotype of the Brugada syndrome are temperature dependent. Circ Res 1999;85(9):803–9.
11. Morita H, Kusano-Fukushima K, Nagase S, et al. Atrial fibrillation and atrial vulnerability in patients with Brugada syndrome. J Am Coll Cardiol 2002; 40(8):1437–44.
12. London B, Michalec M, Mehdi H, et al. Mutation in glycerol-3-phosphate dehydrogenase 1 like gene (GPD1-L) decreases cardiac Na+ current and causes inherited arrhythmias. Circulation 2007; 116(20):2260–8.
13. Watanabe H, Koopmann TT, Le Scouarnec S, et al. Sodium channel beta1 subunit mutations associated with Brugada syndrome and cardiac

conduction disease in humans. J Clin Invest 2008; 118(6):2260–8.

14. Hu D, Barajas-Martinez H, Burashnikov E, et al. A mutation in the beta 3 subunit of the cardiac sodium channel associated with Brugada ECG phenotype. Circ Cardiovasc Genet 2009;2(3):270–8.

15. Hu D, Barajas-Martinez H, Pfeiffer R, et al. Mutations in SCN10A are responsible for a large fraction of cases of Brugada syndrome. J Am Coll Cardiol 2014;64(1):66–79.

16. Antzelevitch C, Pollevick GD, Cordeiro JM, et al. Loss-of-function mutations in the cardiac calcium channel underlie a new clinical entity characterized by ST-segment elevation, short QT intervals, and sudden cardiac death. Circulation 2007;115(4): 442–9.

17. Burashnikov E, Pfeiffer R, Barajas-Martinez H, et al. Mutations in the cardiac L-type calcium channel associated with inherited J-wave syndromes and sudden cardiac death. Heart Rhythm 2010;7(12): 1872–82.

18. Delpon E, Cordeiro JM, Nunez L, et al. Functional effects of KCNE3 mutation and its role in the development of Brugada syndrome. Circ Arrhythm Electrophysiol 2008;1(3):209–18.

19. Ohno S, Zankov DP, Ding WG, et al. KCNE5 (KCNE1L) variants are novel modulators of Brugada syndrome and idiopathic ventricular fibrillation. Circ Arrhythm Electrophysiol 2011;4(3):352–61.

20. Giudicessi JR, Ye D, Tester DJ, et al. Transient outward current (I(to)) gain-of-function mutations in the KCND3-encoded Kv4.3 potassium channel and Brugada syndrome. Heart Rhythm 2011;8(7): 1024–32.

21. Verkerk AO, Wilders R, Schulze-Bahr E, et al. Role of sequence variations in the human ether-a-go-go-related gene (HERG, KCNH2) in the Brugada syndrome. Cardiovasc Res 2005;68(3):441–53.

22. Itoh H, Sakaguchi T, Ashihara T, et al. A novel KCNH2 mutation as a modifier for short QT interval. Int J Cardiol 2009;137(1):83–5.

23. Hu D, Barajas-Martinez H, Terzic A, et al. ABCC9 is a novel Brugada and early repolarization syndrome susceptibility gene. Int J Cardiol 2014; 171(3):431–42.

24. Priori SG, Napolitano C, Gasparini M, et al. Natural history of Brugada syndrome: insights for risk stratification and management. Circulation 2002;105(11): 1342–7.

25. Brugada R, Campuzano O, Sarquella-Brugada G, et al. Brugada syndrome. Methodist Debakey Cardiovasc J 2014;10(1):25–8.

26. Okamura H, Kamakura T, Morita H, et al. Risk stratification in patients with Brugada syndrome without previous cardiac arrest. Circ J 2014;79(2):310–7.

27. Priori SG, Wilde AA, Horie M, et al. HRS/EHRA/ APHRS expert consensus statement on the diagnosis and management of patients with inherited primary arrhythmia syndromes: document endorsed by HRS, EHRA, and APHRS in May 2013 and by ACCF, AHA, PACES, and AEPC in June 2013. Heart Rhythm 2013;10(12):1932–63.

28. Priori SG, Gasparini M, Napolitano C, et al. Risk stratification in Brugada syndrome: results of the PRELUDE (PRogrammed ELectrical stimUlation preDictive valuE) registry. J Am Coll Cardiol 2012;59(1): 37–45.

29. Cordeiro JM, Barajas-Martinez H, Hong K, et al. Compound heterozygous mutations P336L and I1660V in the human cardiac sodium channel associated with the Brugada syndrome. Circulation 2006; 114(19):2026–33.

Iron Overload Leading to Torsades de Pointes in β-Thalassemia and Long QT Syndrome

 CrossMark

Marwan M. Refaat, MD, FHRS, FESC[a,b,c,d,1],
Lea El Hage, MD[e,1], Annette Buur Steffensen, MSc, PhD[f,1],
Mostafa Hotait, MD[a], Nicole Schmitt, MSc, PhD[f],
Melvin Scheinman, MD[e], Nitish Badhwar, MD, FHRS[e,*]

KEYWORDS

• Long QT • β-thalassemia • Iron overload

KEY POINTS

• This is a unique case of torsades de pointes in a β-thalassemia patient with early iron overload in the absence of any structural abnormalities as seen in hemochromatosis.
• Genetic testing showed a novel KCNQ1 gene mutation 1591C >T [Gln531Ter(X)]. Testing of the gene mutation in Xenopus laevis oocytes showed loss of function of the IKs current.
• We hypothesize that iron overload combined with the KCNQ1 gene mutation lead to prolongation of QTc and torsades de pointes.

INTRODUCTION

Cardiomyopathy due to iron overload from chronic blood transfusions is a known complication in β-thalassemia (BT) patients. Congestive heart failure from iron overload is the leading cause of morbidity and mortality in BT patients. Serum ferritin levels (marker of intracellular iron) have been shown to correlate with QT prolongation in acutely ill patients.[1] Sudden death in the setting of early iron overload has been described in animals.[2] A unique case of torsades de pointes (TdP) as the only presentation of iron overload in a patient with BT is presented.

Disclosure: None.
[a] Cardiology Division, Department of Internal Medicine, American University of Beirut Medical Center, Beirut, Lebanon; [b] Department of Biochemistry and Molecular Genetics, American University of Beirut Medical Center, Beirut, Lebanon; [c] Cardiac Electrophysiology, Cardiology, Department of Internal Medicine, American University of Beirut Faculty of Medicine and Medical Center, 3 Dag Hammarskjold Plaza, 8th Floor, New York, NY 10017, USA; [d] Department of Biochemistry and Molecular Genetics, American University of Beirut Faculty of Medicine and Medical Center, 3 Dag Hammarskjold Plaza, 8th Floor, New York, NY 10017, USA; [e] Division of Cardiology, Department of Medicine, University of California San Francisco Medical Center, 500 Parnassus Avenue, MUE-431, San Francisco, CA 94143-1354, USA; [f] Department of Biomedical Sciences, Faculty of Health and Medical Sciences, Danish National Research Foundation Centre for Cardiac Arrhythmia, University of Copenhagen, Copenhagen, Denmark
[1] These authors contributed equally to this work.
* Corresponding author. Cardiac Electrophysiology Training Program, Cardiac Electrophysiology, Cardiology, University of California San Francisco, 500 Parnassus Avenue, MU East 431, Box 1354, San Francisco, CA 94143.
E-mail address: badhwar@medicine.ucsf.edu

Card Electrophysiol Clin 8 (2016) 247–256
http://dx.doi.org/10.1016/j.ccep.2015.10.037

CASE

A 23-year-old woman with a history of diabetes mellitus type II, hypothyroidism, deep venous thrombosis, and long-standing BT major presented with her first syncopal episode. Electrocardiogram (ECG) imaging showed prolonged QTc interval with T-wave alternans (**Fig. 1**A) associated with nonsustained and sustained TdP (**Fig. 1**B). She was initially treated with magnesium, lidocaine, and isoproterenol; however, external defibrillation was required to terminate the TdP episode. Echocardiogram showed normal left ventricular (LV) function with no wall motion abnormality or LV hypertrophy. She was previously started on deferiprone (chelator therapy) for iron overload associated with chronic transfusion therapy. Monitoring for iron overload was done through MRI of the liver that had shown gradual increases in her liver iron levels. Serum ferritin on presentation was 1688 µg/L (normal levels: 8–125 µg/L). Previous ECGs showed stable QTc interval (**Fig. 1**C) with prolongation in her QTc interval (**Fig. 1**D) thereafter that paralleled the increase in iron stores. There was no family history of long QT syndrome (LQTS) or sudden death. She was treated with β-blockers and underwent implantation of a dual-chamber implantable cardioverter-defibrillator (ICD) with atrial pacing at 80 beats per minute to shorten the QT interval.

GENETIC TESTING

Genetic screening of the proband was performed at Familion (New Haven, CT, USA) analyzing the genes *KCNQ1*, *KCNH2*, *SCN5A*, and *KCNE1*. The control group consisted of 400 healthy Caucasian and African American ancestry subjects. Direct DNA sequencing of the probands' DNA revealed a novel mutation c.1591C>T in the *KCNQ1* gene introducing a premature stop-codon $K_V7.1$-Q531X in the channel protein (**Fig. 2**A). A novel variant c.967G>A in the *KCNH2* gene leading to $K_V11.1$-D323N was also identified.

Point mutations Q531X in $K_V7.1$ (GenBank Accession Number NM_000218) and D323N in $K_V11.1$ (NM_000238) were engineered using mutated oligonucleotide extension polymerase chain reaction from plasmid templates harboring the cDNA of interest. After verification of the generated plasmids by sequencing, cRNA was synthesized and injected into *Xenopus laevis* oocytes.

The authors assessed the functional effects of the mutation by measuring currents conducted through wild-type versus mutant channels in an established heterologous expression system. To this end, they expressed wild-type $K_V7.1$ alone, $K_V7.1 + K_V7.1$-Q531X, and $K_V7.1$-Q531X in *X laevis* oocytes and recorded currents using the 2-electrode voltage-clamp technique (TEVC), as shown in **Fig. 2**B. Data were analyzed using Igor

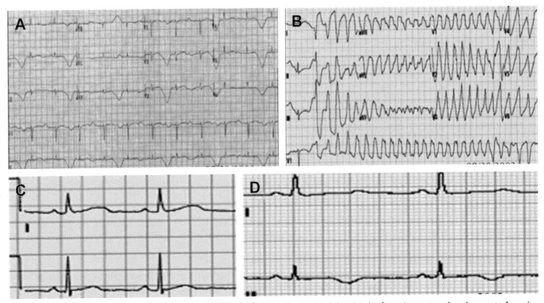

Fig. 1. (*A*) ECG showing electrical alternans, (*B*) ECG showing TdP, (*C*) ECG before iron overload onset showing stable QTc interval (QTc = 447 ms), (*D*) ECG showing an increase in QTc interval after iron overload (QTc = 520 ms).

(HEKA Elektronik, Lambrecht/Pfalz, Germany) and Prism (GraphPad Software, GraphPad Software Inc, La Jolla, CA, USA) software. Mean ± SEM values are shown, and statistical significance (*P<.05) was evaluated by 2-way ANOVA followed by a Bonferroni posttest.

Expression of K_V7.1-WT resulted in small, slowly activating voltage-dependent potassium currents. Expression of the mutant K_V7.1-Q531X resulted in a complete loss of function. Summary data depicted in **Fig. 2C** show that coexpression of K_V7.1 with K_V7.1-Q531X mimicking the heterozygous state in the patient reduced the current levels by 41% (at +40 mV, P<.05), indicating haploinsufficiency. Coexpression with KCNE1, the accessory β-subunit of K_V7.1, could not rescue the loss of function of the mutant. Expression of K_V11.1-D323N showed that the variant behaved similar to wild-type, indicating that this variant is functionally silent (data not shown).

LONG QT SYNDROME

LQTS is a monogenetic cardiac disorder characterized by prolongation of the cardiac action potential resulting in prolonged QT interval and T-wave abnormalities.[3] The prevalence of the disease reaches approximately 1 in 2500 and accounts for hundreds to thousands of deaths in the young population.[4] This repolarization disease is associated with ventricular arrhythmias resulting in syncope and sudden cardiac death (SCD) predominantly in young subjects. Half of the LQTS patients experience their first cardiac event at age of 12, and by 40 years old, 90% of subjects are diagnosed.[5] Most cardiac events/symptoms are triggered by physical activity or emotional stress in addition to occasional events occurring because of loud noises.[6–8] Autosomal-dominant and autosomal-recessive modes of inheritance have been described with autosomal-dominant being the predominant pattern.

The QT interval reflects ventricular repolarization that results from opening and closing of ion channels at the cardiomyocyte level. Malfunction of any of these cardiac ion channels leads to an increase in action potential duration manifesting macroscopically as QT interval prolongation. LQTS is a heterogeneous disease, and more than 600 mutations in 15 genes have been reported (**Table 1**). These mutations comprise loss-of-function mutations in potassium channel genes (KCNQ1, KCNH2, KCNE1, KCNE2, KCNJ2) or gain-of-function mutations in sodium or calcium channel genes (SCN5A, CACNA1C).[9,10] Based on the affected genes and gene product, LQTS is subtyped with LQT1 (KCNQ1, K_V7.1), LQT2 (KCNH2,

K_V11.1), and LQT3 (SCN5A, Na_V1.5), accounting for most cases. However, because of the genetic heterogeneity, the relationship between symptoms, genotype, and QT interval is not always clear. Thirty percent to 50% of subjects become symptomatic, presenting with syncope, and 3% to 5% of patients present with cardiac arrest as the initial manifestation of the disease.

LQT1 is the most common subtype caused by loss-of-function mutations in the KCNQ1 gene that encodes the voltage-gated potassium channel K_V7.1, the pore-forming subunit of the slow delayed rectifier K^+ current I_{Ks}.[11] This current is crucial for shortening ventricular repolarization duration on adrenergic stimulation, and thus, QT interval adaptation in response to increased heart rate. Both gating alterations and trafficking defects have been described.[12] LQT2 is linked to loss-of-function mutations in the KCNH2 gene, which result in altered trafficking or nonfunctional formation of the potassium channel responsible for the rapidly activating delayed rectifier K^+ current (I_{Kr}).[13] Clinical presentation of syncope or SCD can be triggered mostly by emotional stress or occur at rest because it was reported that 15% of cardiac events occur during sleep or at rest.[12] In addition, auditory stimuli such as sudden loud noises or alarm clock are characteristic triggers for LQT2.[14] In addition to loss-of-function mutations in genes encoding potassium channels, mutations in SCN5A encoding the cardiac sodium channel may lead to persistent sodium current. This gain of function in the sodium current, especially in the plateau phase of action potential, results in AP, and hence, QTc prolongation.[15]

Clinical Presentation and Diagnosis

LQT subtypes have common clinical presentation of palpitation, syncope, and SCD, where history of precipitating factors might help the physician in pointing toward a specific subtype. Knowing that physical examination and imaging are not of significant value in establishing the diagnosis of the syndrome, Schwartz and colleagues[16] were the first to propose diagnostic criteria in 1985. The criteria included corrected QT (QTc), syncope, and family history of the disease as major criteria in addition to other minor criteria for diagnosis.[16] There are currently several correction formulas for the QT and JT intervals for changes in heart rate (**Table 2**). The current 1993 to 2011 diagnostic criteria are based on electrocardiographic findings, clinical history, and family history with a Schwartz score 3.5 points or higher, indicating high probability of LQTS. To start with, QT interval is defined between onset of QRS and end of T

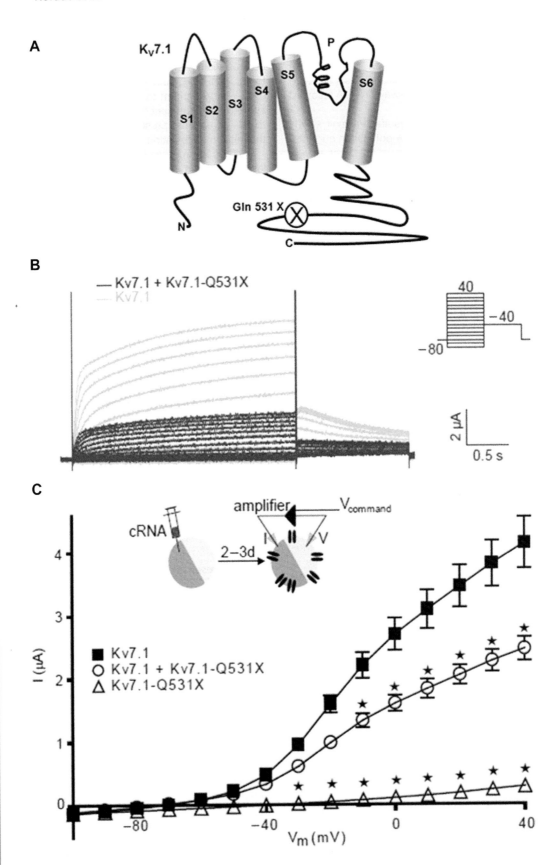

A

$K_v7.1$

S1 S2 S3 S4 S5 S6 P

Gln 531 X

N

C

B

— Kv7.1 + Kv7.1-Q531X
⋯ Kv7.1

40
−40
−80

2 µA
0.5 s

C

amplifier $V_{command}$

cRNA

2–3d

I   V

I (µA)

4

3

2

1

0

■ Kv7.1
○ Kv7.1 + Kv7.1-Q531X
△ Kv7.1-Q531X

−80   −40   0   40

V_m (mV)

Table 1
Subtypes of congenital long QT syndromes

LQTS Subtype	Gene	Protein	Functional Effect
LQTS 1	KCNQ1	$K_V7.1$	Loss-of-function
LQTS 2	KCNH2	$K_V11.1$ annel (hERG)	Loss-of-function (I_{Kr})
LQTS 3	SCN5A	$Na_V1.5$	Gain-of-function
LQTS 4	ANKB	Ankyrin B	Reduction in Na/K ATPase
LQTS 5	KCNE1	KCNE1	Loss-of-function (I_{Ks})
LQTS 6	KCNE2	KCNE2	Loss-of-function (I_{Kr})
LQTS 7	KCNJ2	Kir2.1	Loss-of-function
LQTS 8	CACNA1C	$Ca_V1.2$	Gain-of-function
LQTS 9	CAV3	Caveolin 3	Gain-of-function (sodium channel)
LQTS 10	SCN4B	$Na_V\beta4$	Gain-of-function
LQTS 11	AKAP9	Yotiao	Loss-of-function (I_{Ks})
LQTS 12	SNTA1	Syntrophin-$\alpha1$	Gain-of-function (sodium channel)
LQTS 13	KCNJ5	Kir3.4	Loss-of-function (I_{K-ATP})
LQTS 14	CALM1	Calmodulin 1	Dysfunctional Ca^{2+} signaling
LQTS 15	CALM2	Calmodulin 2	

wave, and its measurement in leads II and V5 was shown to be most predictive for diagnosis.[17] The QTc is considered abnormal when exceeding 450 ms in men and 460 ms in women. Monnig and colleagues[18] showed that 470 ms is a better cutoff value with higher positive predictive value and that QTc greater than 470 ms puts patients at higher risk of developing symptoms. The 36th Bethesda Conference task force recommended that competitive athletes with slightly longer QTc intervals (QTc ≥470 ms in men, ≥480 ms in women) should be restricted to low physical intensity (class IA) sports. The QT interval should be measured using the tangent method on the baseline ECG or during the recovery phase 4 minutes after exercise test when T-P fusion is not observed. In the event of a cardiac arrest, the after-arrest QT interval can be prolonged acutely not due to LQTS, and this QT prolongation can be even greater with the hypothermia protocol. It is important to wait and get the baseline QT

interval after the resuscitation when the patient does not have tachycardia.

The challenging part in diagnosis is subjects who have normal resting ECG who are not risk-free of SCD. In addition to QTc manual measurement, T-wave morphology should also be inspected because some abnormalities are associated with each subtype of the syndrome. Type 1 displays a broad-based T wave; LQTS type 2 is associated with biphasic T-wave pattern, and type 3 displays mostly an isoelectric ST segment followed by a narrow-based T wave.[19] It is important to measure the QT and not the QTu, especially in leads with prominent U waves, such as V1 to V3. It is important as well not to misdiagnose the second component of T (T2) wave in bifid T wave for a U wave.

Exercise testing comes as a powerful tool that helps in uncovering concealed QT syndrome in subjects exhibiting normal resting ECG. On exercise, the normal response to the increase in

Fig. 2. (A) $K_V7.1$ potassium channel with 6 transmembrane segments (S1-S6), pore domain (P), and intracellular N- and C-termini showing the location of the Gln 531 Ter (X) mutation in the C-terminus of the 676-amino-acid-long channel protein. (B) Representative current traces recorded from X laevis oocytes injected with $K_V7.1$ or $K_V7.1$/$K_V7.1$-Q531X. The insert shows the voltage clamp protocol where currents were elicited by clamping the oocytes to test potentials ranging from −100 to +40 mV in 10-mV increments from a holding potential of −80 mV. (C) Comparison of $K_V7.1$-WT (wild-type) and $K_V7.1$-Q531X (mutant) channel currents. To construct I/V relationships for $K_V7.1$ (n = 13), $K_V7.1$/$K_V7.1$-Q531X (n = 13), and $K_V7.1$-Q531X (n = 5), currents were measured at the end of the 2-second test pulse. Expression of the mutant $K_V7.1$-Q531X resulted in a complete loss of function (Δ). Co-expression of $K_V7.1$ with $K_V7.1$-Q531X mimicking the heterozygous state in the patient reduced the current levels by 41% (○). The principle of the TEVC experiments is shown in the inset.

Table 2
The QT/QTc and JT/JTc intervals using the heart rate correction methods

Bazett	QTcB (JTcB) = QT (JT)/RR interval$^{1/2}$
Fredericia	QTcFi (JTcFi) = QT (JT)/RR interval$^{1/3}$
Framingham	QTcFa (JTcFa) = QT (JT) + 154 (1 − 60/heart rate)
Hodges	QTcH (JTcH) = QT (JT) + 1.75 (heart rate − 60)
Nomogram	QTcN (JTcN) = QT (JT) + Nomogram correction factor
Rautaharju QT	(QTcRa) = QT − 155 × (60/HR − 1) − 0.93 × (QRS −139) + k (k = −22 ms for men, and −34 ms for women) Rautaharju JT: (JTcRa) = JT − 155 × (60/HR − 1) + k (k = 34 ms for men, and 22 ms for women)
Wide QRS correction (bundle branch block and intraventricular conduction delay)[46]	QTcc = (QT− (QRS − 120))/RR interval$^{1/2}$ JTc = QTcB − QRS

The exponentially derived equations (such as Bazett's) overestimate the prevalence of the QT interval at HR greater than 100 bpm, and linear methods to correct the QT interval (such as Hodges) is better for clinical use.[47]

Most physicians, including many cardiologists, cannot accurately calculate a QTc and cannot correctly identify a long QT.[48]

heartbeats is QT shortening. LQT1 patients exhibit a paradoxic QT increase instead of shortening, and subjects fail to reach the maximum expected heart rate.[20,21] The QT fails to adapt (ie, shorten) with increasing heart rate due to impaired I_{Ks}. Although LQT2 patients show a mild or no increase in QT interval, LQT3 subjects exhibit the normal physiologic response of QT shortening.[22,23] LQT2 patients could be identified by their steeper QT/HR (heart rate) slope during exercise and their increased QT hysteresis. The QT hysteresis is the difference between QT during exercise and 2 minutes into the recovery phase at similar heart rates (or within 10 beats per minute), when heart rates typically return to approximately 100 bpm.

Pharmacologic/epinephrine stress testing is a supportive diagnostic tool that helps unmasking LQT1 with sensitivity of 92.5% and positive predictive value of 76%[20]; this is mainly due to the I_{Ks} potassium channel sensitivity to sympathetic stimulation and the paradoxic response in the case of channel malfunction. This test might diagnose LQT2 with lower sensitivity, but has no role in diagnosing LQT3 patients.[20] Postural change by standing unmasks reduced repolarization reserve and helps in the diagnosis of LQTS when QT stunning or QT stretching is provoked with an abnormal QT prolongation that persists even as the heart rate returns to normal in patients with LQTS.

Molecular Genetics

Although LQTS syndrome is diagnosed clinically with the aid of surface ECG and exercise stress test, genetic testing helps in completing the clinical picture and categorizing patients. In addition to its significant role in screening family members and detecting affected subjects, it gives a clue on prognosis and aids in risk-stratifying patients. When the clinical diagnosis is certain, 75% of subjects will be genotype positive; thus, a negative test must not rule out the disease. In addition to the 3 most common subtypes (LQT1, 2, and 3) and the genes involved, additional minor mutations have been reported to involve ion channels subunits or interacting proteins.[24] **Table 1** lists all genes reported in LQTS subtypes and the proteins affected behind the clinical manifestations.

Moreover, several modifier gene variants have been reported to play a role in affecting susceptibility to disease. Polymorphisms in coding or noncoding regions linked to the main genes influence QT interval even in the general population. NOS1AP that encodes nitric oxide synthase 1 adaptor protein has been shown to be one of the most significant genes involved in myocardial repolarization. Interestingly, it was demonstrated that variants of NOS1AP modulate risk in LQTS, and half of them were not previously implicated in repolarization.[24,25] Three separate studies were conducted to investigate the link between these gene variants and SCD and identified that 2 intronic variants are associated with SCD even after controlling for QT interval.[25] This association was validated to carry a 30% increase in SCD risk in Caucasian participants, but no significance was observed in African American subjects.[25,26]

Risk Stratification

Knowing that phenotypic expression and clinical presentation of the syndrome varies from asymptomatic to SCD, categorizing LQTS patients based on their risk for major cardiac events is of high significance in the clinical practice. First, as for subtypes, LQT1 patients are the most prone to experience cardiac events, including SCD, where LQT3 experiences the most lethal ones. In addition, patients with Timothy syndrome (LQT8) due to mutations in the voltage-gated L-type calcium channel (LTCC) have very poor prognosis. History of syncope is the strongest personal medical history to predict SCD wherein negative family history of cardiac arrest or sudden death does not infer increased SCD for other family members, in opposite of other arrhythmogenic diseases. As for ECG findings that are proposed to reflect higher risk for sudden death: QTc greater than 480 ms was the highest indicator, TdP, T-wave alternans, notched T wave in lead III, and low resting heart rate. These parameters and risk markers were all included in the updated Schwartz score (in 2011).[27] In a recent study done by Mullally and colleagues[28] in evaluating predictors of life-threatening cardiac events, prior syncope and severe QT prolongation (QTc >500 ms) were associated with 15-fold and 4-fold increase in lethal events, respectively.

Therapy

LQTS patients should be advised to avoid medications that prolong the QT interval (https://www.crediblemeds.org/). Although the approach to start asymptomatic patients on therapy is still controversial, previous studies have shown that 9% of subjects present with cardiac arrest as their first clinical manifestation.[20,29] β-Blockers remain the first line of therapy in all LQTS patients, particularly types 1 and 2.[30] β-Blockers were shown to reduce cardiovascular events up to 64% in LQTS.[31,32] They are mostly effective in LQT1 patients because 23% of LQT2 and 32% of LQT3 patients will still experience symptoms despite treatment.[33] The most used β-blockers are nadolol, propanolol, and atenolol, with doses specified according to the exercise stress test results, making sure to control heart rate not to exceed 130 beats per minute.[20] LQTS type 3 has poor response to β-blockers, and sodium channel blockers (such as mexiletine, ranolazine, and flecainide) were shown to be effective in this subtype, improving heart rate and normalizing QTc interval.[34,35] Many investigators typically target a reduction in peak treadmill heart rate of 30 bpm at peak workload as a practical target for β-blocker effect. According to the 2013 Heart Rhythm Society/European Heart Rhythm Association/Asia Pacific Heart Rhythm Society statement, long-acting β-blocker such as nadolol or sustained-release propranolol is preferred if patients do not suffer from asthma.

From the Rochester-based LQTS Registry, in patients who were prescribed common β-blockers (atenolol, metoprolol, propranolol, or nadolol), the 4 β-blockers are equally effective in reducing the risk of a first cardiac event in LQTS, but nadolol was the only β-blocker associated with a significant risk reduction in patients with LQT2. Patients experiencing cardiac events during β-blocker therapy are at high risk for subsequent cardiac events, and propranolol is the least effective drug in this high-risk group.

In addition to pharmacologic therapy, pacemakers and defibrillators are also used in high-risk patients. Pacemakers are mostly useful in LQTS type 3 patients who are prone to bradycardia and might have high-grade 2:1 atrioventricular block.[20] ICDs are considered in patients experiencing recurrent syncope and episode despite pharmacologic therapy, and a combination of ICD with β-blockers has been shown to decrease SCD.[15,20]

CASE PRESENTATION DISCUSSION

Iron overload leading to SCD has been shown in animals without any effect on the LV contractility.[2] BT patients on transfusion therapy have been shown to have increased QT dispersion on the ECG.[36] Repolarization abnormalities such as prolonged QT interval may be the earliest manifestation of iron overload before the development of cardiomyopathy.[36,37] The authors describe a BT patient with structurally normal heart and iron overload who presented with TdP.

Proposed mechanisms for the TdP include iron overload as a trigger to a patient with abnormal substrate due to a novel $K_V7.1$-Q531X mutation that affected the repolarization reserve:

The trigger includes varied intracellular deposition of iron in the myocardium[38] and influence of iron on the calcium[39,40] and potassium channels.[41] Patchy iron deposition can cause an increase in ventricular late potentials and nonsustained ventricular tachycardia.[42] LTCCs are permeable to calcium, iron, and other divalent cations. High doses of ferric iron have been shown to slow the decay of calcium current, resulting in a prolonged phase 2 of the ventricular action potential that leads to prolonged QT interval.[40] Patients with BT may also be vitamin D deficient, causing an increase in parathyroid hormone (PTH). PTH upregulates the LTCC, thereby increasing iron entry into cardiomyocytes.[39] Accordingly, calcium channel blockers (CCB) have been proven to be beneficial in decreasing or preventing iron-induced cardiomyopathy and/or toxicity. Ferric iron has been shown to suppress voltage-gated potassium currents in murine neural cells.[41] Deferiprone has been used for many years as an iron chelator with no reported case of long QT associated with it.

KCNQ1 encodes $K_V7.1$ protein that forms the α-subunit of the slow delayed rectifier potassium channels.[43] Genetic defects causing loss of function in this gene can lead to LQTS 1 by increasing the duration of phase 3 of the action potential.[44] The authors identified a rare variant c.1591C>T, that introduces a premature stop-codon Gln(Q) 531Ter(X) in the $K_V7.1$ protein. Functional analysis showed that Q531X leads to loss of function of the potassium channel that is likely to prolong the QT interval. The premature stop-codon produces a truncated protein that lacks a large portion of the C-terminus, including the carboxy-terminal assembly domain.[45] In line with this, coexpression of the mutant protein with wild-type protein to mimic the heterozygous state observed in the patient led to 41% reduction of the current. The patient also carried a novel *KCNH2* variant that was functionally silent and also was seen in 5% of healthy volunteers.

The patient's ECG showed prolongation of QT interval that paralleled an increase in iron stores as detected by serum ferritin and increased liver iron concentration on MRI. This case suggests that iron overload could possibly be the precipitating stimulus or trigger for QT interval prolongation and TdP in this patient with a heterozygous *KCNQ1* mutation.

SUMMARY

LQTS represents a serious arrhythmogenic disease that puts patients at high risk for SCD. All family members should be evaluated for the disease after sudden death. Taking a thorough clinical history helps in pointing to patient's subtype by knowing the trigger that induced presenting symptoms. Subjects or family members with high suspicion of the disease should be managed thoroughly and offered genetic testing in addition to exercise testing. Clinical history, family history, exercise stress testing, and genetic testing all aid in risk-stratifying patients, which affect therapy and ICD consideration.

The authors presented a unique case of TdP in a patient with BT without structural heart abnormalities. She had prolonged QTc that paralleled an increase in iron stores. Genetic testing identified a *KCNQ1* gene mutation c.1591C>T, Gln531Ter(X), associated with decreased I_{Ks} current. Based on the chronology of the patient's events, the authors postulate that iron overload could possibly be the precipitating stimulus or trigger for QT interval prolongation and TdP in this patient with an abnormal electrophysiological substrate due to the heterozygous Gln531Ter(X) mutation in the *KCNQ1* gene.

REFERENCES

1. Laudanski K, Ali H, Himmel A, et al. The relationship between serum ferritin levels and electrocardiogram characteristics in acutely ill patients. Exp Clin Cardiol 2009;14(3):38–41.
2. Schwartz KA, Li Z, Schwartz DE, et al. Earliest cardiac toxicity induced by iron overload selectively inhibits electrical conduction. J Appl Physiol 2002; 93(2):746–51.
3. Mizusawa Y, Horie M, Wilde AA. Genetic and clinical advances in congenital long QT syndrome. Circ J 2014;78(12):2827–33.
4. Schwartz PJ, Stramba-Badiale M, Crotti L, et al. Prevalence of the congenital long-QT syndrome. Circulation 2009;120(18):1761–7.
5. Moss AJ, Schwartz PJ, Crampton RS, et al. The long QT syndrome. Prospective longitudinal study of 328 families. Circulation 1991;84(3):1136–44.
6. Moss AJ, McDonald J. Unilateral cervicothoracic sympathetic ganglionectomy for the treatment of long QT interval syndrome. N Engl J Med 1971; 285(16):903–4.
7. Moss AJ, Schwartz PJ, Crampton RS, et al. The long QT syndrome: a prospective international study. Circulation 1985;71(1):17–21.
8. Schwartz PJ, Periti M, Malliani A. The long Q-T syndrome. Am Heart J 1975;89(3):378–90.
9. Napolitano C, Bloise R, Monteforte N, et al. Sudden cardiac death and genetic ion channelopathies: long QT, Brugada, short QT, catecholaminergic polymorphic ventricular tachycardia, and idiopathic ventricular fibrillation. Circulation 2012;125(16):2027–34.
10. Perrin MJ, Gollob MH. Genetics of cardiac electrical disease. Can J Cardiol 2013;29(1):89–99.
11. Wang Q, Curran ME, Splawski I, et al. Positional cloning of a novel potassium channel gene: KVLQT1 mutations cause cardiac arrhythmias. Nat Genet 1996;12(1):17–23.
12. Ackerman MJ, Khositseth A, Tester DJ, et al. Epinephrine-induced QT interval prolongation: a gene-specific paradoxical response in congenital long QT syndrome. Mayo Clin Proc 2002;77(5): 413–21.
13. Schwartz PJ, Priori SG, Spazzolini C, et al. Genotype-phenotype correlation in the long-QT syndrome: gene-specific triggers for life-threatening arrhythmias. Circulation 2001;103(1):89–95.
14. Wilde AA, Jongbloed RJ, Doevendans PA, et al. Auditory stimuli as a trigger for arrhythmic events differentiate HERG-related (LQTS2) patients from KVLQT1-related patients (LQTS1). J Am Coll Cardiol 1999;33(2):327–32.

15. Roden DM. Clinical practice. Long-QT syndrome. N Engl J Med 2008;358(2):169–76.

16. Schwartz PJ. Idiopathic long QT syndrome: progress and questions. Am Heart J 1985;109(2):399–411.

17. Cowan JC, Yusoff K, Moore M, et al. Importance of lead selection in QT interval measurement. Am J Cardiol 1988;61(1):83–7.

18. Monnig G, Eckardt L, Wedekind H, et al. Electrocardiographic risk stratification in families with congenital long QT syndrome. Eur Heart J 2006;27(17): 2074–80.

19. Tester DJ, Ackerman MJ. Genetics of long QT syndrome. Methodist Debakey Cardiovasc J 2014; 10(1):29–33.

20. Medeiros-Domingo A, Iturralde-Torres P, Ackerman MJ. Clinical and genetic characteristics of long QT syndrome. Rev Esp Cardiol 2007;60(7): 739–52 [in Spanish].

21. Takenaka K, Ai T, Shimizu W, et al. Exercise stress test amplifies genotype-phenotype correlation in the LQT1 and LQT2 forms of the long-QT syndrome. Circulation 2003;107(6):838–44.

22. Swan H, Viitasalo M, Piippo K, et al. Sinus node function and ventricular repolarization during exercise stress test in long QT syndrome patients with KvLQT1 and HERG potassium channel defects. J Am Coll Cardiol 1999;34(3):823–9.

23. Schwartz PJ, Priori SG, Locati EH, et al. Long QT syndrome patients with mutations of the SCN5A and HERG genes have differential responses to Na+ channel blockade and to increases in heart rate. Implications for gene-specific therapy. Circulation 1995;92(12):3381–6.

24. Deo R, Albert CM. Epidemiology and genetics of sudden cardiac death. Circulation 2012;125(4): 620–37.

25. Adabag AS, Luepker RV, Roger VL, et al. Sudden cardiac death: epidemiology and risk factors. Nat Rev Cardiol 2010;7(4):216–25.

26. George AL Jr. Common genetic variants in sudden cardiac death. Heart Rhythm 2009;6(11 Suppl):S3–9.

27. Schwartz PJ, Crotti L. QTc behavior during exercise and genetic testing for the long-QT syndrome. Circulation 2011;124(20):2181–4.

28. Mullally J, Goldenberg I, Moss AJ, et al. Risk of life-threatening cardiac events among patients with long QT syndrome and multiple mutations. Heart Rhythm 2013;10(3):378–82.

29. Garson A Jr, Dick M 2nd, Fournier A, et al. The long QT syndrome in children. An international study of 287 patients. Circulation 1993;87(6):1866–72.

30. Priori SG, Wilde AA, Horie M, et al. HRS/EHRA/ APHRS expert consensus statement on the diagnosis and management of patients with inherited primary arrhythmia syndromes: document endorsed by HRS, EHRA, and APHRS in May 2013 and by ACCF, AHA, PACES, and AEPC in June 2013. Heart Rhythm 2013;10(12):1932–63.

31. Moss AJ, Zareba W, Hall WJ, et al. Effectiveness and limitations of beta-blocker therapy in congenital long-QT syndrome. Circulation 2000;101(6):616–23.

32. Hobbs JB, Peterson DR, Moss AJ, et al. Risk of aborted cardiac arrest or sudden cardiac death during adolescence in the long-QT syndrome. JAMA 2006;296(10):1249–54.

33. Priori SG, Napolitano C, Schwartz PJ, et al. Association of long QT syndrome loci and cardiac events among patients treated with beta-blockers. JAMA 2004;292(11):1341–4.

34. Moss AJ, Windle JR, Hall WJ, et al. Safety and efficacy of flecainide in subjects with Long QT-3 syndrome (DeltaKPQ mutation): a randomized, double-blind, placebo-controlled clinical trial. Ann Noninvasive Electrocardiol 2005;10(4 Suppl):59–66.

35. Benhorin J, Taub R, Goldmit M, et al. Effects of flecainide in patients with new SCN5A mutation: mutation-specific therapy for long-QT syndrome? Circulation 2000;101(14):1698–706.

36. Russo V, Rago A, Pannone B, et al. Dispersion of repolarization and beta-thalassemia major: the prognostic role of QT and JT dispersion for identifying the high-risk patients for sudden death. Eur J Haematol 2011;86(4):324–31.

37. Detterich J, Noetzli L, Dorey F, et al. Electrocardiographic consequences of cardiac iron overload in thalassemia major. Am J Hematol 2012; 87(2):139–44.

38. Fitchett DH, Coltart DJ, Littler WA, et al. Cardiac involvement in secondary haemochromatosis: a catheter biopsy study and analysis of myocardium. Cardiovasc Res 1980;14(12):719–24.

39. Otto-Duessel M, Brewer C, Wood JC. Interdependence of cardiac iron and calcium in a murine model of iron overload. Transl Res 2011;157(2):92–9.

40. Tsushima RG, Wickenden AD, Bouchard RA, et al. Modulation of iron uptake in heart by L-type Ca2+ channel modifiers: possible implications in iron overload. Circ Res 1999;84(11):1302–9.

41. Bukanova JV, Solntseva EI, Skrebitsky VG. The effects of ferric iron on voltage-gated potassium currents in molluscan neurons. Neuroreport 2007; 18(13):1395–8.

42. Franzoni F, Galetta F, Di Muro C, et al. Heart rate variability and ventricular late potentials in beta-thalassemia major. Haematologica 2004;89(2):233–4.

43. O'Hara T, Rudy Y. Arrhythmia formation in subclinical ("silent") long QT syndrome requires multiple insults: quantitative mechanistic study using the KCNQ1 mutation Q357R as example. Heart Rhythm 2012; 9(2):275–82.

44. Seebohm G, Strutz-Seebohm N, Ureche ON, et al. Long QT syndrome-associated mutations in KCNQ1 and KCNE1 subunits disrupt normal

endosomal recycling of IKs channels. Circ Res 2008;103(12):1451–7.

45. Schmitt N, Schwarz M, Peretz A, et al. A recessive C-terminal Jervell and Lange-Nielsen mutation of the KCNQ1 channel impairs subunit assembly. EMBO J 2000;19(3):332–40.

46. Patel P, Borovskiy Y, Marchlinski F, et al. Optimal measurement of the QT interval in patients with tachycardia. J Am Coll Cardiol 2015;65(10):A77–8.

47. Patel P, Borovskiy Y, Deo R. QTcc, a novel method for correcting QT interval for QRS duration, predicts all-cause mortality. J Am Coll Cardiol 2015;65(10): A78.

48. Viskin S, Rosovski U, Sands AJ, et al. Inaccurate electrocardiographic interpretation of long QT: the majority of physicians cannot recognize a long QT when they see one. Heart Rhythm 2005;2(6): 569–74.

Printed and bound by CPI Group (UK) Ltd, Croydon, CR0 4YY

03/10/2024

01040376-0004